Drug Safety
Data

HOW TO ANALYZE,
SUMMARIZE, AND
INTERPRET TO
DETERMINE RISK

MICHAEL J. KLEPPER, MD
Cary, North Carolina

BARTON COBERT, MD, FACP, FACG, FFPM
BLCMD Associates LLC
Westfield, New Jersey

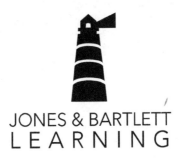

JONES & BARTLETT
LEARNING

World Headquarters

Jones & Bartlett Learning
40 Tall Pine Drive
Sudbury, MA 01776
978-443-5000
info@jblearning.com
www.jblearning.com

Jones & Bartlett Learning
Canada
6339 Ormindale Way
Mississauga, Ontario L5V 1J2
Canada

Jones & Bartlett Learning
International
Barb House, Barb Mews
London W6 7PA
United Kingdom

Jones & Bartlett Learning books and products are available through most bookstores and online booksellers. To contact Jones & Bartlett Learning directly, call 800-832-0034, fax 978-443-8000, or visit our website, www.jblearning.com.

Substantial discounts on bulk quantities of Jones & Bartlett Learning publications are available to corporations, professional associations, and other qualified organizations. For details and specific discount information, contact the special sales department at Jones & Bartlett Learning via the above contact information or send an email to specialsales@jblearning.com.

The authors, editor, and publisher have made every effort to provide accurate information. However, they are not responsible for errors, omissions, or for any outcomes related to the use of the contents of this book and take no responsibility for the use of the products and procedures described. Treatments and side effects described in this book may not be applicable to all people; likewise, some people may require a dose or experience a side effect that is not described herein. Drugs and medical devices are discussed that may have limited availability controlled by the Food and Drug Administration (FDA) for use only in a research study or clinical trial. Research, clinical practice, and government regulations often change the accepted standard in this field. When consideration is being given to use of any drug in the clinical setting, the healthcare provider or reader is responsible for determining FDA status of the drug, reading the package insert, and reviewing prescribing information for the most up-to-date recommendations on dose, precautions, and contraindications, and determining the appropriate usage for the product. This is especially important in the case of drugs that are new or seldom used.

Production Credits

Executive Publisher: Christopher Davis
Special Projects Editor: Kathy Richardson
Editorial Assistant: Sara Cameron
Associate Production Editor: Lisa Cerrone
Associate Marketing Manager: Katie Hennessy
V.P., Manufacturing and Inventory Control:
  Therese Connell

Composition: diacriTech
Cover Design: Kristin E. Parker
Cover Image: © Ron Sumners/Dreamstime.com
Printing and Binding: Courier Stoughton
Cover Printing: Courier Stoughton

Library of Congress Cataloging-in-Publication Data
Klepper, Michael J.
  Drug safety data: how to analyze, summarize, and interpret to determine risk / Michael J. Klepper, Barton Cobert—1st ed.
    p. ; cm.
  Includes bibliographical references and index.
  ISBN-13: 978-0-7637-6912-3
  ISBN-10: 0-7637-6912-6
  1. Pharmacoepidemiology. 2. Health risk assessment. I. Cobert, Barton L. II. Title.
  [DNLM: 1. Pharmacoepidemiology—methods. 2. Data Interpretation, Statistical. 3. Drug Toxicity—prevention & control.
  4. Product Surveillance, Postmarketing. 5. Risk Assessment. 6. Safety Management. QZ 42 K64d 2011]
  RM302.5.K64 2011
  615'.7042—dc22

                                                                                          2010005220

6048

Printed in the United States of America
14 13 12 11 10 10 9 8 7 6 5 4 3 2 1

Dedication

In loving memory of my parents, Shirley and Al. You left us too soon, but your light continues to guide and inspire.

Mike Klepper

To Josiane, my beloved wife.

Bart Cobert

Table of Contents

Introduction

Drug safety and pharmacovigilance have become a major focus for both the medical community and the public. Various drug withdrawals from the market and severe adverse events (*side effects*, to use the older term) including deaths have heightened everyone's awareness that swallowing pills or getting injections is not without the potential for negative consequences.

A drug that reaches the market is no longer simply safe and effective. Rather, it has a positive benefit–risk profile, meaning that there are indeed risks and adverse events, but the benefits (when the drug is used for the labeled disease in the appropriate patients at the approved dosage) outweigh the risks.

There are various textbooks, manuals, and journals that are helping to move the field of drug safety from anecdote to science. We are not aware of any, however, that examine in a step-by-step approach the preparation, analysis, and interpretation of the actual safety data collected in the course of drug development and marketing.

So this book is an attempt to give those people involved in drug development, clinical research, statistics, drug safety, epidemiology, regulatory affairs, and others answers to the question . . . "How?"

HOW to . . .
- Identify safety signals
- Identify red herrings (i.e., false signals)
- Determine a drug effect
- Determine clinical significance
- Determine a drug's risk profile
- Analyze, display, summarize, and interpret safety data

This book is divided into two parts: "Part 1—The Basics," and "Part 2—Approaches to the Analysis, Summary, and Interpretation of Safety Data."

Part 1 provides the fundamental concepts and tools required for risk determination, e.g., the determination of a drug effect and its clinical significance, and understanding what laboratory tests and electrocardiograms measure and what the values mean. Part 1 also includes the processes involved in data collection and data analyses that impact risk determination.

The focus of Part 2 is to provide practical approaches for the analyses, displays, and summary of safety data for an integrated analysis of safety (IAS). An IAS is required for preparation of the Integrated Summary of Safety (ISS) and the Summary of Clinical Safety (SCS)–reports required for drug approval. Part 2 also provides approaches for the preparation of the Periodic Safety Update Report for a Marketed Drug (PSUR). These reports are complex and challenging to prepare. The principles and approaches used in the preparation of these reports can also be used for other documents submitted to health authorities such as clinical study reports and Development Safety Update Reports (DSURs). The chapters in Part 2, with some exceptions, parallel the sections included in the SCS.

One of the unique features of this book is the inclusion of a sample IAS and PSUR for a fictitious drug, Mepro, a nonsteroidal anti-inflammatory drug (NSAID). These sample reports show how the information presented in Part 1 and Part 2 can be applied.

The book is filled throughout with TIPS, CAUTIONS, NOTES, and RED HERRING ALERTS providing helpful and pragmatic advice to help you navigate through the often murky waters of risk determination. TIPS provide useful suggestions of what to do. CAUTIONS are intended to point out areas that can get you into trouble or lead you down the wrong path or to the wrong conclusions. NOTES emphasize or clarify key points of information. RED HERRING ALERTS provide examples of results that can be misleading or represent a false safety signal.

Although *drug* is mentioned throughout the book, the topics discussed are also relevant for biologics, vaccines, OTC products, nutraceuticals, and, in some instances, medical devices.

Lastly, 3 important caveats:

- **Caveat No. 1**—Be sure to follow the regulations and guidance documents relevant to your own country since these can differ across countries.
- **Caveat No. 2**—Regulations keep changing, and new guidances are issued over time. What is relevant today can be outdated tomorrow.
- **Caveat No. 3**—One size doesn't fit all. There are many approaches in the way data can be analyzed, summarized, displayed, and interpreted. Some of the approaches included in this book may not be the best fit for your drug. Or different type of analyses not mentioned in this book will be required. Some may also disagree with the approaches that are recommended. For these reasons, the analysis plan for the IAS should be discussed with the regulatory agency's reviewing division well before you plan to submit your registration dossier.

Both of us have spent decades in drug safety and pharmacovigilance, and this book represents a distillation of the lessons learned during our careers. It is our humble and sincere wish this information will be of value to you.

Michael J. Klepper, MD
Barton Cobert, MD, FACP, FACG, FFPM

Abbreviation List

Abbreviation	Term
ACE	Angiotension converting enzyme
ADR	Adverse drug reaction
AE	Adverse event
AF	Atrial fibrillation
AHQ	*Ad hoc* query
ALP	Alkaline phosphatase
ALT	Alanine aminotransferase
AR	Adverse reaction; Attributable risk
ARDS	Acute respiratory distress syndrome
ARR	Attributable risk ratio
AST	Aspartate aminotransferase
AT	Aminotransferase
ATC	Anatomical Therapeutic Chemical Classification
BMI	Body mass index
BP	Blood pressure
BPM	Beats per minute; Breaths per minute
BW	Body weight
C	Celsius; Cholesterol
Ca	Calcium
CCDS	Company Core Data Sheet
CCSI	Company Core Safety Information
CDC	Centers for Disease Control and Prevention
CHF	Congestive heart failure
CIOMS	Council for International Organizations of Medical Sciences
CK	Creatine kinase
Cl	Chloride
C_{max}	Maximum plasma concentration
CNS	Central nervous system
CO_2	Carbon dioxide
COX	Cyclooxygenase; a fictitious marketed NSAID
CPK	Creatine phosphokinase
CREST	Calcinosis, Raynaud's phenomenon, esophageal dysmotility, sclero-dactyly, and telangiectasias
CRF	Case report form
CS	Clinically significant
CSR	Clinical study report
CT	Combined term; Clinical trial; Computed tomography
CTCAE	Common Terminology Criteria for Adverse Events
CTD	Common Technical Document
CV	Cardiovascular and/or cerebrovascular
DIC	Disseminated intravascular coagulation

DILI	Drug-induced liver injury	MHLW	Ministry of Health, Labour and Welfare (Japan)
DSM	*Diagnostic and Statistical Manual of Mental Disorders*	mmHg	Millimeters of mercury
DSUR	Development Safety Update Report	ms, msec	Millisecond
ECG	Electrocardiogram	MRI	Magnetic resonance imaging
EDC	Electronic data capture	mSMQ	Modified Standardised MedDRA Query
EKG	Electrocardiogram	MSSO	Maintenance and Support Services Organization
EM	Erythema multiforme	N	Normal; Denominator; Number of subjects
EMA, EMEA	European Medicines Agency		
EU	European Union	Na	Sodium
F	Fahrenheit	NASH	Nonalcoholic steatohepatitis
FDA	Food and Drug Administration	NCI	National Cancer Institute
H	Above normal limit (high)	NDA	New Drug Application
Hb	Hemoglobin	NEC	Not elsewhere classified
Hct	Hematocrit	NOAEL	No Observed Adverse Effect Level
HDL	High density lipoprotein	NOS	Not otherwise specified
HLGT	High Level Group Term	NSAID	Nonsteroidal anti-inflammatory drug
HLT	High Level Term		
HR	Heart rate	O_2	Oxygen
GGT	Gamma glutamyltransferase	PADER	Periodic Adverse Drug Experience Report
GI	Gastrointestinal		
IAS	Integrated analysis of safety	PD	Pharmacodynamics
IB	Investigator's Brochure	PI	Package insert
IBD	International birth date	PK	Pharmacokinetics
ICD	International Classification of Diseases	PO_4	Phosphorus
ICH	International Conference on Harmonisation	PR	Pulse rate
		PSUR	Periodic Safety Update Report for Marketed Drugs
ICSR	Individual case safety report		
IND	Investigational new drug	PT	Preferred Term; Premature termination
INR	International normalized ratio		
ISS	Integrated Summary of Safety	PUBs	Perforations, ulcers and bleeds
IT	Information technology	PYE	Person-years exposure
IV	Intravenous	QC	Quality compliance
K	Potassium	QTc	QT interval corrected
Kg	Kilogram	RBC	Red blood cell count
L	Below normal limits (low); Liter	REMS	Risk evaluation and minimization strategy
lb	Pound		
LDL	Low density lipoprotein	s, sec	Second
LFT	Liver function test	SA	Sinoatrial
LLN	Lower limit of normal	SAE	Serious adverse event
LLT	Lowest Level Term	SAP	Statistical analysis plan
LMP	Last menstrual period	SCS	Summary of Clinical Safety
m	Minute	SI	International System of Units
MAH	Marketing authorisation holder	SJS	Stevens-Johnson syndrome
MCHC	Mean corpuscular hemoglobin concentration	SMQ	Standardised MedDRA Query
		SNOMED	Systematized Nomenclature of Medicine
MCV	Mean corpuscular volume		
MedDRA	Medical Dictionary for Regulatory Activities	SOC	System Organ Class
		SPC, SmPC	Summary of Product Characteristics
Mepro	Meproamine dihydroacetate—a fictitious NSAID	SSRI	Selective serotonin reuptake inhibitor
MI	Myocardial infarction		

SUSAR	Suspected, unexpected, serious adverse reaction	US	United States
T	Temperature	VF	Ventricular fibrillation
TBL	Total bilirubin level	VT	Ventricular tachycardia
TdP	Torsades de pointes	WBC	White blood cell count
TEN	Toxic epidermal necrolysis	WD	Withdrawal
TG	Triglycerides	WHO	World Health Organization
TLFs	Tables, listings, and figures	WHO-ART	World Health Organization Adverse Reaction Terms
U/L	Units per liter	WHO-DDE	World Health Organization Drug Dictionary Enhanced
ULN	Upper limit of normal		
URL	Uniform resource locator		

Acknowledgments

It took more than 20 years to transform the dream for this book into reality. Without my friend and co-author Bart, this book would have remained a thought and a desire. Besides his own invaluable contributions to the book's content, Bart's never-ending encouragement and steady hand kept me focused and pulled me out of a period of abject despair when I was ready to walk away from the entire project.

Mike Klepper

We would like to thank James (Jim) Hinson for his review and suggestions for the clinical pharmacology content of the book; Dr. Cecile "Skippy" Berner and Adam Genn for the tedious job of checking many of the tables included in the book; and Ilana Lebowitz for graphic support. A very special thanks is reserved for Dr. Anthony ("Tony") Segreti for his review and suggestions for the statistical content of the book. His gracious help and support were simply invaluable.

Chris Davis, our Editor, who has shown unswerving support throughout this project, has our endless gratitude. We also want to thank our publisher, Jones & Bartlett Learning, for their faith in our vision for this book.

Bart Cobert and Mike Klepper

The Basics

Benefit–Risk

"Primum non nocere—First, do no harm."

■ Benefit Versus Risk

Harold Macmillan, former British prime minister said, "to be alive at all involves some risk."[1] There is risk in everything we do; eating a cheeseburger (high in fat and calories, the risk of choking); driving to work (being hit by a drunk driver, skidding off an icy road). There is even risk in doing nothing (not leaving a dead-end job or staying in a house located on an earthquake fault line).

There are certainly risks involved with drug use. Pharmacologically—or biologically—active substances can disrupt or modify our normal body function and lead to adverse effects. Some risks can be anticipated while others are unexpected. In some cases, the risk is due to an exaggerated response to the drug. An antihypertensive may lower blood pressure too much in a susceptible individual such as an elderly female who becomes dizzy and faints. When she faints, she falls down and fractures her hip. In contrast, some individuals can develop adverse effects that are not based on any known pharmacologic effects but are due to a variety of unique and often poorly understood factors such as an individual's genetic

makeup or capacity to metabolize a drug. These types of unpredictable reactions that are usually rare and serious are referred to as *idiosyncratic reactions*.

But drug risk cannot be evaluated in isolation—the benefit of treatment must also be taken into consideration. A drug can cause adverse effects that can even result in death but still have a favorable benefit–risk profile. For example, suppose there is a new drug being evaluated for the treatment of pancreatic adenocarcinoma with the benefit–risk profile shown in Figure 1-1.

Pancreatic adenocarcinoma is a uniformly fatal disease; the person with this illness has less than a 5% chance of being alive after 5 years, and he has a collective median survival rate of only 4–6 months. Treatment options are few and largely ineffective.[2] Consequently, a drug that decreases pain, tumor size, and hospitalizations while increasing quality of life, survival time, and even curing some would fulfill a significant unmet need for this condition. In evaluating the risk, adverse drug reactions range from nausea and vomiting to potentially life-threatening reactions of agranulocytosis and thrombocytopenia. Agranulocytosis is a condition associated with

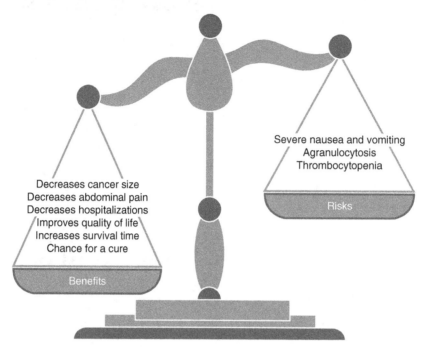

Figure 1-1 Benefit Versus Risk—Theoretical Investigational Drug for Adenocarcinoma of the Pancreas

very low numbers of granulocytes, a type of white blood cell that fights bacterial infection. Patients with agranulocytosis are susceptible to life-threatening infections. Equally worrying is severe thrombocytopenia (low platelet counts), which can result in life-threatening hemorrhage (bleeding). All these risks can, however, be avoided or minimized. Patients with severe nausea and vomiting can be given medication to reduce the nausea and intravenous fluid replacement if vomiting becomes too severe. Patients can also receive granulocyte colony stimulating factor to stimulate white bloods cells, antibiotic therapy to prevent and treat infection, platelet transfusions to minimize the risk of hemorrhage, and blood transfusions for replacement therapy for severe bleeding events. By weighing the benefits versus risks, it is clearly seen that this theoretical drug provides effective therapy for a condition with few treatment options, and the risks can be anticipated, minimized, and treated. For these reasons, the scale tips strongly to the side of benefit, resulting in a favorable benefit–risk profile for this drug.

■ Determining the Benefit–Risk Profile

Throughout preclinical evaluation to clinical development to getting approval and marketing the drug, the drug must show a *favorable benefit–risk profile*. This requires ongoing benefit–risk assessments during the life cycle of the drug.

The *benefit profile* is determined by:

■ Proven efficacy of the drug

■ The unmet need for the drug—the indication for the drug (e.g., cancer versus flatulence) and what alternative treatments, if any, are available

The *risk profile* is determined from the analysis of safety information obtained from nonclinical studies (e.g., animal studies), clinical trials of the investigational drug, and safety information received on the marketed drug.

In the *premarketing setting*, the majority of safety data collected from clinical trials include:

■ Adverse events

■ Laboratory tests

■ Vital signs

■ Physical examinations

■ 12-lead electrocardiograms

■ Other tests depending on the indications, e.g., electroencephalograms in the evaluation of seizure disorders

Once the drug is *marketed*, the majority of safety information comes from spontaneous (unsolicited or voluntary) adverse event (AE) reports primarily from health professionals and consumers. Regulatory authorities, sales people, and other sources can also voluntarily report AEs to the manufacturer. Other postmarketing safety information comes from the literature and information solicited by the manufacturer in the form of postmarketing studies, pharmacoepidemiologic studies, surveys, registries, etc.

■ Adverse Event Versus Adverse Reaction

AEs play the largest role in the determination of risk. The definition of an *adverse event* (formerly referred to as a *side effect*) was established by the International Conference on Harmonisation (ICH).

> An *adverse event (AE)* is any untoward medical occurrence in a patient or clinical investigation subject administered a medicinal product and which does not necessarily have a causal relationship with this treatment. An adverse event can therefore be any unfavorable and unintended sign (for example, an abnormal laboratory finding), symptom, or disease temporally associated with the use of a medicinal product, whether or not considered related to the medicinal product.[3]

AEs where a relationship or causal role to the drug is a reasonable possibility are referred to as *adverse reactions (ARs)* or *adverse drug reactions*.[3,4]

An AE has no implication of causality. It is simply a bad thing that happened—perhaps due to the drug and perhaps not. An AR, however, has some element of possible causality attributed to it. A bad thing may initially be reported as an AE and then become an AR when the evidence accrues there is some level of likelihood that the bad thing was really related to the drug.

■ Mandatory Safety Reporting*

To ensure that a new and clinically important risk is not overlooked or reported too late, health authorities in the United States, the European Union, Japan, and elsewhere require that safety information be reported on both an

expedited (within 7 or 15 day calendar days) and *periodic* (quarterly, biannual, annual, etc.) basis.

Expedited Reporting

A safety finding (i.e., an AE, abnormal laboratory finding, etc.) that meets the following criteria must be reported to authorities expeditiously:

- Results in a *serious* outcome. Serious outcomes include:
  - Death
  - A life-threatening event
  - Inpatient hospitalization or prolongation of existing hospitalization
  - Persistent or significant incapacity/disability
  - Congenital anomaly/birth defect
  - An important medical event
- Is *unexpected*; i.e., the finding is new or the nature or severity of the finding has changed
- Relationship to treatment is *suspected*; i.e., cannot be reasonably ruled out

For investigational drugs, suspected or unexpected safety findings that result in death or are life threatening require reporting to US, EU, Japanese and other regulatory authorities within 7 calendar days; all other suspected serious unexpected events must be reported within 15 calendar days.[3]

The regulations for postmarketing reports are similar but slightly different. For unsolicited (i.e., spontaneously reported without any prompting from the manufacturer) postmarketing AE reports, a causal relationship is assumed, therefore a serious unexpected event must be reported within 15 calendar days. The expedited reporting of serious expected reactions varies among countries. For postmarketing safety findings that are solicited (reported from a study, registry, survey, etc.), reports are submitted within 15 days for events that are serious, unexpected, and a causal relationship cannot be ruled out.[4] That is, for postmarketing solicited information, causality (unlike spontaneous reports) is *not* assumed.

Findings from nonclinical studies that indicate a potential and clinically important risk to humans must also be promptly reported.

Periodic Reporting

Health authorities also require mandatory periodic submission of safety information during clinical development

---

* Be sure to follow the regulations and guidance documents relevant to your own country because these can differ across countries.

and when a drug is marketed. A description of these periodic reports is provided in the next section.

Types of Mandatory Reports Containing Safety Information

The types of mandated reports that contain safety information include:

- **Individual case safety report (ICSR)**—a narrative summary of an AE or other safety finding that occurred in an individual.[4] For investigational drugs, ICSRs are required for serious AEs and other serious safety findings. If the ICSR describes a safety finding that is serious, suspected, and unexpected it must be reported expeditiously to health authorities. Although ICSRs of spontaneous reports of marketed drugs that are serious and unexpected require expedited reporting, the majority of marketed ICSRs are expected and/or nonserious.

- **Investigator's Brochure**—a summary of available nonclinical and clinical study information for investigational drugs in clinical development. The Investigator's Brochure summarizes the known efficacy and safety findings from completed clinical trials and is routinely updated as more information becomes available.[5] If the investigational drug is marketed somewhere, a summary of the postmarketing safety information is also included in the Investigator's Brochure.

- **Clinical Study Report**—a summary of the efficacy and safety results of a clinical study.[6]

- **Periodic reports for drugs under development**—the US IND Annual Report and the EU Annual Safety Report are examples of periodic reports for drugs under development. Each provides a summary of AEs from completed and ongoing studies over a 1-year period.[7,8] These reports are different in content and format and will ultimately be replaced by the ICH-recommended Development Safety Update Report, though local variations from country to country or region to region may be required.[9]

- **The integrated analysis of safety (IAS)**—a comprehensive summary of safety results from every subject who received 1 or more doses of study medication during clinical development. The IAS also includes important nonclinical findings and postmarketing safety information if the drug is already marketed in 1 or more countries. The Summary of Clinical Safety and the Integrated Summary of Safety are both examples of an IAS but differ in format and content.[10,11] An IAS is a requirement for drug approval and must be part of the registration dossier (the documents required for submission and review prior to drug approval). In an IAS, studies are often pooled (combined), enhancing the ability to identify and characterize safety findings that would otherwise go undetected due to the small size or short duration of some of the studies that were done. The results from the IAS form the basis for prescribing information, e.g., the US *package insert,* and the EU *Summary of Product Characteristics.*

- **The 120-Day Safety Update**—a report that is required in the United States 4 months after submission of the IAS and before the drug is approved. The purpose of this update is to summarize safety information received after the data cutoff date of the IAS. This additional information is to determine if the risk profile changed from the time the IAS was submitted.[11]

- **Periodic reports for marketed drugs**—a report that primarily summarizes safety findings of the marketed drug. The purpose of the periodic report is to determine if any new regulatory concerns have emerged, and if the benefit–risk profile of the drug has changed. If so, prescribing information may need to be revised, and risk management activities may need to be initiated or revised to address any newly identified risk(s). The Periodic Adverse Drug Experience Report (PADER) is the periodic report required by the United States, and the Periodic Safety Update Report for Marketed Products (PSUR) is a requirement in the European Union and many other countries.[12–14] The PADER and PSUR are different in format and content. The PSUR is voluntary as of this writing in the United States (though it is expected to become obligatory at some point).

The Story

The objective of a safety report is to answer 3 questions:

1. Is there a drug effect?
2. If so, is the drug effect clinically significant?
3. If clinically significant, is the benefit–risk profile still favorable?

The art and science of a safety report is to take all the available safety data and present it in such a way that the data tell a story about the risk profile of the drug. This story is not something fictional, but fact based. The data that tell the story are like pieces of a jigsaw puzzle that must be correctly interlocked to allow the reviewer to see the risk picture of the drug.

In a report, especially one that summarizes large amounts of data such as an IAS, summary tables of aggregate (group) data and individual data listings and narratives (e.g., information of individual subjects) are often placed in the appendices of the report. The text part of a report should present the data that provides the most relevant findings *extracted* from the information in the appendices. In this way, a reviewer does not have to constantly flip back and forth to the appendices in the back of the report while reading the text to get a picture of the safety profile of the drug. The science of writing a report is to determine what information is important, and the art is the best way to present and display the data. In an IAS summarizing the safety data of several thousand patients, there can be very large volumes of data to go through. Similarly, the PSUR of a widely used drug, marketed in many different countries, can also generate large amounts of data that have to be summarized in the text of the PSUR. Regulations and guidances dictate what information is required. But many gray areas remain regarding the best way to analyze, display, and present the data.

■ Play Detective and Make Preemptive Strikes

Safety results are not always straightforward or black and white. There may be a number of safety findings identified, but whether or not they are real or important is not always clear. Because of this uncertainty, you need to be a detective and gather as many *clues* as the data permit. The clues that point to where the evidence might be are *safety signals*. There are many definitions for a safety signal. The definition that is used throughout this book is any safety finding that serves to flag or alert.

The more clues pointing in the same direction, the greater the likelihood the safety finding is real and not a red herring (false signal). In determining the risk profile, you need to preemptively and proactively state your assessments based on the weight of evidence that you collect. This should be done *before* the health authorities ask you to do so. Not only is this the right thing to do, but it also builds credibility and trust with the health authorities, avoiding the implication that one is trying to hide or downplay a signal. Remember, if you have a question regarding the significance of a finding, it is very likely that the health authority will have the same question.

■ The Journey

Many steps are involved in the determination of risk. The goal of this book is to help guide you in this journey. So let's begin.

References

1. Famous quotes and quotations. http://www.brainyquote.com/quotes/quotes/h/haroldmacm101798.html. Accessed February 18, 2010.

2. Erikson RA, Larson CR, Shabahang, M. Pancreatic Cancer. April 7, 2009. http://www.emedicine.medscape.com/article/280605=overview. Accessed February 18, 2010.

3. International Conference on Harmonisation of Technical Requirements for Registration of Pharmaceuticals for Human Use. *Clinical Safety Data Management: Definitions and Standards for Expedited Reporting E2A* ICH Secretariat, Geneva, Switzerland. October 1994. http://www.ich.org/cache/compo/276-254-1.html. Accessed February 18, 2010.

4. International Conference on Harmonisation of Technical Requirements for Registration of Pharmaceuticals for Human Use. *Post-approval Safety Data Management: Definitions and Standards for Expedited Reporting E2D* ICH Secretariat, Geneva, Switzerland. November 2003. http://www.ich.org/cache/compo/276-254-1.html. Accessed February 18, 2010.

5. International Conference on Harmonisation of Technical Requirements for Registration of Pharmaceuticals for Human Use. *Guideline for Good Clinical Practice E6 (R1)* ICH Secretariat, Geneva, Switzerland. June 1996. http://www.ich.org/cache/compo/276-254-1.html. Accessed February 18, 2010.

6. International Conference on Harmonisation of Technical Requirements for Registration of Pharmaceuticals for Human Use. *Structure and Content of Clinical Study Reports E3* ICH Secretariat, Geneva, Switzerland. November 1995. http://www.ich.org/cache/compo/276-254-1.html. Accessed February 18, 2010.

7. Code of Federal Regulations. PART 312—INVESTIGATIONAL NEW DRUG APPLICATION, Subpart B—Investigational New Drug Application, Sec. 312.33 "Annual reports." April 2009. http://www.accessdata.fda.gov/scripts/cdrh/cfdocs/cfcfr/CFRSearch.cfm?fr=312.33. Accessed April 11, 2010.

8. "Detailed guidance on the collection, verification and presentation of adverse reaction reports arising from clinical trials on medicinal products for human use." April 2006. http://www.gmp= compliance.org/eca_guideline_2673.html. Accessed April 11, 2010.

9. International Conference on Harmonisation of Technical Requirements for Registration of Pharmaceuticals for Human Use. *Development Safety Update Report E2F* ICH Secretariat, Geneva, Switzerland, June 2008. http://www.ich.org/cache/ compo/276-254-1.html. Accessed February 18, 2010.

10. International Conference on Harmonisation of Technical Requirements for Registration of Pharmaceuticals for Human Use. *The Common Technical Document for the Registration of Pharmaceuticals For Human Use—Efficacy—M4E (R1) Clinical Overview and Clinical Summary of Module 2 Module 5: Clinical Study Reports* ICH Secretariat, Geneva, Switzerland, September 2002. http://www.ich.org/cache/compo/276-254-1.html. Accessed February 18, 2010.

11. "Guideline for the Format and Content of the Clinical and Statistical Sections of an Application" July 1988. http://www.fda.gov/downloads/Drugs/ Guidance-ComplianceRegulatoryInformation/ Guidances/UCM071665.pdf. Accessed February 18, 2010.

12. Code of Federal Regulations. PART 314—APPLICATION FOR FDA APPROVAL TO MARKET A NEW DRUG, Subpart B—Applications, Sec. 314.80 Postmarketing reporting of adverse drug experiences. April 2009. http://www.accessdata.fda. gov/scripts/cdrh/cfdocs/cfcfr/CFRSearch.cfm?fr= 314.80. Accessed February 18, 2010.

13. International Conference on Harmonisation of Technical Requirements for Registration of Pharmaceuticals for Human Use. *Clinical Safety Data Management: Periodic Safety Update Reports for Marketed Drugs E2C(R1)* ICH Secretariat, Geneva, Switzerland, November 2005. http:// www.ich.org/cache/compo/276-254-1.html. Accessed February 10, 2010.

14. Volume 9A of The Rules Governing Medicinal Products in the European Union—Guidelines on Pharmacovigilance for Medicinal Products for Human Use—. September 2008. http://www. gmp=compliance.org/eca_guideline_3081.html. Accessed April 11, 2010.

Begin at the End

"Insanity: doing the same thing over and over again and expecting different results" –Albert Einstein

The development of drugs, obtaining marketing authorization, and keeping these products on the market is challenging. There are many steps that are taken before an adequate and full risk assessment is done. These steps are complex, expensive, and time intensive, with many inherent pitfalls and hidden land mines along the way. Previous experience in the various stages of the collection, analysis, display, summarization, and interpretation of safety data provide invaluable lessons. The objective of this chapter is to discuss the realities that are likely to be encountered and the ways to navigate around these inevitable obstacles. Let us begin at the end.

■ What Is the End?

The end is what must be achieved and includes:

- Showing a *favorable benefit–risk profile* throughout the drug's life cycle
- Being in *compliance* with the many regulations and laws governing drug development and marketing
- Getting a drug *approved* and *marketed* in the earliest, most cost-effective way

The first two are requirements applicable throughout the drug's life cycle and are important for ongoing patient safety. If these requirements are not met, drug approval and continued marketing of the drug cannot be achieved. Now that the end is clear, let's take a hard look at reality and the obstacles along the way.

◼ Reality—Pitfalls and Land Mines

Experience shows that:

- ◼ Important safety information will always be missing
- ◼ There is an abundance of lacks

◼ Important Safety Information Will Always Be Missing

Missing safety information has a significant impact on the ability to adequately determine risk in both the pre- and postmarketing setting. This missing information takes many different forms.

Inadequate Number of Patients Exposed to the Investigational Drug Prior to Approval

The recommended number of patients for long-term use for non–life-threatening conditions is a minimum of 1500 patients with 300–600 patients exposed to the drug for at least 6 months and 100 patients exposed for 1 year at an effective dose. For life-threatening conditions, the number of patients evaluated can even be fewer.[1] For rare, adverse drug-related events (adverse drug reactions) the *Rule of 3* needs consideration. The Rule of 3 states there is at least a 95% chance of seeing 1 or more cases of an adverse reaction in $3n$ trial subjects if the true incidence is 1 in n subjects.[2,3] This means if 300 patients are given a new nonsteroidal anti-inflammatory drug and there are no cases of fatal gastrointestinal bleeding, it can be said with 95% confidence that the true incidence does not exceed 3/300 or 1/100 (1.0%). At the 95% confidence level, to say that the incidence of an adverse reaction is less than or equal to 1/10,000 (0.01%), 30,000 patients must be exposed to the drug without observing the adverse reaction. If in 1500–3000 subjects, an adverse reaction does not occur, one can be 95% confident that the true incidence of the reaction is less than or equal to 1/500 (0.2%)–1/1000 (0.1%). This means that during clinical development, drug reactions with a true incidence of < 0.1% cannot be ruled out if only 3000 subjects are exposed to the investigational drug, even if no patients experience the adverse reaction. To put this in perspective, the incidence of toxic epidermal necrolysis, a severe skin reaction that can result in death, is 0.5 per million population per year.[4] With this low incidence, even if 30,000 patients were evaluated (this would be prohibitive from a time and cost perspective prior to drug approval), it would still be highly unlikely to see even one case of toxic epidermal necrolysis during clinical development.

It is also almost certain that there will be differences in the characteristics of the study population who received the investigational drug and the real world population that will take the marketed drug. Patient subgroups historically at greater risk of adverse drug reactions include the young and the elderly and subjects with hepatic or renal impairment. Exposure of adequate numbers of subjects in these various subgroups during clinical development is also typically limited.

The True Incidence of Postmarketing Spontaneously Reported Adverse Events Is Unknown

The true incidence of spontaneously reported adverse events (AEs) cannot be accurately calculated because neither the number of subjects reporting an AE (numerator) nor the number of subjects exposed to the drug (denominator) are known for certain. Not all patients or healthcare providers report all AEs to the company or health authority. It is well known that there is significant underreporting of AEs.[5] Exposure to the marketed drug is an estimate that is calculated in many different ways; e.g., prescriptions written, number of tablets sold, etc. None of these methods is accurate and all methods represent only a sample of all those exposed. It also remains unknown if the patient took all the tablets prescribed. So the spontaneous AE reporting rate does not equal the true incidence rate as it does in clinical trials where (at least in theory) all AEs are reported by the investigator, and the number of subjects exposed is known.

Individual Case Safety Reports Will Have Incomplete Information

Individual case safety reports (ICSRs) provide a narrative summary of AEs and other safety findings. ICSRs that describe serious, unexpected adverse drug reactions must be promptly reported to health authorities. Before marketing, such cases can lead to changes in the protocol and the informed consent, result in a temporary hold on a clinical study, or even end an entire development program. After marketing, a well-documented ICSR or a series of similar cases indicating a new risk can result in changes in prescribing information, the need for new risk management initiatives (e.g., a postapproval safety study, a pharmacoepidemiology study, registry, etc.) or even possible withdrawal from the marketplace. For these reasons, it is essential the ICSR includes complete and accurate information, but this is often not the case as illustrated in the following example.

Toxicoderma

A report was received from a non–English-speaking study site with the diagnosis of toxicoderma. The patient, a 37-year-old Caucasian male was hospitalized because of fever, edema (swelling) around the eyes, and hematoma-like lesions on the extremities (a hematoma is a localized swelling filled with blood) 3 weeks after starting an investigational drug for treatment of depression. No description of the skin lesions was provided regarding size, shape, number of lesions, and location on the extremities including whether the palms and soles were involved (lesions on the palms and soles can help in determining the diagnosis of some types of skin rashes). The study medication was stopped and the patient was seen by a dermatologist and given prednisone (an anti-inflammatory agent) and an antibiotic. The patient eventually recovered. The investigator considered this event to be serious and related to the investigational drug. No other information was provided.

Although this case appears fairly straightforward, there is, in fact, a large amount of critical information that is missing:

- The case was received from a non–English-speaking site where English was not the native language, so much of the written case information was ambiguous.
- Because these lesions were reported as hematoma-like, this could be due to possible bleeding into the skin, but there was no information regarding complete blood count, platelet count, or coagulation test results.
- There was no information regarding the dermatologist's consultation other than the actions taken (prednisone and antibiotics given). Were the lesions truly hematomas? Was there bleeding into the skin? Were the skin lesions suggestive of an infectious process because the patient received antibiotics?
- Was the patient taking a concomitant medication or did the patient have a preexisting medical condition that could be an alternative explanation for this event?

Unfortunately, this lack of important safety information was not discovered until 4 years later at the time the integrated analysis of safety (IAS) was being prepared, and only 8 weeks were left before the drug company's planned submission date. The clinical trial had ended years ago, and the study site was no longer active. The likelihood of getting the missing information was small to none. What was to be done—in fact, very little? Although this case would be included in the IAS, what impact would it have on the risk profile of the drug, on labeling, and on the risk management plan?

The problem here is obvious—the lack of important information should have been addressed in real time—that is, when the event was first received and reviewed by the drug company. If the deficiencies in this case had been dealt with then, a better understanding of this case would have been possible.

The lack of important information at the case level is not limited to clinical development but is even more challenging and pervasive in the postmarketing setting. In theory, all information from clinical trials for each patient should be available (that is the nature of clinical trials). The investigator has a contractual agreement with the drug company to provide complete safety information, and the patient has signed a consent form permitting this. This is not the case for spontaneous postmarketing reports. Many of these reports are received by telephone and "the one chance" phenomenon rules. This means that you will get the best information from the first call, and the likelihood of getting more information diminishes with each follow-up attempt. To prevent this from happening, the person responsible for intake of AE information must be skilled in eliciting relevant case information at all times, but especially during the first call. Sadly, this is often not achieved.

■ An Abundance of Lacks

Throughout clinical development and postmarketing, there is an abundance of things lacking. The major ones are:

- Lack of planning
- Lack of training
- Lack of quality data
- Lack of standards

- Lack of data intimacy
- Lack of time

These lacks are to a large degree interrelated.

Lack of Planning

Lack of planning is a universal problem and is typically at the root of the other *lacks* that are discussed below. Companies often fall into the crisis mode and suffer because proactive steps were not planned for or put into place at the beginning. This usually results in more wasted time and resources, higher costs, and important issues overlooked or inadequately addressed.

Lack of Training

Supporting a drug throughout its life cycle requires multifunctional teams armed with their own technical expertise. For preparation of safety reports (e.g., the Clinical Study Report, the IAS and the Periodic Safety Update Report for Marketed Products), individuals with diverse skills such as data management, programming, statistics, medical writing, and clinical experience are required. The team, to be most effective, should have a *basic* understanding of an investigational drug's pharmacokinetics (how it is absorbed, distributed, metabolized, and eliminated) and pharmacodynamics (how it works). The team should also be aware of the signs and symptoms associated with important adverse drug reactions. In addition, knowing what vital signs, laboratory tests, and 12-lead electrocardiograms measure and what abnormal values signify will lead to more appropriate programs, analyses, and reports that make good medical sense.

RED HERRING ALERT: For example, it is useful for programmers, statisticians, and medical writers to know that hemoglobin and hematocrit are both a measure of red blood cells and should trend in the same direction. Low values are associated with anemia. If one parameter is abnormally high and the other abnormally low, this should be an alert that there is a data, transcription, programming, or analysis error. A well-trained and informed team is more likely to catch this type of error sooner than later.

Lack of Quality Data

Poor quality data take many different forms, including:

- Missing information
- Vague or poorly described verbatim AEs (the terminology used by the reporter)
- Translation and transcription errors
- Data inconsistencies

The determination of risk is dependent on the data collected. If the data are of poor quality, risk assessment is negatively impacted. The saying, "Garbage in…garbage out," applies.

Lack of Standards

The development and maintenance of standards can improve quality and reduce time, resources, and costs. Standards apply to many different things and include, but are not limited, to the following:

- **Standard operating procedures**—These provide a road map of the procedures that should be followed, ensuring consistency of output and compliance with laws governing clinical development and the marketing of drugs. They are obligatory under many countries' regulatory requirements (including the United States and the European Union) and are clearly best practices.
- **Data standards**—These standards (e.g., standard units, standard measurements, standard categories) are applied to the data that are collected and analyzed. An example of a data standard is the use of only 1 unit in the measurement of weight—kilograms or pounds, but not both. In assessing risk, data have to be pooled (combined) in order to increase the chance of identifying a safety signal. To do this, data have to be standardized, e.g., all the data have to be in the same unit. If data standards are not applied early on in the clinical development, the nonstandard data need to be converted to the standards established for data analysis. This results in the inefficient use of time and money and drives up costs and increases the chance of data conversion errors. This is illustrated in the following example.

Nonstandard Categories for Premature Discontinuations

For the IAS, standards as mentioned previously are a requirement for data pooling. An example of this is pooling reasons for premature discontinuation of treatment (dropouts) across studies. Let us say there are 25 studies to be included in the IAS and 4 categories are selected for summarizing reasons for early termination:

1. Lack of efficacy
2. AE
3. Lost to follow-up
4. Other

However, due to lack of up-front planning, the reasons for premature discontinuations were not standardized at the beginning of the clinical development program. Consequently, 8 of the studies had 6 reasons for termination (not just the 4 just listed). Another 5 studies had 7 reasons each. So now, at the time of the IAS (when everyone is rushing to finish the submission) the team will have to figure out how to fit the 6 and 7 reasons into the 4 dropout categories chosen for the IAS. Sometimes this is difficult and can add a level of ambiguity and trouble to the submission, precipitating a request for clarification and reanalysis by the Food and Drug Administration or other health authority. Waiting to standardize data until the preparation of the IAS is costly in terms of time, personnel, programming, quality control…and stress levels.

Lack of Data Intimacy

One of the most interesting and fascinating phenomena observed is companies' avoidance of getting "intimate," with their own data…until they are forced to do so! That is, a careful and thoughtful review of the data to identify potential trends and new safety signals may not be done proactively or on an ongoing basis, but only when required, e.g., for report submissions to health authorities. Evidence of this abounds. Not critically reviewing ICSR information and not aggressively pursuing missing case information as was previously discussed is a disturbing example of this. Another example is absence of thoughtful consideration of problems the data may reveal—both study-related problems (e.g., a multicenter study with a disproportionate number of dropouts from a single investigator site), and the identification and investigation of subtle safety signals.

Lack of Time

Drug companies, not the health authorities, decide the dates for submission of registration dossiers. Submission dates are typically optimistic and often made in a relative vacuum by senior management without close consultation with those responsible for the dossier's preparation. Once established, the timeline often becomes *carved in stone* due to promises to shareholders and investors and the threat of losing a bonus if a submission date is missed.

Experience teaches us, though, that additional time should always be added to the submission date and factored in before a submission date is set. This added insurance is necessary because unpleasant surprises are inevitable. These include the need for reanalysis as well as additional analyses of the data.

■ Need for Reanalysis and Additional Analyses of the Data

Reanalysis of the Data

Data pooling and analysis of integrated data for the IAS require complicated programs, especially if there are many parameters and many measurements to analyze—for example, laboratory tests. Programming and database errors are likely but are often not seen until the data are displayed in tables, listings, and figures.

An example of this is the inconsistencies found in the number of patients who prematurely discontinue treatment due to an AE. This information is usually captured in 2 different places, the end of study case report form page and the AE case report form page; and is displayed in 2 different sections of the submission, the disposition section and the AE section. The AE rates shown in the disposition and AE summary tables must match, but often do not! Because discontinuations due to AEs are important in risk assessment, these data are carefully scrutinized by regulatory authorities and should be correct and consistent in both sections of the submission. If inconsistencies are not discovered before preparation of the IAS, the database has to be corrected and the tables revised (or "rerun," as many refer to this). For an IAS where there are numerous AE tables, such errors can have a tremendous negative impact on time, money, and resources because large volumes of tables have to be reprogrammed and revised. But one of the biggest and most important consequences is that with a fixed submission date, the window for medical review is severely compressed because review cannot be done until the tables are corrected.

Such problems could be entirely avoided if plans are put into place to check for these types of inconsistencies—if the clinical research associate is trained to look for these inconsistencies when reviewing case report forms, and if consistency checks of the data are done on an ongoing basis. But this is often not done and these errors still occur.

Additional Analyses Will Be Required

Once the data are integrated (whether there was planning, whether there were good processes in place, whether the data were standardized), there will always be surprising results (both good and bad) that pop out. These results will not be visible until the analyses of the pooled data are done. These surprises will require further analyses to determine if there is a true drug effect or a false signal (red herring). These additional analyses are referred to as *ad hoc* analyses. The pitfalls are again lack of planning for this eventuality and not starting the integration of studies sooner in the clinical development program. The consequences are predictable—the time for medical review and risk assessment will be further compressed or the submission date may need to be delayed.

If the aforementioned delays are encountered and timelines remain unchanged, there will be insufficient time to do a proper analysis, medical review, and risk determination. The result will be a poor quality and often an inadequate submission. If this occurs, the regulatory agency is likely to do a better analysis of the data, filling in the obvious gaps left by the sponsor. This is even truer now that many submissions are electronic ones, allowing easier data access and analysis by the regulatory agency reviewers. This reflects badly on the sponsor and can raise many questions at the health authority. In the worst case, one might even suspect the company of burying or obfuscating data. Credibility with regulatory agencies and the public will suffer. This can also lead to significant delays in gaining drug approval or even being denied market authorization.

■ Time Is Money

Throughout the chapter examples were given that discuss wasted time and resources resulting in significant financial consequences. The effect of time wasted is illustrated in Table 2-1, which shows the loss of potential revenue when there is a delay in market authorization.

Because of the pitfalls and land mines discussed throughout this chapter, it is easy to see that a delay of a month or more of getting a drug on the market is very

Table 2-1 Time Is Money—Potential Loss of Revenue for a Billion-Dollar-a-Year Drug	
Approval Delay	**Lost Revenue**
1 year	$1,000,000,000
1 month	$83,333,333
1 day	$2,739,726
1 hour	$114,155
1 minute	$1,903
1 second	$32

possible. For a drug with a projected revenue of $1 billion annually, this would translate into more than $80 million in potential lost revenue—money that could be used for reinvestment in research and development or could result in less expensive medicines.

■ The Domino Effect

The various problems described in this chapter are not isolated, and they result in a domino effect of negative consequences. The impact these issues have on achieving the end should now be painfully obvious. But they can be avoided or at least minimized by following the road map to success.

■ The Road Map to Success

The road map to success is to:

- Plan
- Train
- Develop standards and create and maintain an integrated safety database early in the clinical development program
- Aggressively and proactively go after incomplete information in real time
- Commit to quality data
- Commit to thorough and ongoing medical review
- Create documents and submissions that are user friendly, clearly written, and easily understood

With the end clearly in sight, the rest of the book will provide pragmatic approaches to avoid the pitfalls and land mines discussed in this chapter. Time, money, and resources can be saved and quality improved. But most importantly, a better job in determining risk is accomplished...this translates into better patient protection!

References

1. International Conference on Harmonisation of Technical Requirements for Registration of Pharmaceutical for Human Use. *The Extent of Population Exposure to Access Clinical Safety for Drugs Intended for Long-Term Treatment of Non-life-threatening Conditions E1*. Geneva, Switzerland: ICH Secretariat; October 1994 http://www.ich.org/cache/compo/276-254-1.html. Accessed February 18, 2010.

2. *Guidance for Industry Drug-Induced Liver Injury: Premarketing Clinical Evaluation*. Washington, DC: US Department of Health and Human Services, Food and Drug Administration, Center for Drug Evaluation and Research (CDER) Center for Biologics Evaluation and Research (CBER); 2009. http://www.fda.gov/downloads/Drugs/Guidance ComplianceRegulatoryInformation/Guidances/ UCM174090.pdf. Accessed February 18, 2010.

3. Rosner B. The binomial distribution. In: Rosner B, ed. *Fundamentals of Biostatistics*. Belmont, CA: Duxbury Press; 1995:82–85.

4. Chan HL, Stern RS, Arndt KA, et al. The incidence of erythema multiforme, Stevens-Johnson syndrome, and toxic epidermal necrolysis. A population-based study with particular reference to reactions caused by drugs among outpatients. *Arch Dermatol*. 1990;126(1):43–47.

5. Hazell L, Shakir SA. Under-reporting of adverse drug reactions: a systematic review. *Drug Saf*. 2006; 29:385–396.

3

The Dynamic Integrated Safety Database—Something You Shouldn't Live Without

An integrated safety database refers to a database that contains all the safety data collected from all subjects who received 1 or more doses of study medication in a clinical development program. It includes adverse events, laboratory tests, vital signs and electrocardiogram (ECG) data, and any other safety data that were collected during clinical development. It generally excludes postmarketing safety data, which is kept in a separate database (if the drug is already marketed somewhere).

Integration of safety information across clinical trials enhances the ability to identify and characterize drug-related risks. An integrated safety database facilitates an *integrated analysis* and *integrated review* of the data. It is also a requirement for the preparation of the Integrated Summary of Safety (ISS) and Summary of Clinical Safety (SCS) reports—the safety summary documents required before a drug can be approved for marketing.

The creation of the integrated safety database at the end of the clinical development program is too late! Ideally, it should be created at the beginning of clinical development and certainly no later than the beginning of

the Phase 3 program. For this reason, the word *dynamic* is used to underscore that such a database is not static, but is expected to grow as more studies are completed and added to the database.

■ Benefits of Creating and Maintaining a Dynamic Integrated Safety Database

Investing in the creation and maintenance of a dynamic integrated safety database will yield many benefits. In the previous chapter, the importance of planning, the development of standards, a commitment to quality data, and ongoing data review were discussed. The creation and maintenance of a dynamic integrated safety database incorporates all these good practices and avoids the land mines, pitfalls, and negative domino effect (i.e., the cascading negative consequences) that can occur if these practices are not followed. Specific benefits include:

■ Enhancement of ongoing benefit–risk assessments by improving chances of earlier detection of safety signals.

■ Forcing the use of *standardized* data. Standardized data mean that the same unit of measurement is used for a particular data element, or that data are grouped in the same categories across all clinical trials. For example, using only 1 unit for weight, e.g., kilograms across *all* studies, rather than using pounds in some studies. Data standards are required for data pooling (i.e., combining data across different studies). If data standards are used at the beginning of the clinical development program, the need for mapping (converting) nonstandard data into standard categories is avoided.

■ The early development of the statistical analysis plan (SAP) for the integrated analysis of safety (IAS). The SAP is the blueprint for how the data are to be analyzed and displayed. A large part of the SAP developed for an IAS can also be used for individual study reports. This ensures better consistency in the programming, analysis, and display of data across clinical trials.

■ Use in other programs. Many of the data standards and elements of an SAP created for 1 clinical development program are generic (not drug specific) and can be recycled and reused in the clinical development programs for other investigational drugs.

■ Identification of data, programming, and analysis errors. The development of the SAP includes the design of table shells, listings, and figures. When data are displayed in tables, listings, and figures, it is easier to identify data, programming, and analysis errors. Time is saved and data quality is improved when errors are caught and corrected early.

■ Easier review. Displays of pooled data make review easier. This allows the reviewer to become more intimate and familiar with the data, thereby decreasing the risk of missing an important but subtle safety signal.

■ Positive effect on clinical development. Access to integrated data can also affect the ongoing clinical development program. Earlier detection of safety signals can underscore the need for:

  ▫ Revising, putting on hold, or stopping ongoing studies

  ▫ Adding studies to the clinical development program

■ Preview of the ISS/SCS.

  ▫ Data integration increases the likelihood of earlier identification of safety signals, allowing more time to do:

    ▫ Additional (*ad hoc*) analyses that were not originally planned for.

    ▫ Targeted literature reviews to determine the background incidence of a safety finding, e.g., the rate of myocardial infarction (heart attack) in the general population.

  ▫ By starting data integration early, most of the data, programming, and analysis errors should already be identified and corrected before the formal ISS/SCS preparation starts. This ensures that valuable time will not be wasted on correcting errors—time that should be spent on proper medical review.

  ▫ Earlier data integration improves the chances that timelines will be met without compromising quality review time. It also reduces the overall stress associated with the preparation of these reports.

■ Other uses. The integrated safety database can also be used for:

  ▫ Data preparation for external or in-house data safety monitoring committees.

  ▫ Preparation of periodic safety reports—e.g., the US IND Annual Report, the EU Annual Safety Report, the Japanese periodic 6-monthly report, and the International Conference on Harmonisation-recommended Development Safety Update Report.

All these benefits result in better quality data, more efficient use of time and resources, and considerable cost savings. The most important benefit, however, is ultimately to the patient. Earlier and enhanced detection of safety signals, and enough time to do thorough and complete data analysis and review, result in a better understanding of a drug's risk profile!

■ Pooled Versus Integrated Data

In discussing data integration, it is important to make the distinction between *integrated* and *pooled* data. These terms are often used interchangeably but they have different meanings. Integrated data may or may not include data that are pooled.

Integrated data are data that are arranged in such a way that safety information, for example, adverse events, can be reviewed across all clinical studies. Integrated data also includes different safety information, e.g., adverse events, laboratory tests, vital signs, and ECG in 1 database. This aids in the identification of any links or connections in safety findngs. Adverse drug reactions (adverse events that are drug related) seldom occur in isolation and are often linked to other safety findings, e.g., change in vital signs, laboratory, or ECG values. The more links to other safety parameters, the stronger the evidence that the finding is drug related. For instance, epinephrine, an adrenergic receptor agonist, has stimulant properties that cause increases in heart rate and blood pressure. The types of adverse events that are expected with the use of epinephrine are those related to such increases, e.g., tachycardia and hypertension. Measurements of vital signs predictably show an increase in blood pressure and pulse rate values. Assessment of ECGs also show a trend toward increases in heart rate. Three different safety evaluations—adverse events, vital signs, and ECGs all show similar findings, thereby strengthening the weight of evidence that increased blood pressure and heart rate are drug related. An integrated review would therefore require review of different but often related safety parameters. For this reason, it is important that all this information be housed in 1 place, e.g., an integrated safety database.

Pooled data are data obtained from different studies that are combined and then analyzed together. For instance, if there are 5 individual studies with 100 subjects exposed to the investigational drug in each study, the pooled analysis is done on the data from 500 subjects. Some studies should not be pooled because of important differences that confound (confuse) the interpretation of the data. Important factors that can preclude pooling include:

- Different study designs—e.g., a parallel study (where a subject receives only one treatment) versus a crossover study (where a subject first receives a placebo and then the investigational product and vise versa)
- Different doses—e.g., doses considerably lower (1 mg) than doses targeted as the recommended doses (100 mg and 200 mg)
- Different formulations—e.g., topical application—where little systemic absorption is expected versus intravenous administration
- Different study durations—e.g., a 1-day study versus a 1-year study
- Different study populations—e.g., evaluation of an investigational antibiotic in subjects with mild superficial infections versus subjects with life-threatening infections

For many of the reasons listed, data from Phase 1 studies (healthy disease-free volunteers) are usually not pooled with data from Phase 2 or 3 studies (subjects with a disease requiring treatment). Nevertheless, safety data from Phase 1 and Phases 2 and 3 studies, although not pooled, should be included in the integrated safety database.

The following example will help illustrate the difference between pooled and integrated data.

Syncope

A review of adverse events from an integrated safety database revealed 5 cases of syncope (fainting). One case was from a Phase 1 study and the remaining 4 cases were from pooled Phase 2 and 3 studies. All 5 cases occurred in subjects exposed to the investigational drug. Review of each of the 5 cases showed that in 4 subjects, syncope occurred within 1 hour of the first dose of the investigational drug and was associated with systolic blood pressures below 90 mmHg (range of systolic blood pressure values: 60 mmHg–88 mmHg). In the mean change analysis of pooled controlled Phase 2 and 3 studies, systolic blood pressure showed a mean decrease of 5 mmHg from baseline to end point (last measurement on treatment) in the investigational drug group compared to placebo. Furthermore, evaluating marked outliers in controlled Phase 2 and 3 studies showed, a higher rate of subjects in the investigational drug group (6%) compared to placebo (1%) with clinically significant decreases in systolic blood pressure defined as a systolic blood pressure value ≤ 90 mmHg and a decrease of ≥ 20 mmHg from baseline.

In this example, the integrated review of syncope included pooled and nonpooled data and data from different safety evaluations as follows:

- Data from pooled controlled Phase 2 and 3 studies
- Information from Phase 1 studies
- Adverse event data
- Vital signs data

■ How to Create and Maintain a Dynamic Integrated Safety Database

1. The creation and maintenance of a dynamic integrated database is a collaborative effort requiring a multifunctional team with diverse expertise. Teams should include individuals with programming, statistical, database, and clinical experience.

2. Data pooling should be planned early in the clinical development program. Determination of what studies should or should not be pooled should be made on an ongoing basis when studies are added to the clinical development program.

3. Only completed studies should be included—and only after the data are cleaned, verified, and unblinded, and the database for that study locked so no other changes can be made.

4. Data standards should be developed at the beginning of the clinical development program and used throughout drug development.

5. The SAP should also be developed early in the clinical development program and revised as needed. Examples of the content of the SAP include, but are not limited, to the following (specific examples are shown throughout the book):

   ■ Definitions/criteria for:
      ▪ Study periods—baseline, treatment, and posttreatment
      ▪ Treatment-emergent adverse events
      ▪ Clinically significant values/changes
   ■ Conventions used for:
      ▪ Handling missing data
      ▪ Analyses—e.g., what treatment value should be used for categorical shifts and outlier analyses, e.g., end-of-treatment value (last value measured) or any on-treatment value
      ▪ Methods used in determining potential adverse reactions
   ■ Standard analyses for:
      ▪ Rates of adverse events
         ○ Common
         ○ Serious adverse events

         ○ Adverse events leading to discontinuation
         ○ Other significant adverse events or adverse events of interest
      ▪ Laboratory tests, vital signs, ECGs
         ○ Mean/median changes from baseline
         ○ Categorical shifts (shifts from one category to another, e.g., normal to above the normal range, normal to below the normal range)
         ○ Outlier analyses for clinically significant findings
   ■ Data displays
      ▪ Development of table shells, listings, and figures

6. Utilization of the following resources greatly aid in data integration:
   ■ Electronic data capture (EDC) rather than using paper case report forms
   ■ Central laboratories
   ■ Central ECG services

7. Note that if database-to-database transfer is used (e.g., central lab data are loaded directly into the sponsor's database[s]), all appropriate information technology safeguards as well as regulatory requirements such as validated databases and data transfer protocols, data protection, security, etc. must be observed. Care should also be taken to maintain the blind in those studies still underway or where the blind is not broken. Reconciliation of databases (e.g., EDC versus sponsor safety and efficacy databases), source documents, serious adverse event logs, etc. must also be done on an ongoing basis rather than waiting until the end of the trial.

4

Coding Basics

➡ **NOTE:** Throughout the book, MedDRA version 12.0 was used.

In order to determine risk, it is important to review safety data that occurs in groups (aggregates) of people. In order to do an aggregate analysis, data from one individual need to be pooled or combined with data from others. The data collected, however, are not always reported in a uniform way.

■ Why Code?

Coding is a process whereby data are categorized in a standard way so the data can be pooled or combined for analysis. Standardized data also allow various entities such as governments, hospitals, insurance companies, drug companies, and others to exchange data using the same terminology.

In drug safety, coding is typically done for 3 types of data:

1. Adverse events
2. Medical and surgical history
3. Concomitant drugs

These standardized categories or terms can be found in specially designed dictionaries. Examples of dictionaries used for adverse event coding are: the Medical Dictionary for Regulatory Activities (MedDRA), World Health Organization—Adverse Reactions Terminology (WHO-ART), and Systematized Nomenclature of Medicine (SNOMED).[1–3] Dictionaries used to code medical history terms include MedDRA, the International Classification of Diseases, 9th revision, Clinical Modification (ICD-9-CM), and the Diagnostic and Statistical Manual of Mental Disorders, 4th edition (DSM-IV), for psychiatric disorders.[4,5] (The first draft of DSM-V has just appeared and will be available soon.) An example of a dictionary used for concomitant medication terms is the World Health Organization—Drug Dictionary Enhanced.[6]

MedDRA is the dictionary usually used for coding adverse events and medical histories for drugs and biologics. The use of a MedDRA term is required for electronic submissions of individual case safety reports (ICSRs) to regulatory agencies in the European Union, the United States, and Japan.[7] For these reasons, issues specific to MedDRA will also be discussed in this chapter.

Table 4-1 provides examples of adverse events received from various reporters—these events are referred to as *verbatim* or *reported* terms. The reporter is typically a health professional or a consumer but can be someone else or even a different entity such as a regulatory agency or poison control center. In the examples shown in this table, the verbatim terms listed have different names; nevertheless they share the same medical concept of *dyspnoea*. If these terms were not grouped together into 1 standardized term, the rate for dyspnoea would be underestimated. In this example, the verbatim terms were coded to MedDRA terms. MedDRA uses British English spelling rather than American English, which is why the British spelling *dyspnoea* is used instead of the American spelling, *dyspnea*.

In addition to coding adverse events into standard terms, medical history terms should also be coded. This serves 3 purposes:

1. It is important to determine if subjects who participated in a clinical trial are similar/dissimilar to the real world population who will be taking the drug. This determination is done by comparing baseline characteristics of the study population to the population targeted to take the drug once marketed. Medical history is one component of the baseline characteristics of an individual participating in a clinical trial.

2. It is also important to know the baseline characteristics for each treatment group. In clinical trials, differences between treatment groups at baseline can make it very hard to know whether differences at the end of the trial were due to the study drug or due to treatment group differences observed at baseline. This is illustrated by the following example. A higher rate of hypertension (15%) is reported as an adverse event in the investigational group compared to a 3% rate in the placebo group. However, a review of medical histories shows that 5% of the investigational group had a history of hypertension compared to only 1% in the placebo group. This difference in the adverse event rate of hypertension may, therefore, be due to or be influenced by this baseline difference and confounds (confuses) the interpretation of the finding.

3. Medical history is also important in the determination of drug–disease interactions. A drug–disease interaction can indicate a greater risk of developing an adverse drug reaction in subjects with certain medical conditions. An example is the increased risk of stroke in hypertensive women taking oral contraceptives. Table 4-2 illustrates how different verbatim terms in the medical history describing myocardial infarction all get coded to the same standardized term *Myocardial infarction*.

The reasons to code concomitant medications are similar to the rationale for coding medical history; i.e., it is part of a subject's baseline characteristics, needed in the understanding and interpretation of any treatment group differences, and useful in evaluating potential drug–drug interactions. Examples of coded concomitant medications are shown in Table 4-3.

Concomitant medication coding provides a standard term regardless of whether the drug is listed by its proprietary (brand name), Prinivil, or generic name, lisinopril.

■ The Coding Process

Many companies use an autoencoder (a computer program that can provide a coded term automatically if the verbatim term is identified in the program). The autoencoder is used for both *interactive* and *batch* coding. Interactive coding refers to assigning a coded term 1 patient at a time. Batch coding refers to coding the verbatim terms of many subjects at the same time. Interactive coding is usually done for serious adverse events received from clinical trials and spontaneous postmarketing reports that are processed a single patient at a time. The batch method is used to code clinical trial data that are processed in batches.

Table 4-1   Examples of Verbatim Adverse Event Terms Coded to a Standard MedDRA Term

Verbatim Term	Coded Term[a]
Short of breath	Dyspnoea
Heavy breathing	Dyspnoea
Dyspnea	Dyspnoea
Difficulty breathing	Dyspnoea

[a] MedDRA Preferred Term

Table 4-2 Examples of Medical History Terms Coded to a Standard MedDRA Term

Verbatim Term	Coded Term[a]
Heart attack	Myocardial infarction
MI	Myocardial infarction
Myocardial infarction	Myocardial infarction
Myocardial necrosis	Myocardial infarction

[a] MedDRA Preferred Term

Table 4-3 Examples of Coded Concomitant Drugs

Verbatim Drug Name	Coded Term
Propranolol	Beta blockers
Inderal	Beta blockers
Lisinopril	ACE inhibitors
Prinivil	ACE inhibitors

Autoencoders have proven to be very useful, although they cannot be totally relied upon without human review. Most work by looking for matches between the verbatim term and a dictionary term. If a term is found, it is accepted. If the autoencoder does not identify the verbatim term, a coding specialist/drug safety professional has to manually assign a code.

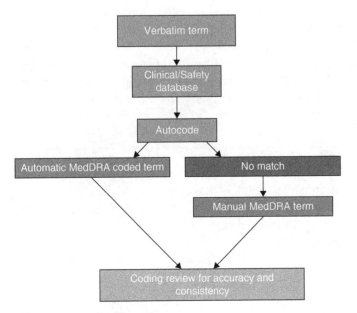

Figure 4-1 Coding Process

Figure 4-1 is a schematic of the process used to code adverse events using the MedDRA dictionary. It shows two paths that can be taken. If the verbatim term is recognized by the autoencoder, a MedDRA term is automatically assigned (path on the left in Figure 4-1). If not, a code has to be assigned manually (the path on the right). With more than 85,000 terms, automatic coding is the preferred method when using the MedDRA dictionary. Moreover, manual coding takes more time and can lead to coding inconsistencies.

> **CAUTION:** Regardless of what path is followed, all coded terms should be reviewed against the verbatim term. Experience shows automatic processes are not infallible and errors can still occur, including technical issues (the autoencoder "was suffering from a case of 24-hour electronic flu"), and much of the output turns out to be gibberish. Review is also important for vague verbatim terms. Such terms may be assigned a code automatically but the coded term is too general and lacks specificity regarding cause and clinical relevance. The term shock is an example of a vague term. The verbatim term shock codes to the same MedDRA term *Shock*. But shock can have many different causes, such as electric, septic, anaphylactic, cardiogenic. A non-healthcare provider may also report severe fright as shock. Shock by itself provides limited insight into what the subject really experienced, and a more specific term should be used instead.

The Quality of the Verbatim Term

The coding process is driven by the quality of the verbatim term. A good quality term is a specific medical term; a poor quality term is often a layman's or nonmedical term or a term that is vague—shock. An example of a nonmedical term is *thick throat*. It is unclear what this term means—does it mean the subject had pharyngitis (sore throat), dysphonia (hoarseness), or laryngeal edema (swelling of the throat and vocal cords)? These 3 conditions fall on different ends of the spectrum of clinical importance—2 are nonserious while the other is life threatening.

Nonmedical terms are unlikely to be matched to a dictionary term, so coding has to be done manually. What term to select can become a guessing game. Coding of clinical trial data is often performed by coding specialists who may have no information other than the verbatim term to code. In a postmarketing setting, a drug safety specialist may code adverse event information received from a call center relying entirely on the case information received by the call center. In the example of thick throat, if a medical term was provided, e.g., pharyngitis, dysphonia, or laryngeal edema, the verbatim term would have been recognized by the autoencoder, and a coded term would have been provided automatically.

To minimize the number of poor quality terms, the following steps can and should be taken.

For Clinical Trials

- At investigator meetings, discuss with the investigator and study coordinator the importance of using medical terminology and the need to avoid vague terms by showing examples like *thick throat* and *shock*.

- The investigator and study coordinator should understand it is their responsibility to put the layman's (patient's) description of the event into a proper medical term. This should be done rather than taking straight dictation from the patient.

- The investigator should be encouraged to provide a diagnosis rather than list individual signs and symptoms of the event. For example, *pneumonia* should be listed rather than fever, productive cough, and infiltrate on chest X-ray.

- Clinical research associates should be trained to recognize verbatim terms that are nonmedical or vague terms so they can get clarification from the investigator and study coordinator as required.

- Batch coding should be performed on a routine basis while the study is still ongoing to identify all terms that don't autoencode. Verbatim terms should also be reviewed for vagueness. If such terms are identified, the study site should be queried for clarification.

For Postmarketing Spontaneous Safety Reports

- Individuals responsible for intake of adverse event information (e.g., call center personnel, drug safety specialists) need to be able to identify nonmedical and vague terms and be trained on questioning the reporter for clarification.

- The reporter, if a healthcare professional, should be asked for a diagnosis if none is given.

Remember, regardless of whether verbatim terms are assigned automatically or manually, *all* coded terms must be reviewed for accuracy and consistency!

■ Coding Conventions

To ensure coding uniformity and consistency, a coding convention document should be established for each clinical development program and marketed product, and the coding specialists should be trained on its contents. Coding conventions should include, but are not limited to:

- How to handle terms listed as both individual signs and symptoms and a diagnosis, e.g., chest pain, elevated cardiac enzymes, myocardial infarction. Should these terms be lumped together and coded to only one term (*Myocardial infarction*) because chest pain and elevated cardiac enzymes are signs and symptoms of myocardial infarction? Or should the terms be split and separately coded to *Myocardial infarction*, *Cardiac enzymes increased*, and *Chest pain*?

  ➡ **NOTE:** It is generally recommended to code the diagnosis and not the individual signs and symptoms—the *lump* approach rather than the *split* approach.

- The approaches to be followed for handling vague and nonmedical terms.
- What MedDRA versions to use and how to handle coding revisions based on the versions selected.
- The process followed for quality control and consistency checks.

TIP: It is recommended that the "Points to Consider" documents developed by the Maintenance and Support Services Organization that supports the MedDRA dictionary be referred to in the development of coding conventions.[8]

■ MedDRA

Because MedDRA is mandated for electronic regulatory submission of ICSRs and is increasingly used in summarizing clinical and postmarketing aggregate data, it is useful to point out its challenges and provide some tips for its best use. MedDRA is organized into 5 levels:

1. System Organ Class (SOC)
2. High Level Group Term (HLGT)
3. High Level Term (HLT)

4. Preferred Term (PT)

5. Lowest Level Term (LLT)

The LLT contains the most specific terms while the SOC contains the least specific terms as is illustrated in Figure 4-2.

Autoencoding usually is done at the LLT level—the level that has the greatest number of terms, including many related and redundant terms. These large numbers of terms increase the chance the autoencoder will identify a dictionary term that can be matched to the verbatim term. LLTs include synonyms (different words with the same meaning) and lexical variants (e.g., the same word spelled differently—*Dyspnea, Dyspnoea,* or the same two words in different word order—*Chest pain, Pain chest*). Once the verbatim term is matched to an LLT, the PT, HLT, HLGT, and SOC are easily determined. Adverse event tables in safety reports typically display the rates of adverse events at the PT level. In electronic reporting of expedited ICSRs to health authorities, the verbatim term, and LLT are included.[7] Given the hierarchical nature of MedDRA, if you have identified the LLT, you will know the unique PT (because it is a one-to-one map of LLT to PT).

■ Multiaxiality

To complicate matters, in many instances, the same MedDRA term can be found in more than one SOC. This is referred to as *multiaxiality*. The MedDRA dictionary flags which SOC is the preferred or primary SOC and which SOC(s) is (are) considered secondary. The PT *Migraine*, for example, can be found in the SOCs *Nervous system disorders* (primary SOC) and *Vascular disorders* (secondary SOC). Because of the possibility of multiaxial terms, a coding convention should be established indicating which SOC should be used; i.e., primary or secondary.

■ Data Retrieval Options

In addition to MedDRA's hierarchy, terms can also be grouped into *Standardised MedDRA Queries (SMQs)*. SMQs are groupings of PTs from one or more SOCs that relate to a defined medical condition or area of interest. They are intended to aid in signal detection. The PTs included in SMQs may relate to signs, symptoms, diagnoses, syndromes, physical findings, laboratory and other physiologic test data, etc., related to the medical condition or area of interest.[9] Examples include but are not limited to the following: *Agranulocytosis, Possible drug-related hepatic disorders—comprehensive search, Rhabdomyolysis/myopathy,* and *Torsade de pointes/QT prolongation.* The SMQ usually contains two categories of PTs—narrow and broad. Broad terms are usually nonspecific and can be found in many different conditions. In contrast, narrow terms tend to be more specific. For example, in the SMQ for *Rhabdomyolysis/myopathy,* one of the narrow terms is *Muscle necrosis,* which is muscle specific; and one of the broad terms is *Blood creatinine increased,* a term that may be due to conditions other than rhabdomyolysis. In using SMQs, whether the broad and narrow terms or only the narrow terms are used should be specified.

In situations where SMQs are not available or are not quite right for the task at hand, other data retrieval options have to be relied upon. In some cases, using a modified SMQ (mSMQ) or an *ad hoc* query (AHQ) is a better option. A modified SMQ refers to an SMQ where PTs have been added to or deleted from the original SMQ. An AHQ refers to a list of PTs the drug company selects to use.

Deciding what terms to include in an AHQ is based on clinical judgment but remains arbitrary and will vary from company to company. For this reason in the methods section of a report, the terms selected should be clearly documented. The reviewer can then decide whether to use as is or revise by adding or deleting terms.

An Example of an Ad Hoc Query

The ad hoc query *Hypotension* was created to identify patients who potentially had decreases in blood pressure and includes the following PTs: *Blood pressure ambulatory decreased; Blood pressure decreased; Blood pressure diastolic decreased; Blood pressure orthostatic decreased; Blood*

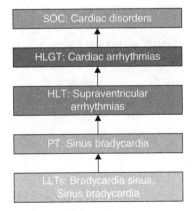

Figure 4–2 An Example of MedDRA's Hierarchy

pressure systolic decreased; Hypotension; Orthostatic hypotension; Presyncope; Syncope; and *Syncope vasovagal.*

MedDRA Challenges

MedDRA use is associated with a number of challenges of which the user must be aware. These include:

- **MedDRA's granularity.** Granularity refers to the number of terms/coding choices in MedDRA— more than 85,000 terms—this makes coding difficult and increases the potential for inconsistencies if manual coding is done. The use of coding conventions (discussed previously) and ongoing review of coded terms are required to minimize coding inconsistencies.

- **Change in versions.** Currently, 2 versions of MedDRA are released each year. In these versions, new codes are introduced, old codes are sometimes retired, or the axiality (hierarchy) is changed. The coded terms affected by the version change will need to be recoded accordingly.

- **Similarity of terms at the PT level.** The PT is supposed to represent a single medical concept, but this is not always true. In MedDRA, different terms are used for diagnoses versus signs/symptoms, but they often represent the same medical condition. Examples include *Blood potassium increased* versus *Hyperkalaemia,* and *Blood pressure decreased* versus *Hypotension.* While it can be argued that *Blood pressure decreased* may be different than *Hypotension* (i.e., blood pressure dropped from baseline values but remained within the normal range, versus a systolic blood pressure < 90 mmHg or a diastolic blood pressure < 60 mmHg), in actual practice, healthcare providers are unlikely to

make this distinction and will use these terms interchangeably. This unintentional dilution (i.e., some events reported as *Hypotension* while other as *Blood pressure decreased*) can lead to underestimation of adverse event rates if these similar terms are not combined in some fashion.

TIP: To avoid this potential dilution, *combined terms* should be used especially for calculating the rates of suspect adverse drug reactions.

➡ **NOTE:** Combined term is our terminology— use whatever word you like, just be sure to define the term you decide to use, so the reviewer understands what the term means.

For example, for a diuretic that can result in decreases in potassium levels, a combined term should be used that incorporates both *Hypokalaemia* and *Blood potassium decreased* to ensure the rate of events related to decreased potassium values is not underestimated. When using combined terms in an adverse event summary table, these terms should be flagged in some fashion and described in the text so the reviewer understands what was done, e.g., *Hypokalaemia**. If the rate for *Hypokalaemia* is 5% and the rate for *Blood potassium decreased* is 3%, the rate for the combined term of *Hypokalaemia** is 8%.

Using a Combined Term

The following is an example of how an explanation of combined terms can be handled in the text and table of a report.

Table 4-4 is a summary of common adverse events (rates ≥ 5%) from placebo-controlled

Table 4-4	Common Adverse Events (Rates ≥ 5%)—Placebo-Controlled Phase 2/3 Studies	
Adverse Event (MedDRA preferred term)	**Placebo** N = 100	**Investigational Drug** N = 100
Headache	25 (25%)	24 (24%)
Nausea	8 (8%)	17 (17%)
Dizziness	10 (10%)	11 (11%)
Myocardial infarction*	6 (6%)	4 (4%)

* Includes: Acute myocardial infarction, Myocardial infarction, and Silent myocardial infarction.

Phase 2/3 studies. Please note that for Myocardial infarction, the terms *Acute myocardial infarction, Myocardial infarction,* and *Silent myocardial infarction* were combined in the calculation of the rate.

Remember, the quality of the verbatim term drives the coding process!

References

1. *Medical Dictionary for Regulatory Activities (MedDRA).* 2010. http://www.meddramsso.com. Accessed February 18, 2010.

2. WHO-ART. http://www.umc-products.com/Dynpage. aspx?id=73589&mn1=1107&mn2=1664. Accessed February 10, 2010.

3. SNOMED. *SNOMED Clinical Terms (SNOMED CT).* 2009. http://www.nlm.nih.gov/research/umls/Snomed/snomed_main.html. Accessed February 18, 2010.

4. *ICD-9-CM.* http://icd9cm.chrisendres.com/icd9cm/. Accessed February 18, 2010.

5. American Psychiatric Association. *Diagnostic and Statistical Manual.* 4th ed. http://psych. org/MainMenu/Research/DSMIV.aspx. Accessed February 18, 2010.

6. *World Health Organization Drug Dictionary Enhanced.* http://www.umc-products.com/graphics/2489.pdf. Accessed February 18, 2010.

7. International Conference on Harmonisation of Technical Requirements for Registration of Pharmaceutical for Human Use. *Revision of the ICH Guideline on Clinical Safety Data Management: Data Elements for Transmission of Individual Case Safety Reports E2B (R3).* Geneva, Switzerland: ICH Secretariat; November 2008. http://www.ich.org/cache/compo/475-272-1.html#E2B(R3). Accessed February 18, 2010.

8. Maintenance and Support Services. *MedDRA term selection: points to consider Release 3.13 based on MedDRA version 12.1.* 2009. http://www.meddramsso.com/subscriber_library_ptc_archive.asp. Accessed February 18, 2010.

9. Maintenance and support services. *MedDRA data retrieval and presentation: points to consider Release 2.1 based on MedDRA version 12.1.* 2009. http://www.meddramsso.com/subscriber_library_ptc_archive.asp. Accessed February 18, 2010.

5

Determining Causality—The Individual Case Safety Report

One of the most challenging aspects of risk assessment is the determination of whether a safety finding is drug related or not. The individual case safety report (ICSR) and safety findings in the aggregate that show a causal association to a drug provide important information in establishing a drug's risk profile. Such assessments are not always clear cut or easy to make, and the methods used in these determinations differ. In this chapter, determining causality for individual cases is discussed; the next chapter is devoted to causal assessments of aggregate data.

➡ **NOTE:** Remember that causality is assumed for spontaneous adverse event (AE) reports of marketed products.

The well-documented ICSR serves 3 important purposes:

1. It is a means of capturing safety information of rare and unexpected events.
2. It provides case details including a narrative description of a safety finding.
3. It is a means of quickly notifying health authorities of safety information that identifies a new and important risk. This new risk can result in a cascade of different consequences ranging from taking no immediate action to stopping a clinical trial program or withdrawing a drug from the market.

■ Information Included in an Individual Case Safety Report

Health authorities require that specific information be collected for ICSRs and reported on designated forms.

The most common are the MedWatch forms used primarily in the United States and the CIOMS 1 form used outside the United States.[1-3] More and more, ICSRs are submitted electronically using prespecified transmission standards.[4] Although there are some differences in format and content among these various forms, they capture similar information. Information specific to the AE includes:

- Patient information, including patient initials and demographic information
- Description of the event—a full, detailed description of the event is required so a narrative of the event can be generated
- Date of onset of the event
- Relevant tests, laboratory data, other diagnostic information
- Relevant medical history and concomitant medications
- Suspect drugs, including dose, frequency, route of administration, and dates of treatment
- Whether or not the AE abated after stopping the drug (this is also referred to as dechallenge), and whether the AE reappeared after the drug was reintroduced (or rechallenged)
- Whether the event had one or more of the following serious outcomes:
  - Death
  - Life-threatening
  - Hospitalization/prolonged hospitalization
  - Disability/incapacity
  - A congenital anomaly/birth defect
  - An important medical event
- Whether the information is an initial report or represents follow-up information

> **CAUTION:** All too often, important case information is missing and follow-up information is not aggressively pursued, leaving large gaps and preventing a complete understanding of the case. This is especially true for postmarketing spontaneous reports.

■ Methods for Determining Causality

There are several methods used to determine causality and none has yet received "official blessing" from the International Conference on Harmonisation or any government agency. Some use computerized algorithms, others use certain predefined criteria, and still others use global introspection (one or more smart and experienced clinicians making a causality determination without a formal algorithm or methodology). One approach is to assign a number to each criterion and calculate a numerical score for each case based on the number and type of criteria met. Another approach is to simply apply these criteria qualitatively, relying on medical judgment to determine if the weight of evidence suggests a causal relationship. It is not clear which method is the best, but most use in some form or variation the criteria established by Sir Austin Bradford Hill, a statistician and epidemiologist.[5] These criteria include:

1. **Temporal association**—In general, the shorter the time interval between taking the drug and the onset of the AE, the stronger the possibility that the event is due to the drug. There are important exceptions, however; for instance, the development of vaginal cancer in daughters whose mothers were exposed to diethylstilbestrol decades earlier. Another exception is a nonallergic type reaction that occurs so soon after drug exposure that it is not pharmacologically likely or biologically possible.

2. **Dose relationship**—The higher the dose, the greater the AE rate is, and/or the worse the severity. A dose relationship suggests a causal relationship. However, a low dose of a product does not by any means rule out the possibility that it caused the event. For instance, idiosyncratic drug reactions (i.e., rare, unpredictable reactions with unknown mechanisms) are often dose independent.

3. **Positive rechallenge/dechallenge**—A positive rechallenge is *strong* evidence the drug caused the event. Conversely, a negative rechallenge essentially rules out a causal relationship. Although rechallenge information is very important to have, it is not always ethical to obtain, especially for AEs that are life threatening or are associated with significant morbidity. For this reason, there may be limited rechallenge information available for causality assessment and a greater reliance on dechallenge information.

4. **Biological plausibility**—The AE can be explained biologically. For instance, hypotension (low blood pressure) and syncope (fainting) are biologically plausible for an antihypertensive drug that dilates blood vessels. The development of lung cancer after 1 month's exposure to a drug is not, however,

CAUTION: Although a positive dechallenge suggests causality, the evidence is not as strong as a positive rechallenge. For instance, a patient was taking an investigational drug and developed nausea and vomiting 24 hours later. The drug was withdrawn and within 24 hours the nausea and vomiting resolved. At the same time a 24-hour flu epidemic passed through the community. Affected flu victims also developed nausea and vomiting with resolution within 24 hours. Without rechallenging the patient, it is unclear whether the nausea and vomiting were drug related or due to the 24-hour flu. If the AEs were flu related, resolution of the nausea and vomiting would also be expected within 24 hours and coincidental to stopping the drug.

biologically plausible because lung cancer takes years to develop.

5. **Specificity**—A specific type of AE is repeatedly observed. An example is the congenital anomaly of phocomelia (the absence of arms and legs with the attachment of hands and feet directly to the body, giving the appearance of seal-like flippers) in children born to mothers who took thalidomide during the first trimester of pregnancy.

6. **Consistency**—The same AE is seen across different studies, across different geographic regions, and across different demographic groups.

7. **No alternate explanation for the AE**—An example would be a boy with a history of peanut allergy taking Drug A for 3 months with no AEs reported. He is sitting on an airplane, and the person next to him opens a bag of peanuts and starts to eat them. Within a minute the boy develops an anaphylactic reaction. Based on the facts of the case, there is an alternative explanation for the anaphylaxis, i.e., the anaphylaxis can be due to the peanuts rather than Drug A.

■ The Narrative

A narrative is the synthesis of all the important aspects of the case and provides *the story* of the event of interest. Weaving all the appropriate information (pertinent positives and negatives) into an informative narrative requires medical knowledge, clinical judgment, and writing skills. If properly done, the narrative will provide all

the available evidence in support of or against a causal association. Although computers can be programmed to generate some simple and straightforward narratives, computers currently lack the functionality or the *fuzzy logic* needed to select, order, and summarize the *relevant* data from a complicated case.

The narrative should include the following information:

- The diagnosis using a MedDRA term
- A case reference number and patient demographic information
- The source of the report
- The suspect drug(s)—dose, frequency, route of administration, and dates of treatment
- Relevant medical history and concomitant medications
- A detailed description of the event, including:
  - When the suspect drug(s) was (were) given
  - The onset of the patient's symptoms in relation to when the suspect drug was given
  - The progression of the event
  - Relevant tests and diagnostic procedures
  - Treatment received
- The outcome of the event
- The reporter's assessment of the relationship to treatment
- The sponsor's assessment of the case

An Example

The following are 2 versions of narratives summarizing the same case information. The purpose of presenting these 2 different versions is to illustrate some of the key issues discussed in this chapter.

Narrative—Version 1

Diagnosis: Intentional overdose

This case, OSTEO-2008-0012, is a report referring to a 64-year-old Caucasian female (Subject 0023/AKB) from the ABC Company sponsored trial 10-10312, "Long-term Safety Evaluation of OSTEO, 5 mg and 10 mg given daily, for the Treatment of Osteoporosis in Postmenopausal Women." An investigator reported the case.

The subject's medical history included an appendectomy in 1974, bunion removal (left foot) in 1986, depression in 1996, and migraines since 2002.

Concomitant medications included rizatriptan benzoate 1 tablet as necessary (prn) for migraine treatment. Allergies were not reported. Habits: no smoking history, consumption of about one glass of wine/week.

The subject was randomized to the 10 mg OSTEO dose group and started treatment on 02-AUG-2006.

On 16-AUG-2006 the subject intentionally overdosed on clonazepam. She reported feeling "down" for about 10 days before overdosing, but could not identify any specific reason. The same day the subject presented to the emergency department (ED). She was treated with activated charcoal given orally and observed. She was released later that day for self-referral to a mental health facility. The next day, 17-AUG-2006, she went to a mental health clinic and was transferred for admission to the psychiatric ward of a nearby hospital. Discharge date was not provided.

On 28-AUG-2006 the subject reported her intentional overdose to the study coordinator and she was discontinued from the study the same day. No further information was reported. Her last dose of study medication was 15-AUG-2006.

The investigator assessed the event of intentional overdose as unlikely related to study drug treatment.

Additional information was requested.

Follow-up received on 7-SEP-2006 indicated patient started rizatriptan in 2002 and that bunion removal was in 1997 rather than 1986.

Follow-up received 30-SEP-2006 indicated the last dose of study medication was received on 16-AUG-2006.

➡ **NOTE:** Providing follow-up information in this sequential fashion is distracting and confusing; *relevant* follow-up information should be incorporated into the body of the narrative.

Narrative — Version 2

In this narrative, the revised information is bolded, with an explanation of revisions in italics.

Event term: Intentional overdose (depression should also be considered—see comments later in this narrative)

This case, OSTEO-2008-0012, is a report referring to a 64-year-old Caucasian female (Subject 0023/AKB) from the ABC Company sponsored trial 10-10312, "Long-term Safety Evaluation of OSTEO, 5 mg, and 10 mg given daily, for the Treatment of Osteoporosis in Postmenopausal Women." An investigator reported the case.

*The subject's **relevant** medical history included: depression in 1996 and migraines since 2002 (omitted appendectomy and bunion removal because they are not relevant to the case). Allergies were not reported. Habits: no smoking history, consumption of about one glass of wine/week. Concomitant medications included rizatriptan benzoate 1 tablet as necessary (prn) for migraine treatment **since 2002** (date of start of treatment is now included).*

The subject was randomized to the 10 mg OSTEO dose group and started treatment on 02-AUG-2006.

*On 16-AUG-2006 this subject with a **history of depression** intentionally overdosed on clonazepam (although depression is mentioned in the medical history it is repeated here since it is an important aspect of the case). She reported feeling "down" for about 10 days before overdosing, but could not identify any specific reason. The same day the subject presented to the ED. She was treated with activated charcoal given orally and observed. She was released later that day for self-referral to a mental health clinic. The next day, 17-AUG-2006, she went to a mental health clinic and was transferred for admission to the psychiatric ward of a nearby hospital. Discharge date was not provided.*

*On 28-AUG-2006 the subject reported her intentional overdose to the study coordinator and she was discontinued from the study on the same day. No further information was reported. Her last dose of study medication was **16-AUG-2006** (the date is now corrected).*

The investigator assessed the event of intentional overdose as unlikely related to study drug treatment.

Sponsor's assessment of the case: *Although the patient had a history of depression, there was no mention that she was depressed at time of entry into the study. The fact that she was taking no antidepressant medication supports the suggestion she was not clinically depressed before starting treatment with OSTEO. The details of the case suggested no other factors that explain her depression. Although the package insert for rizatriptan* *includes depression, she was taking the drug since 2002 with no mention of depression. Furthermore, the subject's depression started within 10 days of starting OSTEO. For these reasons, a causal relationship to OSTEO is considered possible. The sponsor also thinks that because the patient admitted to feeling "down" and subsequently intentionally overdosed, the diagnosis should also include depression; this will be discussed with the investigator.*

➡ **NOTE:** The sponsor should always independently and objectively assess the case information. If the sponsor disagrees with the investigator, the reason(s) should be clearly stated. In general, both the investigator's and the sponsor's assessment are listed, particularly if they differ. For reporting purposes, however, the most conservative assessment is used—that is if one feels the case is related to the drug and the other doesn't, for regulatory reporting purposes, the case is considered related to the drug.

Additional information was requested.

Questions and Answers

1. **What information is missing?**
   Dosage strength, how many pills of clonazepam were taken, and last dose. Whether she took more OSTEO than prescribed. More details regarding her ED visit, e.g., mental status, vital signs, tests taken, and their results. Details regarding her stay in the psychiatric ward.

2. **Do you agree with the diagnosis of intentional overdose?**
   Yes, but depression should be added based on the subject stating she felt "down," which was the probable cause of her intentional overdose.

3. **Is this case serious?**
   Yes. Although the patient was released from the ED and not hospitalized, some would argue that because she was depressed and intentionally overdosed, she should have been directly admitted into the psychiatric ward. She was admitted to a hospital the following day, presumably for her depression that started after 10 days' treatment with OSTEO

and therefore met the serious criterion of hospitalization. Another criterion was that this was an important medical event, because she experienced clinically significant depression that led to her intentional overdose and eventual hospitalization.

4. **Do you agree with the investigator's causality assessment?**
   No. The case meets the following criteria for causality: temporal association to OSTEO; and no alternative explanation for the event is apparent.

➡ **NOTE:** A recommended reference for the proper approach to writing ICSR narratives is *Current Challenges in Pharmacovigilance: Pragmatic Approaches.*[6]

References

1. US Department of Health and Human Services, Food and Drug Administration. *Voluntary reporting* [Form FDA 3500]. http://www.fda.gov/Safety/MedWatch/HowToReport/DownloadForms/default.htm. Accessed February 22, 2010.

2. US Department of Health and Human Services, Food and Drug Administration *Mandatory reporting* [Form FDA 3500A]. http://www.fda.gov/Safety/MedWatch/HowToReport/DownloadForms/default.htm. Accessed February 22, 2010.

3. Council for International Organizations of Medical Sciences. *Suspect adverse reaction* report. http://www.cioms.ch/cioms.pdf. Accessed February 22, 2010.

4. International Conference on Harmonisation of Technical Requirements for Registration of Pharmaceuticals for Human Use. *Revision of the ICH Guideline on Clinical Safety Management: Data Elements for Transmission of Individual Case Safety Reports E2B (R3).* Geneva, Switzerland: ICH Secretariat: November 2008. http://www.ich.org/cache/compo/276-254-1.html. Accessed February 22, 2010.

5. Hill AB. The environment and disease: association or causation? *Proc R Soc Med.* 1965;58:293–300.

6. Report of CIOMS Working Group V. *Current Challenges in Pharmacovigilance: Pragmatic Approaches.* Geneva, 2001.

6

Determining Causality— Aggregate Data

In the previous chapter, determining causality of individual case safety reports (ICSRs) was discussed. The objective of this chapter is to focus on the approaches used in determining causality when dealing with aggregate data. Aggregate data refers to data from a group of patients rather than the data from a single individual. The methods used in the determination of drug-related effects differ in the aggregate analysis of data from clinical trials and spontaneous postmarketing adverse event (AE) reports. These differences will be discussed.

■ The Randomized, Controlled Clinical Trial

In clinical trials, the determination of causality is based on observed differences between treatment groups. The gold-standard study design to show this is the *randomized, double-blinded, controlled* study. In this type of study, subjects are allocated to a treatment group based on a computer-generated list where treatment assignment is randomly (by chance alone) determined. If treatment allocation is truly random, the different treatment groups should be similar with respect to demographics and other baseline characteristics. Any differences in safety findings between treatment groups are then presumed to be drug related. If the treatment groups differ with respect to demographics and baseline characteristics, this baseline difference can confound (confuse) interpretation of the safety finding. For instance, suppose a higher rate of strokes is observed in patients receiving Drug A compared to placebo. There are, however, considerably more elderly individuals in the Drug A group who, by age alone, are at greater risk of stroke. This difference in age confounds (or confuses) the determination of whether the difference in the rate of stroke is due to Drug A, due to more elderly subjects in the Drug A group, or a combination of both Drug A and age.

Double-blinded means that neither the subject nor the investigator knows what treatment is assigned.

TIP: Randomization should minimize the risk of large baseline differences from occurring. If striking differences are seen, be suspicious that treatment assignments were not made according to the computer-generated randomization list.

In reality, these types of studies are triple-blinded, because the drug company's (sponsor's) team running the study is also blinded to treatment until study completion. Blinding decreases or may even eliminate most bias because the treatment is unknown to all. Sometimes blinding fails. For example, a placebo-controlled study of a beta-adrenergic blocker (e.g., propranolol) may be fully and adequately double blinded. But it may become very clear which patients are on the beta-adrenergic blocker because a normal and expected pharmacologic response to treatment is a slowing of the pulse. Thus a *blinded* patient may be strongly suspected of being on the beta-adrenergic blocker if his or her pulse drops after the drug is started.

In a *controlled* study, 1 group of subjects is given a control (i.e., placebo or an active comparator drug), and another group is given the investigational drug. In some studies, there are 2 control groups—a placebo group and an active comparator group. Placebo is a dummy product with no apparent medicinal effects but is identical in appearance to the investigational product. An active control or active comparator is a marketed drug, already approved for the indication that the investigational drug is being evaluated for. When possible, the appearance of the active control is made to look like the investigational drug. In this way, the subject and investigator usually cannot identify which treatment is being received. The active comparator and investigational drug are usually from the same drug class, e.g., angiotensin-converting enzyme inhibitors for treatment of hypertension. Alternatively, for new chemical entities when the investigational drug is first in its class, the active control can be from a different drug class, e.g., thiazide diuretics. The use of a placebo control allows the results of each treatment to be objectively compared, because there is usually some degree of "background noise" (safety findings that are not drug related) found in the general population at all times. For instance, a headache may be due to a drug effect, but people not exposed to the drug may also experience headache. The magnitude of difference between the rate of headache in the investigational drug group compared to the placebo rate helps to determine whether the drug does or does not cause headaches. The greater the difference in the rates of headache between the placebo and the investigational drug groups, the greater the likelihood the headaches are drug related.

The objective of active-controlled studies is usually to show no difference in safety (and efficacy) findings between the investigational and active-controlled groups if they are from the same drug class. Even if the investigational drug looks better than the active control (i.e., it has a lower rate of headache), a claim cannot be made that the investigational drug is safer than the active control because the study is usually not strong enough (powered) to detect that such a difference is not due to chance alone. The observed lower headache rate in this case is hypothesis generating, i.e., the results suggest the investigational drug *might* cause fewer headaches, but remains unproven. To prove that the investigational drug causes fewer headaches than the active control, a *prospective*, randomized, active-control study would have to be done. *Prospective* means the objective of the study is stated up front or specified; e.g., "the objective of the study is to determine if investigational Drug X decreases the risk of headache by $\geq 50\%$ compared to the marketed Drug Y." The study would then have to be adequately powered (have enough patients) to be able to show this magnitude of difference.

Some clinical studies do not have a control group and are referred to as uncontrolled studies. A lack of a control limits the ability to determine a causal relation to a drug because of the background noise of AEs found in the general population, e.g., headache, as discussed previously. This can cause confusion because it is difficult to determine without a control whether an AE is drug related or is simply background noise. If a new safety signal is identified from an uncontrolled study, there are options that can be used to determine if the finding is drug related.

■ One option is to do a thorough literature review, hoping to identify the rate of the AE reported in the population with the disease being evaluated (e.g., the rate of myocardial infarction in diabetic patients). The AE rate found in the literature is then compared to the rate observed in the study. This is often challenging for the following 2 reasons: the AE rate in the general diabetic population cannot be found; or the rates cannot be easily compared due to differences between the study population and the general diabetic population, e.g., age and gender differences, medical history, concomitant drug use, etc.

■ Another option is to use historical control subjects—subjects who were treated in a different study in an earlier period of time. This option also has important limitations. Because these evaluations are retrospective (i.e., the results are already known) and treatment assignment is also known, potential bias can be a problem in selecting the historical control group to use. Baseline differences in the historical control group and the investigational group are also possibilities that can confound (confuse) interpretation of findings. For instance, there may be different inclusion/exclusion criteria that were used in the historical control group (e.g., subjects > 65 years old were excluded) compared to the group receiving the investigational drug (subjects > 65 years were not excluded from the study). These differences can impact study results.

For these reasons, the randomized, double-blinded controlled study remains the best source of determining causality. The results from these studies receive prominent attention in the integrated analysis of safety.

■ Determining Meaningful Differences

The determination of a drug effect is largely based on observed rate differences between treatment groups. This simple or crude rate is calculated for AEs and other safety findings of interest, e.g., the rate of subjects with clinically significant laboratory changes. The formula is straightforward:

Rate of safety finding of interest (%) = $(n/N) \times 100$

where n is the number of subjects who reported the safety finding of interest (the numerator), and N is the number of subjects who were exposed to treatment (the denominator). Based on this formula, if 10 subjects reported dizziness and 100 subjects were exposed to Drug B, the rate of dizziness in the Drug B group is: $(10/100) \times 100 = 10\%$.

Quantitative and qualitative approaches are then used to determine *meaningful* differences between treatment groups, using one or more of the following methods:

■ *Statistical* method—Testing hypotheses; e.g., utilizing p values of ≤ 0.05, to test the null hypothesis of no difference in the rate of a safety finding for the investigational drug versus placebo is not advised, especially if the study is not powered adequately to detect important safety

differences. However, using 95% confidence intervals around the difference between the rate in the investigational drug group and the placebo group can be informative. The 95% confidence interval provides a best estimate of the difference between the investigational drug and placebo for the safety parameter along with an interval estimate that displays the precision of the estimate. As with any statistical assessment, the use of confidence intervals must be interpreted using clinical judgment, because there may be real differences identified through statistical methodology that are not of clinical importance.

■ **Rule of thumb method**—Specifying the rate in the investigational group *and* the magnitude of difference that is observed between the investigational group and control group. For instance, a rate of $\geq 5\%$ in the investigational group and $\geq 2 \times$ the rate in the placebo group.[1]

■ **Eyeballing the data method**—Looking at the difference in rates between treatment groups and making a clinical judgment call whether these differences are clinically meaningful even if the rates do not reach statistical significance (*Statistical* method) or meet specified criteria (*Rule of thumb* method). The pattern of the data can also suggest a potential drug effect, e.g., a dose response is seen.

RED HERRING ALERT: Always be on the alert for the unexpected. There are 2 interesting findings shown in Table 6-1. One is the lower rate of headache in the investigational group compared to placebo. The other interesting finding is the 5% rate of increased hair growth observed in the investigational group (with no cases noted in the placebo group). The lower rate of headache in the investigational group can be an indication that the investigational drug has some analgesic (painkiller) property or other effect that may be beneficial in pain control or headache treatment. Increased hair growth, although reported as an adverse event may really be a benefit for someone who is bald! Such findings can be early clues of undetected benefits and new indications. Minoxidil, a vasodilator, originally intended for treatment of hypertension, showed hair-growth properties. A topical formulation was developed and tested, and minoxidil was subsequently shown to be efficacious in the treatment of male pattern baldness, and is now on the market for this indication.[2]

Table 6-1	Summary of Adverse Events with a Rate of ≥ 5% in the Investigational Drug Group	
Adverse Event[a]	Placebo N = 100	Investigational Drug N = 100
Dyspepsia	5 (5%)	12 (12%)
Headache	24 (24%)	10 (10%)
Insomnia	8 (8%)	7 (7%)
Dizziness	5 (5%)	6 (6%)
Nausea	2 (2%)	5 (5%)
Hair growth increased	0	5 (5%)

[a] MedDRA Preferred Terms

All these methods have their own pros and cons and the best methodology to use should be decided in consultation with a statistician. The method(s) of choice should be clearly documented in the methodology section of the report. Most importantly, the limitation(s) of the selected method should be fully understood.

The following example illustrates the application of the *Rule of thumb* approach. Table 6-1 is a summary of AEs from a placebo-controlled study with a rate of ≥ 5% in the investigational drug group.

The AEs that are shaded in gray are considered *potential* adverse drug reactions (ADRs) based on the *Rule of thumb* criteria of a rate of ≥ 5% in the investigational drug group and ≥ 2× the rate of placebo.

Safety analyses are usually descriptive—they describe and compare the differences between treatment groups. Large differences between treatment groups are *suggestive* of a drug effect but do not *prove* one. To prove a finding, a prospective study (with the objectives specified) and adequately powered as discussed previously would have to be done. Although such studies are sometimes done for risk determination, e.g., studies evaluating the risk of death, strokes and/or myocardial infarctions, prospective studies are usually conducted to demonstrate efficacy.

Because a drug effect is usually inferred rather than proven, the term *potential adverse reaction* is often used until there is further evidence to support a causal relationship.

Findings that are statically significant do not always prove causality. Whenever *multiple comparisons* are done, for example, comparing the rates of hundreds of different AEs, statistically significant results can occur by chance alone. The more comparison testing, the greater the chance of spurious statistically significant findings. Also be aware of interim analyses that may suggest significance initially, but not in later analyses. On the other hand, rare and infrequent AEs may be adverse reactions—that is, be treatment-related , but are simply too few in number to analyze statistically.

A drug effect that is statistically significant is not necessarily clinically significant. In studies that are highly powered (i.e., have a very large sample size and are thus able to detect true drug effects), small differences (e.g. 0.5 mm Hg mean increase in systolic blood pressure), may result in statistically significant findings. Such a small change, even if sustained, is unlikely to harm the patient.

The nature of clinical trials may produce some very strange results. For example, many studies begin collecting data during the screening period before the study drug is given. This period may be used to:

- Determine if a prospective patient qualifies for the study (i.e., meets the study protocol's requirements).

- Acclimate to procedures that will be used in the study, e.g., treadmill walking, to eliminate any potential training effect before baseline measurements are taken. This is sometimes referred to as the *wash-in* period. This is seen in angina and intermittent claudication studies, among others.

- Stop (wash-out) drugs excluded by the study protocol before the study drug is started.

AEs that occur in the screening or pretreatment period should *not* be included in the AE analysis or included in AE summary tables. This information, however, should be captured and tracked since AEs reported during screening may indicate unsafe protocol-specific procedures. For example, a study protocol states that beta-adrenergic blocking drugs (e.g., propranolol) should be stopped during the screening period, and a patient develops a myocardial infarction because the protocol did not include a warning that the drug's dose should be tapered and not stopped abruptly. The only time pretreatment AEs should be included in the analyses of AEs is if the AE is present at baseline and worsens in severity during treatment or during the residual effect of the drug (i.e., the period after the last dose when drug levels are still detectable).

Another anomaly occurs if several unusual AEs are all reported from the same study site and from no others. One needs to play detective and investigate the site for anything odd. Although clustering of events at 1 site can happen, this is *fishy*, and one should be suspicious. If there is a true drug effect observed, similar findings should be seen across sites and not seen at 1 site alone. This is sometimes called a *drug-investigator* or *drug-site interaction*.

Play Detective

Even though all the methods described previously can fall short in proving a causal relationship to the investigational drug, meaningful differences between the investigational and control groups raise the suspicion of a drug effect and underscore the need for further detective work. A true safety finding rarely occurs in isolation. For these reasons, one should proactively look for patterns, links, and trends in the data. For example, if Drug C has a higher rate of bradycardia (slow heart rate) compared to placebo, and this is a true finding, a trend toward decreases in heart rate should also be seen in the analysis of vital sign data and the analysis of electrocardiographic data where heart rate is also measured. Identifying similar patterns and trends in the data and linking these to different but related safety parameters increases the likelihood that observed differences are real and not *red herrings* (false signals). The next chapter is devoted to identifying these patterns and links.

Once a potential adverse reaction is identified, further characterization of the finding is required. This is to determine whether other factors such as dose, age, renal function, etc. impact the adverse reaction in some fashion, i.e., make it worse or better. This topic is further discussed in subsequent chapters.

■ How to Determine Causality— Postmarketing Safety Data

The process for determining causality for postmarketing spontaneously reported AEs involves:

- Identification of new safety signals
- Review of cases
- Additional evaluation

Identification of New Safety Signals

Depending on the volume of cases, looking for new signals is done manually, or automatically by employing data mining techniques.

The Manual Method

In the manual method, the following data should be reviewed for identification of new signals:

- ICSRs, for serious adverse reactions not previously reported, or cases of special interest. Special interest cases are those that include AEs that are historically linked to drugs, e.g., hepatotoxicity, anaphylaxis, aplastic anemia, seizures, renal failure, etc.
- Unlisted events, i.e., those AEs that were not previously included in the company's core safety information (CCSI).
- Summary tabulations of AEs to get an overview of the most common AEs reported as shown in Table 6-2. This information should be compared across earlier *reporting* periods to see if the most commonly reported events have changed over time.
- Line listings to have a capsule view of the cases. The listings provide a means of identifying patterns of events without having to read the details of each ICSR and should include the following information:
  - Marketing authorization holder case reference number
  - Country in which case occurred

Table 6-2 — Summary of Postmarketing Reports by Adverse Event Terms[a]

Adverse Event Term by MedDRA SOC/PT	Spontaneous/ Regulatory Bodies	Postmarketing Studies	Literature	Total
Blood and lymphatic system disorders				
Ecchymosis	98 (5)	15	5 (2)	118 (7)
Anemia	47 (3)	4	5 (2)	56 (5)
Leukocytosis	19 (2)	10 (1)	0	29 (3)
Neutropenia	1	1	0	2
Thrombocytopenia	1 (1)	0	0	1 (1)
Cardiac disorders				
Palpitations	40	27	10	77
Hypertension	10 (2)	1 (1)	5 (2)	16 (5)
Tachycardia	9	7	4 (1)	20 (1)
Myocardial infarction	3 (3)	0	1 (1)	4 (4)
Nervous system disorders				
Insomnia	20	16	1	37
Depression	5 (1)	2 (1)	1	8 (2)
Anxiety	3	3	0	6

[a] The number in ( ) represents the number of terms considered serious. The *italicized* events are unlisted AEs.

- Source (e.g., clinical trial, literature, spontaneous, regulatory authority)
- Age and sex
- Daily dose of suspected drug (and, when relevant, dosage form or route)
- Date of onset of the reaction. If not available, best estimate of time to onset from therapy initiation. For an ADR known to occur after cessation of therapy, estimate of time lag if possible (may go in Comments section).
- Dates of treatment. If not available, best estimate of treatment duration.
- Description of reaction as reported, and when necessary as interpreted by the market authorization holder (English translation when necessary).
- Patient outcome (at case level) (e.g., resolved, fatal, improved, sequelae, unknown). This field does not refer to the criteria used to define a serious ADR. It should indicate the consequences of the reaction(s) for the patient, using the worst of the different outcomes for multiple reactions.
- Comments, if relevant (e.g., causality assessment if the manufacturer disagrees with the reporter; concomitant medications suspected to play a role in the reactions directly or by interaction; indication treated with suspect drug[s]; dechallenge/rechallenge results if available).[3]
- Change in the *frequency* of reports over time. Unlike clinical trials where rates can be calculated because the numerator (number of patients reporting an AE) and denominator (the number of subjects exposed to the drug) are known, neither the numerator nor the denominator is known with certainty. To determine increased frequency the *reporting rate* should first be calculated.

The reporting rate is calculated using the following formula:

$$\text{Reporting rate} = \text{number of cases/exposure estimate}^4$$

This is illustrated in Table 6-3 for 2 events, syncope and anaphylaxis.

Once the reporting rate is calculated for each AE for each period, the reporting rates can be compared to see if the pattern has changed, i.e., whether the reporting rate is the same, increased, or decreased over time, as shown in Table 6-4.

Table 6-3 **Number of Cases and Exposure Estimates per Period**

	Period 1	Period 2
Number of anaphylaxis cases reported in each period	8	6
Number of syncope cases reported in each period	2	0
Exposure estimate for each period based on million tablets sold	2	6
Reporting rate of anaphylaxis (cases/million tablets sold)	4	1
Reporting rate of syncope (cases/million tables sold)	1	0

Table 6-4 **Cases per Million Tablets Sold**

Adverse Events	Period 1	Period 2	Period 3	Period 4	Total
Anaphylaxis	4	1	3	0	8
Syncope	1	0	5	10	16

Table 6-4 shows the frequency of anaphylaxis cases has changed little over time, while the frequency of syncope appears to be increasing. This change in reporting rate for syncope is a safety signal that requires further evaluation. Statistical tests to determine increased frequencies are sometimes utilized—check with your statistician to determine the best method to use.

Automatic Method—Data Mining

For large volumes of events, data mining techniques should be employed. Data mining is the process of searching and analyzing large databases by using mathematical and statistical methods to identify previously undetected data patterns. One method utilizes a form of proportional (also called *disproportional*) analysis where the ratio of the number of an AE of interest (e.g., cases of renal failure) is divided by all AEs reported for a given suspect drug. This is then compared to the ratio of the same AE of interest—cases of renal failure—for all other drugs in the database (excluding the study drug) relative to all AEs reported for all these drugs. If the ratio for cases of renal failure for the suspect drug is

greater than the ratio seen for all other drugs in the database combined, a signal may be generated. For example, suppose 3 of 15 AEs for Drug X were for renal failure. This gives a proportion (ratio) of 3/15. For all other drugs in the database (Drug X is now excluded), there were 70 renal failure cases in the 2000 total AEs giving a proportion (ratio) of 70/2000. This is calculated as [3/15]/[70/2000], which equals 5.7. This is a fairly strong suggestion (signal) that renal failure is more common with Drug X compared with the rest of the drugs in the database and should be investigated further.

One problem here, though, is that normal variation means that just about every AE for the study drug will either be higher or lower than the ratio for all the other drugs. It is highly unlikely that an exact equal ratio will occur. Thus one might expect that of all the AE categories, half would be above the ratio for the rest of the drugs and half below. Obviously the entire half above is not a signal nor is the entire half below suggestive that the drug in question protects against these AEs. Thus many reviewers will require at least a

> **CAUTION:** It is important to emphasize the need for caution when determining increased frequency. Incomplete information, the absence of a control, the effect of the media, AE underreporting,[5] inaccurate exposure information, and many other factors can lead to false conclusions.

> **CAUTION:** Data mining is a useful tool that helps identify cases that warrant further review. Data mining can generate many false signals or miss important ones and therefore cannot be a substitute for proper case review. Nevertheless, data mining is a useful first-line tool when it is used appropriately and its limitations are understood.

two-fold higher ratio for the suspect drug before calling it a signal.

Review of Cases (Creating a Case Series)

Once a signal is identified, further exploration is required. In addition to reviewing all the cases with the same diagnosis (including cases from clinical trials, the literature, etc.), it is useful to expand the search and include cases that may have different diagnoses but may still be medically related (i.e., similar mechanism of disease). To do this, a *case definition* needs to be established.

Case Definition

A case definition prospectively establishes the criteria to be used in searching and identifying cases of interest. What criteria to use are dependent on the safety signal. This is often subjective and requires clinical judgment. Attempts have been made to try to standardize case definitions with the development of Standardised MedDRA Queries (SMQs). SMQs, as discussed in Chapter 4, are groupings of AE terms that relate to a defined medical condition or area of interest. The AEs included in SMQs may relate to signs, symptoms, diagnoses, syndromes, physical findings, laboratory and other physiologic test data, etc. SMQs were developed for important medical conditions known historically to be drug related. However, SMQs are not available for many important adverse reactions. In certain instances, established SMQs require modifications (terms need to be added or deleted). In the absence of an SMQ, search criteria have to be established; this is referred as an *ad hoc query* (AHQ). For instance, if a signal for hypotension is identified, AEs that are related to hypotension should also be included in the case definition. The selection of these terms should be based on common pathophysiology (similar underlying mechanism) and/or similar signs and symptoms. Because there is no SMQ for hypotension, an AHQ query has to be created. In Chapter 4, an example of suggested terms to be included in an AHQ for *Hypotension* is provided.

Because of the subjective nature of case definitions and the clinical judgment involved, individuals with clinical training/experience should either establish the search criteria or review the case definition established by others to ensure clinical comprehensiveness and relevance.

Examples of criteria used in case selection include but are not limited to the following:

- Source of cases—e.g., postmarketing spontaneous reports, literature, clinical studies, etc., or all sources.
- Time period—specific time reported (e.g., only cases from 1998 to 2008) or no time limit.

- Adjudicated versus nonadjudicated cases— diagnosis confirmed by an independent source versus including any case of interest regardless of whether the diagnosis was confirmed or not.
- Start and end date of the suspect drug—therapy dates for use in determining if a temporal association exists between the suspect drug and the adverse event(s) of interest.
- AE terms—a list of different but related AE terms to be part of the case definition (e.g., the SMQ or AHQ) as discussed previously.

Depending on the results of the initial search, expanding the case definition (if the search criteria are too restrictive) or narrowing the search criteria (if the criteria are too broad and nonspecific) may be required. The cases meeting these criteria become part of a *case series*.

Case Series

The cases are then reviewed looking for overlying patterns that might tie the cases together. Unfortunately, there are no clearly accepted standard methods or algorithms for doing this. One common method involves making a spreadsheet or line listing with each case summarized on one line and then scanning and totaling commonalities among the cases. Similarity of findings across cases strengthens a causal association, while little to no similarities among cases weakens the evidence for a causal relationship. The following is a recommended list of key information that should be included in the line listing:

- Patient identifier
- Demographic information—age, gender, race
- Source and geographic location
- Start and end dates of suspect drug
- Dose of suspect drug
- Reported (verbatim) AE term, MedDRA Preferred Term
- Other AEs reported for the same subject
- Onset and end dates of the AE of interest as well as for any other reported AE
- Coexistent illnesses
- Concomitant medication

For example, Drug Z is suspected of increasing the risk for myocardial infarction. Search criteria are established, which includes identifying all cases that have one or more terms found in the SMQ *Myocardial infarction*. Cases from all sources (e.g., premarketing clinical trials, postmarketing spontaneous reports, the literature, etc. covering the years 2003–2008 are also part of the search criteria. The search is done and 30 cases are identified and displayed in line listings as described previously. Review of the cases reveals that 25 of 30 cases involved hypertensive males over 55 years and that in 22 of these 25 cases, the patients were also obese; all but one (21) were also diabetic.

From this review, it can be concluded that hypertensive obese male diabetics > 55 years of age may be at increased risk for myocardial infarction. Further evaluation, e.g., additional analyses; a literature search looking at the risk of myocardial infarction in obese diabetic males > 55 years old; a study, etc. may be required to determine if this signal is real or not (see "Additional Evaluation").

Case series provide useful information but have limitations that include:

- Poor quality and incomplete case information
- Potential case selection bias due to selecting unblinded cases retrospectively
- Potential confounding because there is no control group

Additional Evaluation

For verification of a causal relationship to the drug, additional clinical or epidemiologic studies may have to be done (e.g., a large simple safety study or a case control study). This is especially true for AEs associated with a high degree of morbidity and mortality. The type of study selected depends on a number of factors, including whether the event is rare (e.g., toxic epidermal necrolysis—a rare [0.5 per million population per year][6] but severe and serious skin condition) or an event that has a high background rate in the population (e.g., hypertension). It is also important to understand the strength and limitations of each type of study. Consultation with an expert in the area of interest, as well as an epidemiologist, and a statistician is recommended to help determine the best type of study to do.

References

1. *Conducting a Clinical Safety Review of a New Product Application and Preparing a Report on the Review.* Washington, DC: US Department of Health and Human Services, Food and Drug Administration, Center for Drug Evaluation and Research (CDER); 2005. http://www.fda.gov/downloads/Drugs/GuidanceComplianceRegulatoryInformation/Guidances/UCM072974.pdf. Accessed February 23, 2010.

2. Olsen EA, Whiting D, Bergfeld W, et al. A multicenter, randomized, placebo-controlled, double-blind clinical trial of a novel formulation of 5% minoxidil topical foam versus placebo in the treatment of androgenetic alopecia in men. *J Am Acad Dermatol.* 2007; 57(5):767–774.

3. International Conference on Harmonisation of Technical Requirements for Registration of Pharmaceuticals for Human Use. *Clinical Safety Data Management: Periodic Safety Update Reports for Marketed Drugs E2C(R1).* ICH Secretariat, Geneva, Switzerland, November 1996. http://www.ich.org/cache/compo/276–254–1.html. Accessed February 23, 2010.

4. Report of CIOMS Working Group V. *Current Challenges in Pharmacovigilance: Pragmatic Approaches.* Geneva, 2001.

5. Hazell L, Shakir SA. Under-reporting of adverse drug reactions: a systematic review. *Drug Safety* 2006; 29: 385–396.

6. Chan HL, Stern RS, Arndt KA, et al. The incidence of erythema multiforme, Stevens-Johnson syndrome, and toxic epidermal necrolysis. A population-based study with particular reference to reactions caused by drugs among outpatients. *Arch Dermatol.* 1990; 126(1):43–47.

Determining the Weight of Evidence— Patterns and Links

S ometimes identification of a safety signal is so obvious that a person would have to be comatose to miss it. But signal identification is often subtle and can be overlooked if the safety finding is viewed in isolation. For this reason, it is important to determine the *weight of evidence*—all the safety findings (evidence) that point to a causal relationship to the drug. Safety data can often appear as a jumble of information that is overwhelming to sort out. But safety review can actually be fun and rewarding if you know what to look for. Identifying the various patterns and links that exist is one key to unlocking the mystery of the data.

The objective of this chapter is to help train your eyes to see these *patterns* and *links*. The more patterns and links that are identified, the greater the *weight of evidence* that a safety finding is real and not a *red herring* (false signal).

■ Patterns

Data patterns take many different forms and include:

- Change from baseline
- Differences observed between treatment groups
- Trends
- Even distribution versus clustering of findings

■ Change From Baseline

In determining a drug effect, it is important to see if anything changed for the patient from the time just before the patient received the study medication (baseline) to the time during treatment (treatment period) and the period following treatment (posttreatment period). Any change from baseline should be considered a possible drug effect (this assumes the baseline measurement is stable—i.e., is truly representative of the patient's condition before treatment was received). This is illustrated in Figure 7-1, which shows the change in serum creatinine

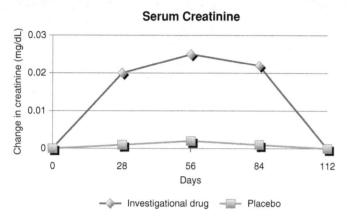

Serum Creatinine

Figure 7-1   Mean Change in Serum Creatinine

(a measure of renal function) for an investigational drug and placebo. Baseline is Day 0, the treatment period is Days 1–84, and the posttreatment period is up to Day 112 (28 days after the last dose of study medication).

This figure shows there is little change from baseline in the mean (average) serum creatinine values in the placebo group, which is quite different from the pattern seen for those taking the investigational drug. In the investigational group, serum creatinine increases from baseline and stays elevated during the treatment period. After treatment is stopped, the serum creatinine value returns to baseline. This pattern is highly suggestive of a drug effect.

Differences Between Treatment Groups

In clinical trials, having a comparator is invaluable in the determination of a drug effect. Placebo and active comparators, however, tell you different things. A difference in findings between placebo and the investigational group *suggests* a drug effect as discussed previously in

Chapter 6 and illustrated in Figure 7-1. In comparing an investigational drug and an active control (i.e., a marketed drug in the same drug class and/or used for the same indication as the investigational drug), no difference between treatment groups is looked for. Sometimes the results *suggest*, but do not prove, the investigational drug is better or worse than the active comparator. This is shown in Table 7-1.

Based on these findings, nausea and clinically significant increased creatinine values appear to be related to treatment with the investigational drug and active control. But a greater rate of nausea appears to be associated with the active control compared to the investigational drug.

Trends

Identification of data trends is very useful in determining risk. Some safety parameters such as laboratory tests, vital signs, and electrocardiogram (ECG) data are analyzed in several different ways, including:

- Measuring central tendency; i.e., determining mean or median changes of the group.
- Categorical shifts; i.e., the number (%) of subjects with values that shift from one category to another; e.g., a shift from normal to above normal values.
- Identification of outliers; i.e., the number (%) of subjects with potentially clinically significant values whose values are very different or divergent from other subjects' values.
- Looking at the rates of adverse events that are related to these quantitative measurements. For instance, a statistically significant decrease in mean heart rate is noted in the investigational group compared to placebo. If this is a real finding, some of these patients may have much greater decreases in heart rate than the mean, and in some cases these decreases will be reported as adverse events

Table 7-1	Treatment Group Comparisons		
	Placebo N = 100	Investigational Drug N = 100	Active Control N = 100
Nausea	3 (3%)	20 (20%)	40 (40%)
Pharyngitis	3 (3%)	2 (2%)	3 (3%)
Clinically significant creatinine values	1 (1%)	8 (8%)	7 (7%)
Clinically significant sodium values	1(1%)	1(1%)	1 (1%)

(*Bradycardia* or *Heart rate decreased*), resulting in a higher rate of these adverse events in the investigational group compared to placebo.

Similar trends observed from these separate and different analyses increase the *weight of evidence* that a safety finding is real. This is illustrated in Table 7-2, showing the results of different analyses evaluating changes in white blood cell counts (WBCs).

This example shows that even though the data are analyzed in a variety of ways, each analysis shows a similar trend, strengthening the *weight of evidence* of a drug effect. In the real world, trends are often more subtle, but this example illustrates the importance of data trends. The way the results from different analyses are grouped together in the *dashboard display* shown in Table 7-2 also makes trend identification easier. Dashboard displays refer to user-friendly displays of different types of data that when viewed together allow the reviewer to get a quick picture/understanding of the information.

Table 7-2 is an example of trends noted in a group of patients. Identifying a trend in the data for an individual patient is also important. Table 7-3 shows how the same platelet count obtained at the same visit (gray shaded areas) can tell different stories based on the trend in each patient's platelet counts.

In Scenario 1, a patient has an isolated, clinically significant value. With no other information available, it is surmised that either the investigational drug caused the drop in platelet count, the low value was a lab error, or perhaps the finding was caused by another drug or concomitant illness. Even if the low platelet count was drug related, it was transient and normalized with continued treatment. The platelet count values in Scenario 2 paint a very different picture. In this case, the patient has clinically significant low platelet counts pretreatment, on treatment, and posttreatment. The pattern remains essentially unchanged, suggesting no drug effect since there is really no change from baseline. The pattern of platelet counts is very different in Scenario 3. In this example the patient has normal values at screening and baseline. Once treatment starts, platelet values progressively decrease until a clinically significant low value as noted on Day 56 is

---

Table 7-2 **Summary of White Blood Cell Data**
(normal range = 4–10 × 10^9/L; clinically significant values ≤ 2.8 × 10^9/L)

	Placebo	Investigational Drug
Mean change from baseline (× 10^9/L)	+0.05	−0.75
Rate (%) of patients with an above normal or normal baseline WBC value and a below normal treatment value	1%	10%
Rate (%) of patients with a normal baseline WBC value and a clinically significant low WBC treatment value	0	2%
Adverse event rate:		
WBC decreased	0	1%
Leukopenia	0	5%

Table 7-3 **Platelet Counts**
(normal range = 150–400 × 10^9/L; clinically significant values ≤ 75 × 10^9/L)

Visits	Scenario 1	Scenario 2	Scenario 3
Screening (Day 7)	225 × 10^9/L	71 × 10^9/L (L, CS)	175 × 10^9/L
Baseline (Day 0)	178 × 10^9/L	69 × 10^9/L (L, CS)	225 × 10^9/L
Visit 1 (Day 28)	180 × 10^9/L	74 × 10^9/L (L, CS)	100 × 10^9/L (L)
Visit 2 (Day 56)	70 × 10^9/L (L, CS)	70 × 10^9/L (L, CS)	70 × 10^9/L (L, CS)
Final visit (Day 84)	312 × 10^9/L	73 × 10^9/L (L, CS)	65 × 10^9/L (L, CS)
Posttreatment visit (Day 91[a])	281 × 10^9/L	71 × 10^9/L (L, CS)	125 × 10^9/L (L)

[a] 7 days since last dose.
L = below normal value; CS = clinically significant value.

reached. The platelet count is still clinically significantly low at the next visit. However, 7 days after the last dose of the drug is given, the platelet count starts to rise and approaches the normal range. Unless there is an alternative explanation for these findings, this pattern is very suggestive of a drug effect based on temporal association and dechallenge; that is, the changes occur after treatment is started, and start to normalize after treatment is stopped, respectively. In each scenario, although the patient has the same clinically significant low value at the same visit, the different trends in platelet counts for each patient suggest very different things.

■ Even Distribution Versus Clustering of Findings

Real safety findings in general should be evenly distributed. For clinical trials, similar safety findings should be seen as follows:

■ Across different study sites in a multicenter trial

■ Across geographic areas in international multicenter studies

■ Across multicenter studies evaluating the same investigational or marketed drug

For drugs that are approved in more than 1 country, similar types of adverse events should be seen in each country where the drug is marketed in proportion to the amount of drug sold in that country (all things being equal) unless there is a good reason to suspect that the patients are different, the practice of medicine is different, or that there are some other local factors that produce such effects. This is illustrated in the following example.

TIP: Suspicions should be raised if there is a clustering of findings at only 1 site, in a multicenter study; or in only 1 geographic location in a multi-country study. Clustering of results can indicate nothing (e.g., a chance finding), or it can be a true safety signal. It can also indicate that a site is not following the protocol, or it can represent a unique group of patients (different from those seen at other sites) who might be more susceptible to a drug effect. It may even indicate fraud (i.e., manufactured data). When clustering is identified, the data should be very carefully scrutinized.

Drug A and Pancreatitis

Pancreatitis (inflammation of the pancreas) is an expected event associated with marketed Drug A. Suppose Drug A is marketed in 5 countries at the same dose, and similar amounts of the drug are sold in each of the 5 countries. However, it is discovered that in France, the number of pancreatitis cases is 3 times the number of cases of pancreatitis reported in the other 4 countries. This can be due to several different reasons, 4 of which are summarized next:

■ **Scenario 1:** One of France's independent university drug safety units is doing a study to determine the mechanism involved in the development of pancreatitis after exposure to Drug A. The safety unit sends a letter to all licensed physicians requesting case information of any patient who was given Drug A and developed pancreatitis. (This information is solicited rather than spontaneously reported, so a greater number of cases is expected.)

■ **Scenario 2:** All cases of pancreatitis and Drug A are reviewed by the manufacturer, and it is discovered that alcohol consumption of French patients who developed pancreatitis is on average 3 times greater than consumption by patients with pancreatitis from other countries. (Alcohol consumption is a confounder since alcohol use can cause pancreatitis. There may also be an interaction between alcohol and Drug A, resulting in a greater risk of pancreatitis.)

■ **Scenario 3:** No further geographic imbalances are seen in the subsequent 12 months of marketing the drug. (The increased number of cases seen initially represents a clustering of reports due to chance alone during 1 reporting period that is not seen subsequently.)

■ **Scenario 4:** The local newspaper and radio and TV stations announce that the wife of a prominent local French celebrity is suing the manufacturer of Drug A because her husband died from complications of pancreatitis after taking Drug A. (Increased reports may be due to the influence of the media—so-called secular effects.)

This example shows that there may be many reasons for the cluster of pancreatitis cases in France … and it can be that none are important or mean anything. What is important is that a change in pattern—a cluster of cases—should serve as a *flag*, alerting the manufacturer that this finding deserves further investigation.

■ Links

In clinical studies, sources of safety information include:

- Adverse events
- Laboratory tests
- Vital signs
- 12-lead ECGs
- Physical examinations

Once a drug is marketed, the majority of safety information comes from spontaneous reports of adverse events. Adverse events, whether from clinical trials or spontaneous reports, are reported in different ways, including the following:

- As a *symptom*—an abnormal feeling or complaint reported by the patient, e.g., flank pain
- As a *sign*—objective evidence of a finding, e.g., hematuria (blood in urine) or a kidney stone

identified on an intravenous pyelogram (a type of X-ray of the kidneys, ureters, and bladder)

- As a *diagnosis*—a disease or syndrome (a collection of specific symptoms and signs associated with it). For example, the diagnosis of *Nephrolithiasis* includes the following signs and symptoms:
  - Symptoms—severe flank pain, nausea, red urine
  - Signs:
    - On *physical exam*: Punch tenderness of the flank in question but a soft and nontender abdomen.
    - On *laboratory tests* and *scans*: hematuria and a computed tomography scan showing a kidney stone.
    - *Other findings*: an actual kidney stone (if passed and retrieved).

Not everyone with nephrolithiasis will have all the signs and symptoms just summarized, but the more of these specific signs and symptoms there are, the greater the *weight of evidence* there is in support of the diagnosis.

Links refer to the relationship of certain safety findings to other safety findings. These links may be related

Table 7-4   A Patient With Acute Blood Loss—Links in Safety Findings[a]

Adverse Eents[b] MedDRA Preferred Term	Laboratory Tests	Vital Signs Analyses	ECG Analyses	Physical Exam
Symptoms: *Fatigue; Dizziness; Dyspnoea* **Signs:** *Haemoglobin decreased; Haematocrit decreased; Red blood cell count decreased; Blood pressure decreased; Blood pressure diastolic decreased; Blood pressure orthostatic decreased; Blood pressure systolic decreased; Heart rate increased; Hypotension; Hyperhidrosis; Orthostatic hypotension; Pallor; Syncope; Tachycardia* **Diagnoses:** *Anaemia; Duodenal ulcer haemorrhage; Shock haemorrhagic*	Decreased Hb, Hct, and/or RBCs	Decreased systolic blood pressure; decreased diastolic blood pressure; increased pulse rate; blood pressure decreases upon standing (orthostatic changes)	Increased heart rate	Diaphoretic, pale

[a] These are the main terrms—more can be added to the table. [b] Adverse events in the table are *italicized*. ECG = 12-lead electrocardiogram; Hb = hemoglobin; Hct = hematocrit; RBC = redblood cell count.

signs, symptoms, and diagnoses. Links also exist between certain safety measurements and assessments. For example, hemoglobin (Hb), hematocrit (Hct) and red blood cells (RBCs) are different laboratory tests that measure different things about RBCs but they are closely linked to each other. If for instance RBC values are very low, low values of Hb and Hct are also expected. '

If these parameters fall below a certain level, anemia results. Many different signs and symptoms can be associated with anemia e.g., pallor (paleness), fatigue, and dyspnea (shortness of breath). If anemia results from sudden blood loss, due to a bleeding duodenal ulcer, then diaphoresis (sweating), dizziness, hypotension (low blood pressure), orthostatic hypotension (blood pressure decreases that occur with changes in position), tachycardia (fast heart rate), syncope (fainting) and hemorrhagic shock (inadequate blood flow to vital organs resulting in organ dysfunction/failure) can also occur. In addition to these adverse events, vital sign measurements should also reveal an increased pulse rate and low blood pressure. If an ECG is obtained at the same time, an increased heart rate should also be seen on the ECG tracing. On physical examination, the patient with acute and

significant blood loss would be pale and diaphoretic. In this example, summarized in Table 7-4, we see that not only are the laboratory tests—RBCs, Hb, and Hct—linked to each other, but there are also links to other safety measurements/assessments, including adverse events, changes in vital signs, and ECG and physical examination findings. Not all safety findings will be as obvious as this example. But the more links identified, the greater the *weight of evidence* that there is something real going on.

Understanding the various links in safety data requires medical knowledge. A basic understanding of the links and patterns associated with common and/or important adverse drug reactions, however, should be part of the training of all members of the multifunctional team responsible for risk determination—e.g., programmers, statisticians, medical writers, drug safety and regulatory professionals, and medical reviewers. The more trained eyes there are, the greater the chance of discovering safety signals.

Other examples of data patterns, links, and dashboard data displays that enhance signal identification and strengthen the *weight of evidence* are provided throughout the book.

Determining Clinical Significance ... and Then What?

In the determination of risk and the importance and significance of adverse events and safety issues, the following 3 questions need to be answered:

1. Is there an adverse drug effect or safety issue?
2. If so, is this drug effect or issue clinically significant?
3. If so, is the overall benefit–risk profile still favorable?

Answers to the first 2 questions are an integral part of determining the drug's benefit–risk profile—something required throughout the development and marketing of a drug. Whether implicitly or explicitly stated, the determination of what the drug effect means clinically must be determined on an ongoing basis. To put it another way, many drugs have effects—both good and bad—but these effects have no clinical significance. Sometimes determining whether there is a real drug effect is devilishly difficult, but the clinical significance part is easy. Sometimes just the reverse is true. This is one of the things that make drug safety so interesting and challenging.

The determination of a drug effect is discussed in many chapters throughout the book. The objectives of this chapter are to:

- Define clinical significance
- Provide approaches to be used in determining clinical significance
- Determine what to do with clinically significant findings that are drug related

■ The Definition of Clinical Significance

One of the major goals of this book is to help you navigate through the gray areas of uncertainty that are associated with the determination of risk. One of the grayest areas is the determination of clinical significance.

It would be useful to have a standard definition and specific criteria for determining clinical significance, but none exists. The next best thing is to provide a working definition that can be used as a framework in assessing clinical significance. *Clinical* is something that applies to patients, and *significance* means something of importance—presumably, importance refers to the health of the patient, but sometimes it refers to other things, such as the effects on the family (e.g., a drug makes a patient snore, producing nocturnal marital discord) or on society (e.g., extending a terminal patient's life 2 weeks at enormous cost). For the purposes of this book, we will avoid the societal and political aspects and consider importance to the patient as our guiding principle.

So we see that something important to the patient is central to the understanding of the clinical significance of an adverse drug effect. When we expand this concept of something important to the patient, a useful working definition emerges; i.e., "any drug effect that interferes with a person's ability to perform the activities of daily living." Examples of drug effects that result in outcomes that can impact the performance of these activities include the following:

■ If you die or develop an immediate life-threatening event due to drug-induced anaphylaxis, you can't attend your own wedding (outcome = *death* or *immediately life threatening*)

■ If you are hospitalized due to a drug-related bleeding ulcer, you can't participate in your company's summer picnic festivities (outcome = *hospitalization*)

■ If you had a stroke due to drug-induced malignant hypertension and the left side of your body is paralyzed, you can no longer earn a living as a carpenter (outcome = *disability*)

■ If you are born blind due to drug-related congenital blindness, it is more difficult to handle the activities of daily living (outcome = *congenital abnormality*)

■ If you need to go to an outpatient clinic for a blood transfusion to treat your severe drug-induced anemia, you have to take time off from work (outcome = *medically important*)

These clinically significant outcomes should look familiar, because these are the criteria used for defining *serious adverse events*. Although serious criteria are used for regulatory reporting purposes, we see that these criteria are also useful in determining clinical significance.

TIP: Any event that results in a serious outcome is usually clinically significant!

A drug effect that does not meet serious criteria can still be clinically significant if it still negatively impacts a person's ability to perform the activities of normal living. For example:

■ If you have episodes of frequent and explosive diarrhea, you don't want to go mountain climbing (nor do your friends want to hike with you!).

■ If you develop persistent, flu-like symptoms such as sneezing, runny nose, and malaise (commonly seen with interferons) that don't resolve in a week or 10 days as most other nondrug flu-like diseases do, you won't be at your best, or won't even be able to run the marathon for which you been training for the last 6 months.

These examples are less *black and white*, i.e., less clear and straightforward, and some degree of medical judgment is required in assigning clinical significance to these events.

Still other findings may be initially asymptomatic with the patient unaware of anything going on. With continued exposure and the problem left untreated, the risk of developing a clinically significant outcome increases. For instance, suppose a drug causes a mean increase in diastolic blood pressure of 10 mmHg. If this condition is sustained and untreated, a patient who is taking that drug has an increased risk of cardiovascular, cerebrovascular, and renal disease.

This example illustrates that a drug effect may not result in a serious outcome in the short term, but the risk is potentially clinically significant in the future and must not be ignored.

■ Approaches Used in Determining Clinical Significance

Determining clinical significance requires consideration of a number of different factors. The following is a list of these factors … the more factors present, the greater the clinical significance.

■ The drug effect resulted in a serious outcome.

■ It was severe in intensity.

■ It led to discontinuation of treatment.

■ It was sustained rather than transient.

■ It put the patient at risk for developing a clinically significant outcome.

■ The drug effect was large (e.g., a 10 mm Hg mean increase in diastolic blood pressure versus a mean increase of 0.5 mm Hg).

- The outcome of the drug effect was permanent (caused total blindness) or resulted in sequelae (e.g., decreased visual acuity).
- The drug effect could not be prevented or minimized (e.g., by reducing the dose).

For situations that are not clear, i.e., fall into the *gray zone*, the determination of clinical significance depends heavily on clinical judgment. Judgment, however, is not infallible or necessarily objective or reproducible (e.g., how many times have you witnessed 3 health professionals give 3 different assessments of the same case, or 3 economists give 3 totally different opinions on where the stock market is heading?) Judgment is an *opinion*—hopefully an informed opinion. This opinion is reached in many different ways and covers a wide spectrum of approaches from the most scientifically rigorous and objective to the least scientific and subjective. These approaches include the following, in descending order of objectivity:

- Evidence-based medicine
- Expert opinion
- Experience
- Intuition ("gut feeling")
- Bias

Evidence-Based Medicine

Evidence-based medicine is the most objective and scientific approach in forming a clinical opinion. The gold standard in decision making relies on results from prospective, randomized, controlled studies, but such studies are rarely done for safety as discussed in Chapter 6. Results of safety analyses typically *suggest*, but do not *prove*, a drug-related safety finding. Remember too—what is statistically significant is not necessarily clinically significant. Conversely, what is clinically significant is not necessarily statistically significant. This is seen with rare or infrequent adverse events that are too few in number to analyze statistically.

For these reasons, determining clinical significance based on scientific evidence has its limitations.

Expert Opinion

Without scientific data available, the determination of clinical significance often depends on the clinical opinion of experts. Experts who have done research or are very well versed in the research results in the area of concern can render a useful opinion based on their knowledge and experience. The problem with this approach is that such opinions may be somewhat subjective and biased.

There are innumerable examples of court cases where very qualified experts of opposing counsels give opposite opinions on the same data! Many instances of conflicts of interest in which experts have some financial interest in the outcome of a case are also emerging. In fact, few people are without bias of one sort or another and perhaps the best we can hope for is that all biases and potential conflicts of interest are made public and thus taken into account when judging an expert's opinion.

Experience

The determination of clinical significance can also be based on the experience of the health professional. This is similar to the opinion of the expert but carries a bit less weight since the health professional's sphere of experience may lack the depth and breadth of experience of the expert.

There is an interesting offshoot of this seen in the determination of treatment-related serious adverse events (SAEs) as judged by an investigator during a clinical trial. In a large trial with many patients, a particular SAE may be quite rare and seen only in a handful of patients. Any individual investigator might think that this rare and bizarre SAE is not related to the drug. Only someone (e.g., the sponsor or health authority) seeing the totality of the cases and seeing the same rare and bizarre event occurring in multiple sites is able to conclude that the SAE is related to the drug and is significant.

Intuition

Physicians will often tell you of their experience in *trusting their gut (i.e., trusting a feeling or an intuition)*, and some of these anecdotes sound remarkably similar. For example, a man goes to the emergency department with vague and nonspecific complaints, saying, "I just don't feel well." All objective measurements, e.g., vital signs, laboratory tests, and a 12-lead electrocardiogram are normal, except the patient is anxious and appears "green around the gills" (translation: the patient doesn't look well). Even though there is little objective evidence of a problem, the physician's *gut* (intuition) is alerting him that the patient may have a potentially serious problem unfolding. The physician, without clear objective evidence of a particular diagnosis, decides to *trust his gut* and admits the patient for observation. One hour later, the patient has a cardiac arrest in his hospital room. Intuition may turn out to be our internal supercomputer processing information that is currently beyond our level of awareness or comprehension, sending us alerts of potential problems. For these reasons, computers lacking this *fuzzy logic* to process and evaluate subjective feelings have not as yet replaced health professionals. Determining clinical significance based on intuition, however, has its limitations, especially among reviewers who have not actually physically seen a patient and have only the patient's case report form to review.

Bias

Bias plays a powerful role as the basis of clinical opinions. Even if evidence-based data are presented to health professionals, it does not mean the health professional will be convinced of the data or follow the recommendations from such evidence. This is shown in the results of a Canadian study evaluating risk of teratogenicity and drug labeling. In this study, health professionals were shown reassuring labeling that explicitly stated that certain drugs did not cause fetal malformations when used in pregnancy. Nevertheless, the health professionals still rated these drugs as having some risk of causing birth defects.[1]

So we see that all these approaches, even the most scientific and objective, have limitations in determining clinical significance.

Another big challenge is that clinical significance must be determined on *snapshots* of data taken over time. These data can be limited with respect to both the depth and breadth of information that is provided. For these reasons, stating the clinical significance of the data is really a *conditional* assessment that can change when more information is available.

Even with these restrictions, whenever a drug effect is observed or cannot be ruled out, some statement of its clinical significance needs to be made based on the composite of factors discussed previously. If the finding is considered clinically significant, the basis for this should be included. The following are some examples of statements that can be made depending on what is found:

- Scenario 1: There is a drug effect, but there is no evidence of any clinically important findings (e.g., no deaths, SAEs, notable laboratory changes, etc.). *Statement*: "A drug effect is seen but based on the data to date, no clinically significant findings are identified."
- Scenario 2: There is a drug effect, but you are uncertain whether or not the findings are clinically significant. *Statement*: "A drug effect is seen, but the clinical significance, if any, is unknown at this time."
- Scenario 3: There is a drug effect, and the vast majority of patients have no clinically significant findings, but there are a few patients who do have questionable findings. *Statement*: "A clinically significant drug effect cannot be ruled out at this time based on ..."(provide the basis for this, e.g., two subjects who developed increased serum creatinine values and concomitant fluid retention, etc.)
- Scenario 4: There is a drug effect, and it is clinically significant. *Statement*: "There is (or use the term *appears to be* if you are less certain) a clinically significant drug effect, based on ..." (provide the reasons, e.g., increased rate of deaths, increased risk of acute renal failure, etc.).

CAUTION: Even if a drug-related finding is not *initially* considered clinically significant, the finding needs to be put on your radar screen and closely monitored to see what happens after longer exposure to the drug. Further evaluation to better understand the basis of this finding is also required. This is illustrated in the example discussed at the end of the chapter.

■ ... and Then What?

If a clinically significant drug effect is identified, the next important step is to determine if the benefit–risk profile tilted from favorable to unfavorable. This is based on the following:

- The extent of the finding, e.g., common or rare, only found in a subgroup of patients, e.g., those with renal impairment, etc.?
- Can the risk be minimized or avoided?
- Is the condition being treated clinically important, e.g., cancer versus flatulence?
- Is there safer therapy available?

If the benefit–risk profile is still considered favorable after the identification of a clinically significant drug effect, the following steps should be taken:

- Monitor patients closely to determine if the finding is changing over time (e.g., the finding is becoming more frequent, more severe, etc.).
- Do further evaluations to better understand and characterize the finding.

Range of Options for an Investigational Drug

If the benefit–risk profile is determined to be unfavorable, there is a range of options that can be implemented. What options are chosen is dependent on what the risk is and whether the risk can be avoided or minimized. The options for an investigational drug include:

- Revise the study protocol and informed consent: Two types of problems are frequently seen:
  1. A risk is dose related. In this case, a simple reduction in the dose may suffice to correct the problem.
  2. The risk is seen within a particular group (e.g., diabetics). Excluding these patients may be sufficient to eliminate the problem (though, of course, it means the drug will not be approved for marketing in this group of patients).
- Evaluate further; e.g., do additional nonclinical studies, do more testing in ongoing clinical studies, start new clinical studies, etc.
- If possible, recommend a treatment for the adverse event. For example, if diarrhea occurs in the study of a new antibiotic used in patients with life-threatening infections where no other antibiotic is effective, adding a drug to treat the diarrhea may suffice and allow the patient to complete the course of treatment.
- Place the study on temporary hold.
- Put the study on permanent hold.
- Stop development.

Range of Options for a Marketed Drug

The options for an unfavorable risk–benefit profile for a marketed drug include:

- Revise the product labeling.
- Initiate new risk management strategies; e.g., create/revise medication guides; design a limited access program.
- Evaluate further; e.g., conduct a large, simple safety study; do a pharmacoepidemiologic study.
- Take the drug off the market.

The following is an example of a safety finding that highlights some of the key concepts discussed in this chapter.

Change in Serum Creatinine

Investigational Drug X is a drug under development for the treatment of hypertension. The drug is a member of a class of antihypertensives already on the market. A small but consistent increase in mean creatinine values is seen in the investigational drug group compared to placebo. This difference is statistically significant (p-value = 0.01). The greatest mean change is 0.025 mg/dL observed at Day 56. This change is considered small and clinically insignificant. Figure 8-1 shows the mean changes in creatinine from baseline (Day 0) that persists during the treatment period (Days 1–84), and returns to baseline posttreatment as shown on Day 112 (i.e., 28 days posttreatment).

The number (%) of subjects with creatinine values that shifted from below normal or normal range at baseline to above the normal range during treatment is small and no different than placebo (investigational drug = 1%; placebo = 1%). There are no subjects in either treatment group with values that reach clinically significant values, i.e., > 2.0 mg/dL. There are no trends seen for increases in serum urea nitrogen, decreases in serum albumin or increases in urinary levels of protein. In addition, no renal-related adverse events were reported. Similar serum creatinine findings are seen in 3 other studies, i.e., statistically significant increased mean creatinine values but no other findings.

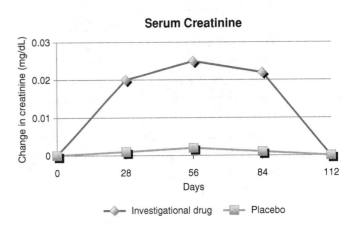

Figure 8-1 Mean Changes in Serum Creatinine Values

Questions

1. **Is there a drug effect?**

   Yes, based on the pattern and consistency of results seen across 4 studies.

2. **Is this drug effect clinically significant?**

   Based on the data to date, no clinically significant findings are identified.

3. **What should be the next steps?**

   This requires a safety signal investigation. Prepare a list of hypotheses for this finding, and gather information to confirm or reject these hypotheses. Gather information from other completed clinical and animal studies to see if similar effects were seen.

The following is a list of hypotheses and the action plan to prove or disprove them:

- **Hypothesis No. 1**: The reagent used for the serum creatinine test interacts with the investigational drug, causing a false positive. Action plan:
  - Discuss with director of central laboratory.

- **Hypothesis No. 2**: The drug causes muscle injury with release of creatine from the muscle, resulting in increased creatinine levels (creatinine is formed from muscle creatine). Action plan:
  - Review muscle-related adverse events.
  - Review creatine kinase (CK) values.

- **Hypothesis No. 3**: The drug causes renal injury. Action plan:
  - Review animal data to determine if renal injury was noted and discuss with an independent animal toxicologist.
  - Do a literature search to determine if similar findings were reported for other drugs.
  - Discuss the findings with a nephrologist who is expert in the field of drug-induced renal toxicity.

- **Hypothesis No. 4**: The drug causes changes in creatinine values but is not nephrotoxic. Action plan:
  - Wait to see the results from the other investigations. If hypotheses 1–3 are negative, this is the most likely hypothesis.

Follow-up reveals the following:

- The central lab investigated the possibility of interference with the reagent/tests, and none was found. (If you still think there is some interference with the lab test and disagree with the central lab's findings, have a different lab do an investigation to ensure that the lab that investigated itself did a fair and unbiased investigation.)

- Review of all animal data revealed no renal-related findings. This was confirmed by an independent animal toxicologist.

- No increases in CK values or increases in muscle-related adverse events were seen in clinical trials.

- A nephrologist whose specialty is drug-induced nephrotoxicity reviewed the data. She indicated these findings were similar to 2 other drugs that ultimately had to be withdrawn from the market after long-term drug exposure. Renal lesions were not seen for at least 6 months and then some patients ($< 0.5\%$) started to show signs of renal toxicity that led in some cases to irreversible renal failure. The nephrologist reminded the company that the longest exposure to the investigational drug was 3 months. She recommended collection and analysis of the following urinary biomarkers: kidney injury molecule (KIM-1), albumin, total protein, β2-microglobulin, urinary clusterin, urinary trefoil factor 3, and urinary cystatin C. She also proposed a study in 2 species of rats (Wistar and Sprague Dawley rats) with exposure to high doses of the investigational drug for 6 months and measurement of the same urinary biomarkers recommended for the clinical studies.

- The literature search confirmed what the nephrologist said—2 drugs with initial findings similar to the investigational drug were withdrawn from the market due to nephrotoxicity.

The results of the rat study and the additional measurements of urinary biomarkers both in the clinical and rat study revealed the following:

- Both species of rats as well as patients in clinical studies showed small but consistent increases in KIM-1 values.

■ Examination of the kidney tissue of sacrificed rats revealed subtle but abnormal cellular findings suggestive of early toxicity.

Two other expert nephrologists were also asked to review the data. All 3 nephrologists concluded that the risk of the investigational drug causing nephrotoxicity in humans after longer term treatment was high. These findings were presented to the company's in-house safety committee, and the consensus of the committee was to stop the development of the investigational drug, and the drug was "killed."

➡ **NOTE:** Although the findings of small but consistent increases in serum creatinine did not appear to be initially clinically significant, further evaluation revealed evidence that with prolonged exposure, there was a real risk of renal toxicity. This case underscores the importance of continuously monitoring and reevaluating drug-related findings that may not at first appear clinically significant. In this case, the investigational drug was a "me-too" drug under development for a condition that was already saturated with other efficacious and safer treatments. All these factors led to the assessment that the benefit–risk profile was unfavorable. If, instead, the investigational drug was under development for the treatment of pancreatic cancer—a condition uniformly fatal with little treatment options available, and showed promising efficacy but had the same risk profile—it is likely development would continue, provided patients were closely monitored for renal dysfunction.

On another note, in real life, the results of the findings summarized in this example are rarely this straightforward or consistent. It is not uncommon to have conflicting results. For instance, only 1 of the 2 other nephrotoxic drugs reported in the literature was withdrawn from the market; and 2 of the 3 nephrologists felt the drug might be toxic but the third didn't. For these reasons, what to do varies and should be based on the weight of available evidence, with measures put into to place to do ongoing reevaluation until there is confirmation that the signal is real, and the clinical significance of the finding is determined.

Reference

1. Pole M, Einarson A, Pairaudeau N, et al. Drug labeling and risk perceptions of teratogenicity: a survey of pregnant Canadian women and their health professionals. *J Clin Pharmacol.* 2000;40: 573–577.

Clinical Laboratory Tests—What Is Measured; What It Means

The objective of this chapter is to provide a basic understanding of what laboratory tests measure and what changes in these labs mean from a drug perspective. This information will provide the foundation for Chapter 17—The Analysis of Laboratory Data. A basic knowledge of laboratory tests will also aid in understanding laboratory abnormalities described in individual case safety reports.

> ➡ **NOTE:** This chapter is written for individuals with little or no clinical training. General references are provided for those interested in learning more about the topic and are organized for those with[1-5] and without[6,7] clinical experience.

◼ Laboratory Tests

The laboratory parameters (also referred to by some as *analytes*) that are measured in clinical trials fall into 3 main categories: hematology, clinical chemistry, and urinalysis.

Hematology (Blood) Parameters

Hematology parameters include 3 basic components: erythrocytes or red blood cells (RBCs), white blood cells (WBCs), and platelets. Platelets are not cells but fragments from a cell called the *megakaryocyte*. The production of RBCs, WBCs, and platelets is referred to as *hematopoiesis*. Hematopoiesis occurs in the bone marrow, and the cascade of cells involved in the process is illustrated in Figure 9-1.

One of the key concepts in understanding drug-induced injury is knowing that all blood elements come from one cell—the *multipotential hematopoietic stem cell*. (The word *multipotential* means that this stem cell can

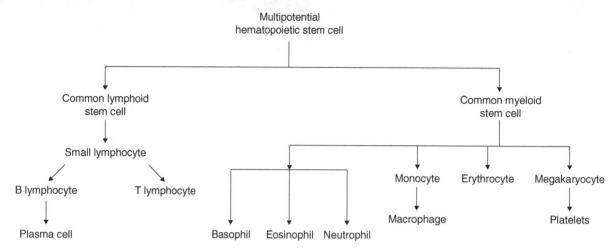

Figure 9-1 Hematopoiesis—Simplified

differentiate into any one of the other cells shown in Figure 9-1). Injury to this cell will adversely affect all 3 blood lines and result in a condition called *aplastic anemia* resulting in *pancytopenia* (decreases in RBCs, WBCs, and platelets). Aplastic anemia is a life-threatening condition that can result in death due to severe anemia (low RBC counts), infection due to low WBC counts, and hemorrhage (bleeding) due to low platelet counts. Chloramphenicol (an antibiotic) and phenylbutazone (a nonsteroidal anti-inflammatory drug [NSAID]) are examples of 2 drugs that can cause aplastic anemia. Aplastic anemia can also be caused by a *hypersensitivity* reaction or an *autoimmune disease*, in which the bone marrow is attacked and injured by the body's own *immune system*.

A *complete blood count* is a test that measures:

- The number of RBCs
- Hemoglobin (Hb), hematocrit (Hct), mean corpuscular volume (MCV), and mean corpuscular hemoglobin concentration (MCHC)
- The number of WBCs, which are made up of different types of cells—neutrophils, lymphocytes, eosinophils, basophils, and monocytes
- The number of platelets

The complete blood count also provides information on the microscopic appearance of RBCs, WBCs, and platelets.

Red Blood Cells

The purpose of the RBC is to carry oxygen (O_2) to the various cells in the body and to carry carbon dioxide (CO_2) away. *Hemoglobin* is a protein found in RBCs that is responsible for the transport of O_2 and CO_2. O_2, in combination with Hb, gives blood its bright red color while CO_2 and Hb give blood a dark red/purplish color. *Bilirubin* is a breakdown product of Hb (see "Hepatic Profile" for further discussion of bilirubin).

Blood is made of 2 components—a cellular component and a liquid component—*plasma* (or *serum*). The cellular component is predominantly made up of RBCs but also includes WBCs and platelets. Plasma contains glucose, proteins, lipids, hormones, minerals, clotting factors, and other components (see "Clinical Chemistry"). When blood is centrifuged (spun at high speeds), the cells and plasma separate. If the clotting factors and fibrinogen (a protein that is converted to fibrin, which, along with platelets, form a *clot* or *thrombus*) are removed from plasma, the resulting liquid is referred to as *serum*. Some tests are done with serum and some with plasma. To obtain plasma, an anticoagulant is added to the test tube to prevent clotting and the using up of clotting factors and fibrinogen. The tube is then centrifuged and the clear liquid portion of the contents of the tube, which is the plasma, is carefully poured off. Serum is obtained by letting the blood in the test tube clot, producing a solid and a liquid component in the test tube. The liquid (obtained by centrifuging) is the serum.

Hematocrit is the percentage of the blood (by volume) that is composed of RBCs. An Hct value of 45% means that the RBCs make up 45% of the total volume of blood, and the remaining 55% is plasma. Sometimes people leave off the percent sign when reporting this value and just refer to a hematocrit of 45. *Anemia* is a condition in which the RBC count, Hb, and Hct values are below normal.

Conditions associated with elevated RBC, Hb, and Hct values (*erythrocytosis* or *polycythemia*) can result in an increased risk of thrombosis (blood clots).

Drug-induced anemia results from:

- Bone marrow toxicity—destruction of any of the cells in the red cell line shown in Figure 9-1.

- Deficiency, impaired absorption, blocking or increased loss of the essential components for normal RBC production, such as iron, vitamin B_{12}, and folate (folic acid). For example, metformin (an antidiabetic drug) can block B_{12} absorption.[8] Many drugs are folate antagonists, including phenytoin (an anticonvulsant) and methotrexate (an antineoplastic/immunosuppressant drug). Alcohol is also an important folate antagonist. Aspirin and NSAIDs can lead to iron loss due to bleeding.

- Increased destruction—referred to as *hemolysis*—where RBCs rupture and are destroyed. This is typically due to a hypersensitivity or immunologic reaction. Examples of drugs that can cause hemolysis include methyldopa (an antihypertensive), quinidine (an antiarrhythmic agent), and penicillin (an antibiotic).

- Increased blood loss by adverse effects on coagulation factors and platelets, or direct damage to blood vessels. Warfarin and heparin inhibit coagulation factors. Aspirin and NSAIDs inhibit the platelet's property of adhesiveness necessary for normal clot formation and can also cause ulcers, which can damage blood vessels and cause bleeding. Sometimes the effects on coagulation factors are desirable and are the reason for the patient's use of the drug. Heparin and warfarin are given to patients with blood clots to dissolve the clot or to prevent recurrences. Too much of these drugs can result in severe bleeding.

Examination of different RBC components and other laboratory tests are necessary in the evaluation of anemia and provide clues to its medical cause. These include:

- **Mean corpuscular volume (MCV)**—The mean corpuscular volume is the measurement of the RBC's size. RBCs with low, normal, and increased MCV values are referred to as *microcytic, normocytic,* and *macrocytic,* respectively.

- **Mean corpuscular hemoglobin concentration (MCHC)**—The mean corpuscular hemoglobin concentration is a measurement of the average Hb

TIP: Anemia can occur due to nondrug-related causes (e.g., bleeding, cancer, etc.). Also note that drugs rarely cause an increase in these parameters. One drug that does is erythropoietin, commonly referred to as EPO and used in the treatment of anemia. This increase in RBCs is a desired effect and not an adverse event! A word of caution though … other drugs that increase RBCs are anabolic steroids. Both erythropoietin and anabolic steroids are misused as performance-enhancing drugs, and their use is not permitted in competitive sports.

concentration of RBCs. *Hypochromic* and *normochromic* are terms that indicate low and normal MCHC values, respectively.

- *Reticulocytes*—Reticulocytes are immature RBCs found in blood. Increased numbers indicate more rapid turnover of RBCs and are seen with hemolysis or blood loss.

- *Ferritin*—Ferritin levels reflect the body stores of iron. Iron is one of the key components of hemoglobin.

- *B_{12} levels*—B_{12} is a vitamin that is essential for RBC formation.

- *Folate*—Folate (folic acid) is necessary for the production of healthy RBCs.

- *Haptoglobin*—Haptoglobin is a protein that binds with *free* hemoglobin (hemoglobin that is released from damaged or hemolyzed RBCs).

- *Coombs test*—A Coombs test detects antibodies that adhere to RBCs. The presence of antibodies can trigger an immune response, resulting in hemolysis.

- *Indirect bilirubin*—Indirect bilirubin is indicative of increased bilirubin formation. Bilirubin is a breakdown product of hemoglobin. Increased levels of indirect bilirubin are seen with increased release and destruction of hemoglobin (see "Hepatic Profile" for more on bilirubin).

Table 9-1 provides a summary of laboratory clues that help determine the cause of different types of drug-induced anemias.

White Blood Cells

White blood cells (WBCs) are made up of several different cell types—*neutrophils, bands* (which are immature neutrophils), *lymphocytes, eosinophils, basophils,* and *monocytes.* The main purpose of WBCs is to fight infection and other foreign intruders in the body.

Table 9-1	Different Types of Drug-Induced Anemias—Laboratory Clues [1-3]				
	Aplastic Anemia (Bone Marrow Toxicity)	Hemolytic Anemia	Iron-Deficiency Anemia	Anemia Due to Acute Hemorrhage	Anemia Due to B_{12} or Folate Deficiency
MCV	Normal	Normal	Decreased	Normal	Increased
MCHC	Normal	Normal	Decreased	Normal	Normal
Reticulocyte count	Decreased	Increased	Decreased	Normal (initially). Increased after 3–4 days	Decreased
Ferritin	Decreased	Increased	Decreased	Normal initially	Increased
B_{12}	Normal	Normal	Normal	Normal	Decreased* in B_{12} deficiency
Folate	Normal	Normal	Normal	Normal	Decreased* in folate deficiency
Coombs test	Negative	Positive	Negative	Negative	Negative
Haptoglobin	Normal	Decreased	Normal	Normal	Decreased
Indirect bilirubin	Normal	Increased	Normal	Normal	Increased

* May be normal in some subjects

Source: Adapted from Fischbach F, Dunning MB. *A Manual of Laboratory & Diagnostic Tests.* 8th ed. Philadelphia PA: Lippincott; 2009.

Sometimes, WBCs can attack our own cells and tissues and cause damage—this occurs in hypersensitivity reactions and autoimmune diseases. Each WBC has specific functions:

- Neutrophils (including bands) defend against bacterial infections but also are involved in inflammatory disorders.

- Lymphocytes play a part in the immune response. The B lymphocytes produce antibodies, and the T lymphocytes attack body cells that are invaded by viruses or become cancerous.

- Eosinophils defend against parasitic infections but also play a role in allergic disorders.

- Basophils, like eosinophils, defend against parasitic infections and are involved in allergic disorders.

- Monocytes possess phagocytic properties; i.e., they can ingest foreign substances and are involved in immune defense and inflammatory processes.

Granulocytes refer to WBCs with granules and include neutrophils, eosinophils, and basophils. These granules contain substances that fight infection but can also cause harm to our tissues by causing inflammation and tissue injury. *Mast cells* are cells that also have granules. They are very similar to basophils and can cause tissue injury and life-threatening allergic reactions. Mast cells are located in tissues and do not circulate in the blood. *Leucopenia* (or *leukopenia*) refers to low WBC counts. This finding is associated with an increased risk of infection.

Drug-induced leucopenia is usually caused by injury to the cells in the bone marrow that produce WBCs or by increased destruction due to hypersensitivity reactions. An increase in WBCs is referred to as *leucocytosis* (or *leukocytosis*) and occurs in many conditions such as infection, inflammation, and leukemia (WBC cancer).

The values of the different types of WBCs in a complete blood count are presented as a percentage (%) of the total WBC count; as an absolute count, or both. To calculate absolute values, simply multiply the WBC count and the percentage (%) of the specific WBC. For example, if the percentage (%) of neutrophils is 50%, and the WBC count is 5,000 cells/mm³, the absolute neutrophil count is 5,000 cells/mm³ × 50% = 2,500 cells/mm³.

TIP: The percentage of neutrophils, lymphocytes, eosinophils, basophils, and monocytes should equal 100%; if not, there is an error somewhere, although rounding can produce a total of 99 or 101.

Platelets

Platelets are fragments from megakaryocytes (Figure 9-1). Platelets are involved in *hemostasis* or the stoppage of bleeding. A low platelet count is referred to as *thrombocytopenia*, and an elevated platelet count is referred to as *thrombocytosis*. Thrombocytopenia is associated with an increased risk of bleeding while thrombocytosis is associated with an increased risk of clot formation.

Drug-induced thrombocytopenia typically results from injury to the megakaryocyte or cells in the bone marrow that form the megakaryocyte. Drug-induced thrombocytopenia can also be due to a hypersensitivity reaction.

Clinical Chemistry

Clinical chemistry is composed of a number of different tests that measure various substances that are found in the plasma.

TIP: For the analyses of clinical laboratory tests, it is useful and more reviewer friendly to group clinical chemistry into the subcategories of *hepatic profile, renal profile, metabolic and muscle profile,* and *lipid profile,* because many laboratory tests are interrelated and trends found in certain groupings of laboratory tests aid in identifying potential safety signals, e.g., liver injury or renal problems.

Hepatic Profile
The laboratory tests that typically make up the hepatic profile include: *alanine aminotransferase (ALT), aspartate aminotransferase (AST), total bilirubin (TB),* and *alkaline phosphatase (ALP).* Abnormal test results suggest potential liver- and/or gallbladder-related problems.

ALT and AST, are enzymes found within the *hepatocyte* (liver cell). When the hepatocyte is damaged, these enzymes leak out of the hepatocyte and into the blood, causing elevated blood values.

TIP: ALT is the enzyme most specific to the liver. AST is found in many tissues and other organs such as the heart and skeletal muscle. If the source of blood elevation is an injured liver, both the ALT and AST values should be elevated. If only the AST value is elevated, a nonhepatic source is more likely. *Gamma glutamyltransferase (GGT)* is another enzyme found in the liver and is very sensitive to alcohol. If GGT is elevated along with ALT and AST, alcohol may be the culprit alone, or may indicate an adverse interaction between alcohol and the drug.

Bilirubin, as mentioned previously, is the breakdown product of hemoglobin. There are 3 types of bilirubin measurements—*indirect (unconjugated), direct (conjugated),* and *total bilirubin* (indirect + direct bilirubin values). Indirect bilirubin is not soluble in water, and therefore only low values are usually found in the blood. In the liver, the bilirubin is conjugated with a substance called *glucuronic acid,* which makes bilirubin soluble in water, and therefore higher levels of direct bilirubin are observed in the blood compared to indirect bilirubin. In clinical trials, TB is typically measured. If TB is elevated, then the blood is examined further to determine the direct bilirubin levels. Indirect levels are not directly measured but derived by subtracting the direct bilirubin levels from the TB values. With hemolysis, elevation of TB and indirect bilirubin is usually seen. If there is injury to the hepatocyte, or biliary obstruction, the TB as well as the direct bilirubin values are elevated. Elevated bilirubin values cause *jaundice*—a yellow discoloration of the skin and the sclerae (white part) of the eyes. The presence of bilirubin in the urine (*bilirubinuria*) is also associated with elevated plasma bilirubin levels.

ALP is an enzyme predominantly found in liver and bone. Children have ALP values considerably higher than adults due to bone growth. When there is obstruction to the biliary tract such as in gallstones blocking or irritating the bile ducts, ALP values increase.

TIP: The liver is a prime target for drug-induced injury. Liver injury can take different forms. One form of injury, hepatocellular injury, which involves the hepatocyctes, is of particular concern. Clinically significant increases in ALT and/or AST associated with concomitant increases in total bilirubin levels (TBLs) with little or no increase in ALP is referred to as *Hy's law.* Liver function tests meeting Hy's law criteria may be a signal of significant hepatocellular disease that can lead to liver failure.[9] This topic is discussed further in Chapters 11 and 17. The *clue* for this type of liver injury is the abnormal ALT/AST/TBL values while ALP is normal or only mildly elevated.

Renal Profile
The laboratory tests associated with kidney function include: *creatinine, blood urea nitrogen (BUN), total protein,* and *albumin.* The analysis of urine also provides information about kidney function (see "Urinalysis").

Creatinine is a by-product of energy metabolism in muscle. Normal kidneys are able to excrete creatinine; however, in renal disorders, creatinine excretion is impaired and creatinine blood levels rise.

BUN is formed in the liver and is a waste product of protein metabolism. Like creatinine, BUN is excreted by the kidney and is elevated if kidney function is impaired. Unlike creatinine levels, elevated BUN levels can be due to nonrenal factors. Low levels of BUN can result from liver failure, malnutrition, and overhydration. Elevated levels can occur with bleeding in the gut (where blood is broken down to BUN), excessive protein intake, or rapid protein (tissue) breakdown from conditions such as burns.

Total protein is made up of various proteins in the plasma, one of which is albumin. Normal renal function prevents the loss of total protein/albumin from the body and little, if any, total protein/albumin is found in the urine. In renal disease, especially in a condition called the *nephrotic syndrome*, large amounts of total protein/albumin are excreted in the urine.

Total protein/albumin act like sponges keeping fluid in the blood vessels. Low protein levels are associated with fluid shifts within the body and may result in fluid accumulation in tissues (*edema*) and the abdomen (*ascites*). Because proteins are synthesized in the liver, low protein/albumin levels can also occur with liver disease.

> ➡ **NOTE:** If the cause for low protein/albumin values is due to abnormal liver function rather than kidney problems, these analytes should be included in the hepatic profile discussed in the previous section.

TIP: In renal disease, *both* creatinine and BUN are typically elevated. If only BUN is elevated, this may be due to a nonrenal cause, a laboratory error, or mild dehydration due to fasting before the patient took the blood test.

Metabolic and Muscle Profile

The metabolic and muscle profile includes a diverse group of analytes: *glucose, electrolytes* (*sodium, potassium, chloride, bicarbonate,* and *calcium*) *inorganic phosphorus, uric acid,* and the muscle enzyme *creatine kinase*. Abnormalities in these laboratory parameters can signal many different medical conditions.

Glucose is a simple sugar and a very important source of energy for the brain and many of the body's functions. Glucose comes primarily from carbohydrate metabolism (the breakdown of carbohydrates), but protein and fats can also be converted into glucose. Too little glucose (*hypoglycemia*) or too high values (*hyperglycemia*) can result in significant symptoms including coma. *Diabetes mellitus* is a common disease associated with elevated blood glucose levels. Glucocorticosteroids (e.g., prednisone) and thiazide diuretics (e.g., hydrochlorothiazide) are examples of drugs that can increase blood glucose levels in some patients. Glucose should ideally be measured during fasting conditions because food can affect glucose levels.

Electrolytes are particles that have a positive or negative charge in solution. A positively charged particle is referred to as a *cation* (pronounced *kat eye on*); a negatively charged particle is an *anion*. Examples of electrolytes include sodium (Na^+), potassium (K^+), chloride (Cl^-), bicarbonate (HCO_3^-), and calcium (Ca^{2+}). Calcium also exists in a nonelectrolyte form (see discussion on calcium later in this section). Electrolyte movement causes an electric current, and these currents stimulate various electromechanical or electrochemical events within the body, such as conduction of a nerve impulse and skeletal and cardiac muscle contraction. Some electrolytes are also involved in acid-base balance, energy-producing biochemical reactions, and fluid balance.

Sodium (Na^+) carries a positive charge and is mainly found outside the cell (extracellular) during resting conditions. The flow of sodium into a cell and back out of it again is a requirement for many essential biochemical and biomechanical reactions such as nerve conduction. The kidney, along with various hormones such as *aldosterone* and *vasopressin* (*antidiuretic hormone*), is responsible for maintaining normal sodium levels. High sodium levels often result in fluid retention; e.g., swollen fingers and ankles after eating too many salty potato chips. If extreme, *hyponatremia* (low sodium levels) and *hypernatremia* (high sodium levels) can cause seizures and coma. Diuretics are often used to rid the body of excess sodium and fluid, but hyponatremia can occur with too much diuretic use.

Potassium (K^+) carries a positive charge and is found mainly inside the cell (intracellular) during resting conditions. The flow of potassium out of a cell and back into it again is also a requirement for essential biochemical and biomechanical reactions. The kidney is responsible for maintenance of plasma potassium levels, and high potassium levels (*hyperkalemia*) can occur with renal impairment. Another cause of hyperkalemia is *metabolic acidosis*, where intracellular potassium moves outside the cell as a response to the acidosis (see discussion on metabolic acidosis later in this section). *Hypokalemia* (low blood levels) can result from severe vomiting and diarrhea, or inadequate dietary potassium. Hypokalemia can cause cardiac irritability and if severe enough can induce life-threatening arrhythmias such as *ventricular tachycardia* and *ventricular fibrillation* (see Chapters 10 and 11). On the other hand, *cardiac arrest* (the stopping of the heart) can occur if potassium levels become too high. Thiazide and loop diuretics can cause hypokalemia. Triamterene, amiloride, and spironolactone are examples of diuretics that are potassium sparing and can result in hyperkalemia.

> **RED HERRING ALERT:** Red blood cells are a rich source of intracellular potassium, and if left too long before processing, the cells can rupture (hemolyze) and release potassium into the plasma. This can result in a spuriously high potassium value (false result) that may mislead one into thinking the patient is at risk of going into cardiac arrest. If the patient has normal creatinine and BUN values (normal renal function), and no evidence of metabolic acidosis, hemolysis due to a lab processing error is a likely culprit.

Chloride (Cl^-) is an electrolyte that carries a negative charge and is mainly found outside the cell in the extracellular space. Chloride is involved in water and acid-base balance. The kidneys control chloride levels. Conditions sometimes associated with hypochloremia (low chloride levels) include loss of fluids (from prolonged vomiting, diarrhea, and sweating) and diuretic abuse, especially with loop diuretics.

Some causes of hyperchloremia (elevated chloride levels) include a certain type of renal disease referred to as *renal tubular acidosis*, diarrhea resulting in the loss of bicarbonate, and the use of carbonic anhydrase inhibitor diuretics.

Bicarbonate (HCO_3^-) is an electrolyte with a negative charge. It plays a unique role as an essential buffer in maintaining *acid-base balance*. Acid-base balance refers to the levels of acidity or alkalinity of the blood, and the correct balance necessary for survival. The *pH* is a measure of how acidic or basic (alkaline) a solution is. A pH of 7.0 is considered the neutral point on the pH scale. The pH is inversely proportional to how acidic a solution is. The lower the pH, the more acidic a solution is and vice versa. A pH of between 7.35 and 7.45 is considered normal. Mechanisms are in place in the body to ensure pH maintenance in the normal range. One of these mechanisms is the presence of buffers such as bicarbonate, which helps to raise the pH in conditions where the pH is

decreased and lowers the pH if it is too high. Another mechanism to maintain pH is by controlling the respiratory (breathing) rate. CO_2 acts like an acid. High CO_2 levels are associated with a low pH, and low CO_2 levels can result in a high pH. In conditions where the pH is low, the respiratory rate increases and more CO_2 is eliminated by way of the lungs. CO_2 levels then go down, thereby increasing the pH. In conditions where the pH is high, slower breathing occurs, raising CO_2 levels and decreasing the pH. If buffers and respiratory mechanisms fail or are overwhelmed, *metabolic acidosis* (low blood pH) or *metabolic alkalosis* (high blood pH) can occur. Examples of conditions causing metabolic acidosis are *shock* (inadequate blood flow to vital organs) and *diabetic ketoacidosis*. Severe vomiting is an example of a condition that can result in metabolic alkalosis. In either severe acidosis or severe alkalosis, the enzymes required for the many biochemical and biomechanical reactions necessary to support life cannot function maximally. Death will result if the underlying conditions are not promptly and adequately treated and the pH corrected.

Calcium exists in 2 forms in the body. About 50% is bound to protein (albumin), and the rest is unbound and in ionized form (it has a positive charge–Ca^{2+}). In low protein states, e.g., the nephrotic syndrome, malnutrition, and liver disease, albumin and consequently protein bound calcium are reduced. Calcium has an inverse relationship to inorganic phosphorous; the higher the inorganic phosphorous levels, the lower the calcium values and vice versa. Calcium is involved in many different bodily functions that range from being the main component of bones and teeth to blood coagulation (clot formation), heart and muscle contraction, and nerve conduction. Low levels of calcium (*hypocalcemia*) are associated with *tetany* (sustained muscle contraction) and convulsions (seizures); and high levels (*hypercalcemia*) may result in coma, cardiac toxicity, and arrhythmias. Thiazide diuretics inhibit calcium excretion by the kidneys while loop diuretics (e.g., furosemide) have the opposite effect and enhance excretion.

The majority of inorganic phosphorus is found combined with calcium in bone. The remainder is involved in acid-base balance, various biochemical reactions such as glucose and lipid metabolism, and the storage and transfer of energy. In solution, it is ionized (carries a negative charge–PO_4^{3-}). As mentioned previously, inorganic phosphorus levels are inversely related to calcium levels. Increased inorganic phosphorus levels occur in renal insufficiency.

Uric acid is a breakdown product of *purines* (building blocks of DNA and RNA). Purines are found in many foods, especially organ meats (e.g., kidney, liver), certain fish such as sardines and salmon, and yeast (used in beer and bread making). The kidneys remove most of the uric acid from the body; the rest leaves the body via the stool. Uric acid levels increase whenever there is rapid production and destruction of cells such as in leukemia (cancer of the WBCs); excessive tissue breakdown (catabolism); diets rich in purines and protein; or in renal impairment. Increased blood uric acid levels also occur with thiazide and loop diuretic use. Uric acid crystals can form and deposit in the joints, causing *gout*, a painful inflammation of the joints. High levels of uric acid in the urine (*hyperuricosuria*) can also result in kidney stones (*nephrolithiasis*).

Creatine kinase is an enzyme that is found in cardiac and skeletal muscle. Elevated levels may indicate skeletal muscle injury, cardiac injury, or a myocardial infarction (heart attack). Some drugs, for example cocaine and HMG-CoA reductase inhibitors (statins), can cause *rhabdomyolysis*. Rhabdomyolysis is a condition that occurs with skeletal muscle injury. Creatine kinase leaks out of the injured cell into the blood, resulting in high plasma creatine kinase levels. In some severe cases, *myoglobin* (a protein similar to hemoglobin that binds O_2) also leaks out of the muscle cell. Myoglobin can injure the kidneys and cause renal failure.

Lipid Profile

The lipid profile usually includes: *cholesterol, high-density lipoprotein cholesterol, low-density lipoprotein cholesterol,* and *triglycerides*. An increase in *cardio- and cerebrovascular risk* (risk of heart attacks and strokes, respectively) is associated with abnormal lipid levels.

Cholesterol is found in animal fats and oils. It is widely distributed throughout the body and is an essential component of cell membranes. Cholesterol is also found in bile acids, sex and other hormones, and myelin sheaths (the envelope covering of nerve fibers). Hereditary factors and diet influence blood levels. Cholesterol is not soluble in the blood and is transported in the body as either high-density lipoprotein ("good") cholesterol, or low-density lipoprotein ("bad") cholesterol. Elevated levels of cholesterol and low-density lipoprotein cholesterol are associated with an increased risk of cardio- and cerebrovascular disease, while high-density lipoprotein cholesterol is associated with a decreased risk. Blood samples should be obtained during fasting conditions because eating can affect test results.

Triglycerides are the chemical form of fat found in foods and fat stored in the body. High levels are associated with an increased risk of coronary artery disease.

Urinalysis

Urinalysis refers to the examination of the urine. Urine abnormalities provide clues to both renal and nonrenal problems. The urine is examined for specific gravity, pH, protein, blood, glucose, ketones, and bilirubin. It is then centrifuged, and the sediment (the solid part found in the bottom of the centrifuging tube) is examined under the microscope for RBCs and WBCs, casts, crystals, and bacteria. The presence of blood in the urine is determined by both a chemical test and microscopically.

Specific gravity is a measurement of the concentration of particles in the urine. The more particles, the more concentrated the urine and the higher the specific gravity. Specific gravity is also an indicator of the kidney's ability to concentrate urine by reabsorbing water. During dehydration, the healthy kidney will reabsorb water, limiting the volume of water excreted and thereby increasing the urine concentration and specific gravity.

The urine pH measures how acidic or basic (alkaline) the urine is, and it is influenced by certain foods. For instance, a diet rich in citrus fruits, legumes, and vegetables is associated with urine that is alkaline, while acidic urine is more likely found in nonvegetarian diets. Control of the urine pH is important in the management of urinary tract infections, kidney stones, and drug treatment. Bacteria responsible for urinary tract infections make the urine more alkaline by making ammonia and other alkaline waste products. Uric acid, cystine, and calcium oxalate stones precipitate in acidic urine, while alkaline urine increases the risk of calcium phosphate, calcium carbonate, and magnesium phosphate stones. Certain antibiotics such as streptomycin, kanamycin, and neomycin are more effective in the treatment of urinary tract infections if the urine is alkaline.

Blood in the urine (either measured chemically or microscopically) may be due to many different conditions including kidney trauma, kidney stones, genitourinary system malignancy, infection, or coagulation disorders.

Bile indicates potential hepatocellular disease or obstructive biliary disease.

Generally there should be no *glucose* in the urine (*glucosuria*). In diabetes mellitus, high levels of blood glucose overwhelm the kidneys' ability to reabsorb glucose, and this

RED HERRING ALERT: One of the most common reasons for *hematuria* (blood in the urine) in women of childbearing potential is menstruation. The blood in this case is not from the urinary tract but from the reproductive system. Due to the anatomical closeness of these 2 systems in females, menstrual blood can easily contaminate urine during the collection of a urine sample. Menstrual status should be checked in a woman of childbearing potential, anytime blood in the urine is reported.

excess *spills* (is excreted) into the urine. Urine glucose is inversely related to glucose control in diabetics; the higher levels of glucose in the urine, the less diabetic control.

The healthy kidney, as discussed previously, prevents the passage of *protein* from the blood to the urine and little to no protein should be found in urine. *Proteinuria* (protein in urine) or microproteinuria (very small amounts of protein in the urine) can be seen in kidney disease, such as the nephrotic syndrome, where large amounts of protein are excreted in the urine, resulting in low plasma levels. Although proteinuria is usually seen in renal disease, proteinuria can also occur with fever and exercise.

Ketones result from the metabolism of fatty acid and fats. In diabetics where glucose utilization is impaired, more fatty acids and fats are metabolized and ketone levels increase. Ketones are also found during starvation and with high-fat, low-carbohydrate diets.

The urine sediment where bacteria, white and red blood cells, casts, and crystals are found (if present) provides further clues to renal and nonrenal problems.

A properly obtained urine specimen contains no bacteria, unless the patient has a urinary tract infection. The presence of bacteria with no evidence of infection indicates a contaminated urine specimen.

The presence of large numbers of WBCs is usually indicative of a urinary tract infection, although the presence of WBCs can be due to other causes such as renal disease. Evidence of bleeding or RBCs in the urine was discussed previously.

Casts are cells or other material that are found in the urine sediment that are clumped together and have the shape of the renal tubule (the tubular structure found in the kidney). Casts include RBC casts, WBC casts, epithelial casts, waxy or broad casts, hyaline casts, and granular casts. The presence of up to 2 hyaline or granular casts per high-powered field is considered normal; anything more or the presence of other casts usually signifies kidney problems.

The presence of crystals may cause no problems or increase the risk of kidney stone formations.

■ Laboratory Clues

Some laboratory tests, as previously discussed in this chapter, can measure the function of more than 1 organ system. Table 9-2 is a summary of the *clues* that can help determine the source of the lab abnormality.

Table 9-2	**Other Laboratory Clues**	
Laboratory Finding	**Potential Etiology for Abnormal Finding**	**Clues**
Elevated ALP	Liver disease, bone disease	Likely bone-related if other liver function tests are normal.
Elevated AST value	Liver disease, heart disease, muscle disease	Likely due to a muscle/cardiac disorder if ALT is normal.
Low albumin/Low total protein	Liver disease, kidney disease, malnutrition	Likely kidney-related if creatinine, BUN, and urine protein are increased.
Increased bilirubin	Liver disease, increased destruction of red blood cells (hemolysis), gallbladder disease	Likely due to hemolysis if Hb and Hct are decreased, indirect bilirubin levels are elevated, and other liver function tests are normal.

References

1. Fischbach FT, Dunning MB. *A Manual of Laboratory & Diagnostic Tests*. 8th ed. Philadelphia, PA: Lippincott; 2009.

2. Sacher RA, McPherson RA. *Widman's Clinical Interpretation of Laboratory Tests*. 11th ed. Philadelphia, PA: F. A. Davis Company; 2000.

3. Goldman L, Ausiello DA, Arend W, et al. *Cecil Medicine: Expert Consult-Online and Print (Cecil Textbook of Medicine)*. Philadelphia, PA: Saunders; 2008.

4. Fauci AS, Kasper DL, Longo DL, et al. *Harrison's Principles of Internal Medicine*. 17th ed. New York, NY: McGraw-Hill Professional; 2008.

5. eMedicine. http://emedicine.medscape.com/. Accessed March 15, 2010.

6. WebMD. http://www.webmd.com. Accessed March 15, 2010.

7. Mayo Clinic Diseases and Conditions http://www.mayoclinic.com/health/DiseasesIndex/DiseasesIndex. Accessed March 15, 2010.

8. Andrès E, Noel E, Goichot B. Metformin-associated vitamin B12 deficiency. *Arch Intern Med*. 2002; 162:2251–2252.

9. *Guidance for Industry Drug-Induced Liver Injury: Premarketing Clinical Evaluation*. Washington, DC: US Department of Health and Human Services, Food and Drug Administration, Center for Drug Evaluation and Research (CDER) Center for Biologics Evaluation and Research (CBER); July 2009. http://www.fda.gov/downloads/Drugs/GuidanceComplianceRegulatoryInformation/Guidances/UCM174090.pdf. Accessed March 15, 2010.

12-Lead Electrocardiograms— What Is Measured; What It Means

An electrocardiogram (ECG, or EKG) is a graphic display of the *electrical* events involved in the cardiac cycle. Heart rate, heart rhythm, and other important information regarding heart function can be determined from the ECG. The ECG can be diagnostic in many cardiac conditions including myocardial infarction (heart attack); arrhythmias (atrial fibrillation, torsades de pointes, ventricular fibrillation, and other important arrhythmias); and conduction abnormalities such as 3rd-degree atrioventricular heart block (complete heart block), a condition where electrical impulses necessary in stimulating the heart muscles to contract are blocked, resulting in the need for a pacemaker.

A basic knowledge of what ECG parameters are and what they measure is necessary to understand the best way to analyze and interpret ECG findings.

➡ **NOTE:** This chapter is written for individuals with little or no clinical training. General references are provided for those interested in learning more about the topic and are organized for those with[1-3] and without[4-6] clinical experience.

■ Basic ECG Concepts

An electrical current exists within our bodies due to the flow of electrolytes (particles that have either a positive or negative charge) in and out of the various cells within our bodies. The change in electrolyte flow from the resting state is referred to as *depolarization*. *Repolarization* is the process where electrolyte flow is reversed and the cell is returned to its resting state. Examples of electrolytes include sodium, potassium, calcium, and chloride and were discussed in Chapter 9.

The function of the heart (which is a muscle) is to pump blood throughout the body. To accomplish this, the heart is made up of *myocardial cells* that, when they contract, provide the basic pump action of the heart. Before the mechanical event of contraction occurs, the myocardial cells receive an electrical impulse that results in depolarization of the myocardial cell. This electrical process of depolarization stimulates the myocardial cells to contract. Depolarization is followed by repolarization, or a return to the resting state of the myocardial cell. Contraction of the myocardial cells requires exquisite coordination among the millions of myocardial cells so they all contract in unison. *Atrial fibrillation (AF)* and *ventricular fibrillation (VF)* are examples of arrhythmias where individual myocardial cells or groups of myocardial cells in the atria and ventricles, respectively, contract haphazardly rather than together, giving the appearance of a *bag of worms*. This results in inadequate cardiac contraction and can have dire consequences including sudden death in the case of VF. The coordinated contraction of myocardial cells is dependent on 2 other types of specialized cardiac cells—the *pacemaker* and *conducting cells.*

Pacemaker cells are specialized cells that spontaneously generate an electrical impulse. This impulse then travels along special pathways made up of conducting cells that deliver the impulse from the pacemaker cells to the rest of the cells of the heart. The heart actually has several different pacemaker cells located throughout the heart. The dominant pacemaker of the heart is called the *sinoatrial node (SA node)* and normally discharges at a rate of 60 to 100 impulses per minute. *Normal sinus rhythm* refers to the normal heart rhythm controlled by the SA node. The process of impulse generation from the pacemaker cells and conduction of this impulse along the conducting pathways allows the uniform delivery of electrical impulses to the myocardial cells, ensuring a coordinated contraction and maximal pumping of the heart.

■ The Basic ECG

The ECG traces the electrical impulse from the SA node through contraction and relaxation of the ventricles (the major pumps) of the heart. Figure 10-1 shows an example of 3 leads from a normal 12-lead ECG.

The 12-lead ECG captures the electrical activity from different parts of the body and provides 12 different views of the electrical activity (the electrical vectors) of the heart. The ECG is obtained by placing leads on each limb and on 6 different chest surface (precordial) positions over the

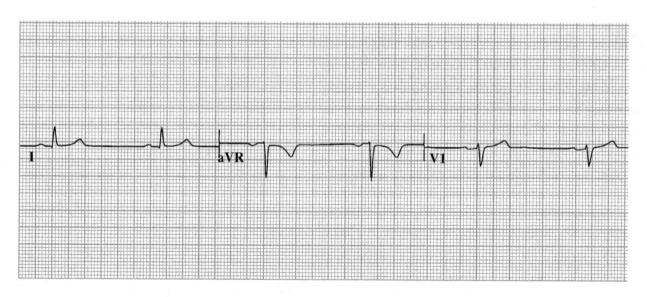

Figure 10-1 Normal Electrocardiogram*

* This shows 3 leads from a normal 12-lead ECG of a 32-year-old male. The heart rate is 45 bpm. Although the normal range for heart rate is 60–100 bpm, lower heart rates are normal (and expected) in healthy males who exercise regularly.
Source: O'keefe JH, Hammill SC, Freed MS, Pogwizd SM. *The Complete Guide to ECGs.* 3rd ed. Sudbury; MA: Jones and Bartlett; 2008.

heart. The limb leads, so called because they measure the impulses from the leads on the arms and legs, are referred to as leads *I, II, III, aVR, aVL,* and *aVF*. The 6 chest leads are referred to as *V1* through *V6*, with V1 being the 1st chest lead on the subject's right side of the sternum (breast bone) and V6 being the last lead located on the left side of the chest at the midaxillary line (midpoint line of the armpit). ECG paper (or its computer equivalent) is composed of 1-mm squares or boxes. Each 1-mm square on the horizontal axis measures a unit of time; i.e., 1 mm = 0.04 second or 40 milliseconds, when the ECG paper moves at a rate of 25 mm/second. Each 1 mm box on the vertical axis represents 0.1 millivolt and measures the height (voltage) of the waveform. Increased voltage waveforms (that is, higher spikes on the ECG) are seen when the atria or ventricles hypertrophy (increase in size) (for example, left ventricular hypertrophy that results from sustained hypertension). Low-voltage waveforms may be observed with *cardiomyopathies* (disorders of the heart muscle), where muscle tissue is abnormal, damaged, or destroyed, e.g., cardiac toxicity associated with doxorubicin use. The *isoelectric line* refers to the flat line of the ECG and represents the baseline, or 0-voltage point. The ECG shown in Figure 10-1 is composed of a number of waveforms and lines (intervals) connecting each waveform. Waveforms above and below the isoelectric line are referred to as positive and negative waveforms, respectively. The ECG waveforms and intervals are shown in Figure 10-2.

The following is a brief description of what these various waveforms and intervals represent:

- **P wave**—depolarization of the atria.
- **PR interval**—the time it takes for the impulse to go from the SA node to the ventricles.

First-degree heart block is defined as a PR interval of > 210 milliseconds (ms).

- **QRS complex**—depolarization of the ventricle.
- **T wave**—repolarization of the ventricles.
- **ST segment**—time from the end of ventricular depolarization to the end of ventricular repolarization.
- **QT/QTc interval**—time from depolarization of the ventricle to the end of repolarization of the ventricle. The QT interval is inversely related to heart rate (i.e., the QT interval is longer at slower heart rates and shorter with faster heart rates). For this reason the QT interval has to be corrected for heart rate differences—this is referred to as the *QTc*. Various formulas are used to calculate the QTc—2 of the more popular correction formulas used are Bazett and Fridericia.[7] Other factors can also affect the QT interval, for example, gender—females have longer QTc intervals than males.
- **U wave**—is a wave that follows the T wave. What causes the wave is not clear nor is the U wave always seen.

These waveforms and intervals parallel the path the electrical impulse takes from its start in the SA node to stimulation and relaxation of the ventricles. The electrical activity measured by the ECG precedes the mechanical event of contraction of the myocardial cells. Problems in the heart can be electrical and are usually easily picked up by the ECG or other more sophisticated electric measuring techniques.

Table 10-1 provides the normal ranges for ECG parameters.

With this information we can now interpret the ECG shown in Figure 10-1 by looking at the waveforms and counting ECG squares. Remember that each ECG square on the horizontal axis = 40 ms (5 squares = 200 ms) and each 25 mm = 1 second (s).

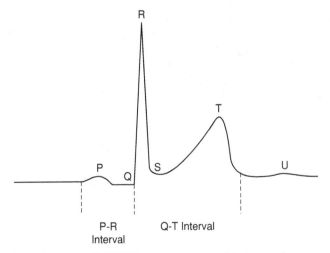

Figure 10-2 ECG Waveforms and Intervals

Table 10-1	ECG Parameters—Normal Ranges[2,8]
ECG Parameter	**Normal Range**
Heart rate	60–100 beats/min
PR interval	120–200 ms (0.12–0.20 s)
QRS complex	70–110 ms (0.07 to 0.11 s)
QTc (QT-corrected)	<430 ms (< 0.43 s) (Males)
	<450 ms (< 0.44 s) (Females)

- The heart rate is 45 beats per minute (bpm). This is calculated by counting the squares between 1 QRS complex and another (which is one heart beat). The distance between the 2 QRS complexes is approximately 33 mm or 33 squares. The heart rate is calculated as follows:

  $$HR = (25 \text{ mm/s})/(33 \text{ mm/beat}) = 0.76 \text{ beat/s};$$
  $$0.76 \text{ beat/s} \times 60 \text{ s/minute} = 45 \text{ bpm}$$

- The rhythm is sinus bradycardia (i.e., the impulse comes from the SA node because the P wave and PR interval are normal; and bradycardia because the heart rate is below 60 bpm).

  ➡ **NOTE:** The normal range for heart rate as shown in Table 10-1 is 60–100 bpm. Heart rates below this range are normal (and expected) in healthy males who exercise regularly. Just as your muscles get stronger with weight lifting and training, the heart (also a muscle) becomes stronger with exercise. A different clinical picture would be seen in a frail 90-year-old female with a heart rate of 45 bpm—the patient would likely be dizzy, hypotensive, or even unconscious.

- The PR interval is 200 ms (5 squares).
- The QRS complex is 70 ms (< 2 squares).
- The QT interval is 400 ms (10 squares). Using the Fridericia correction formula,[7] QTc is 365 ms.

■ Drug-Induced ECG Changes

Drug-Induced QTc Prolongation

QTc prolongation is an electrical problem in the heart associated with an increased risk of developing life-threatening ventricular arrhythmias that can result in sudden death. That is, the electrical disturbance can lead to a mechanical pumping problem and death. The longer the QTc prolongation, the greater the risk. Many drugs have been removed from the market or "killed" in development because they cause QTc prolongation. Examples of drugs that prolong the QTc interval include Class Ia and III antiarrhythmics, cisapride, and terfenadine. Both terfenadine and cisapride were withdrawn from the market due to QTc prolongation.[9]

Figures 10-3 and 10-4 show ECG tracings of the life-threatening ventricular arrhythmias torsades de point (TdP) and VF, respectively. These ECG patterns are very different from those of the normal ECG seen in Figure 10-1.

In Figure 10-3, the waves (which are abnormal QRS complexes) vary in amplitude, which is characteristic of TdP.

No discernible ECG pattern is seen in Figure 10-4, just chaotic and nonuniform waves, which is characteristic of VF.

TdP and VF are the most dire rhythm disturbances. They are medical emergencies that can rapidly (within minutes) lead to death if not immediately treated. For these reasons, the potential for QTc prolongation is of prime concern in the development of a new drug or in

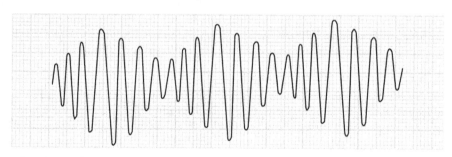

Figure 10-3 Torsades De Pointes
Source: Holler T. Cardiology Essentials. Sudbury, MA: Jones and Bartlett; 2008.

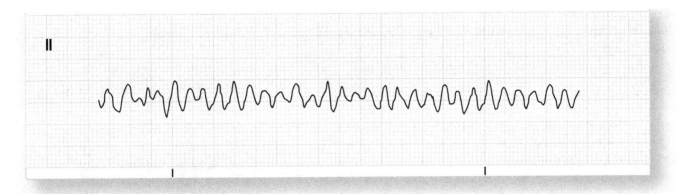

Figure 10-4 Ventricular Fibrillation
Source: From *Arrhythmia Recognition: The Art of Interpretation*, courtesy of Thomas B. Garcia, MD.

the use of an older drug in susceptible patients. There are specific nonclinical and clinical evaluations that must be done prior to drug approval, and these are summarized in *The Non-Clinical Evaluation of the Potential for Delayed Ventricular Repolarization (QT Interval Prolongation) by Human Pharmaceuticals S7B*[10] and *The Clinical Evaluation of QT/QTc Interval Prolongation and Proarrhythmic Potential for Non-Antiarrhythmic Drugs E14*[7] respectively. A specific study evaluating QT/QTc prolongation in humans, known as the *thorough QT/QTc study*, is often a requirement for drug approval. Whether or not this study should be done is based on several factors that include:

- Findings from nonclinical evaluations suggesting a risk for QT prolongation
- Whether it is feasible to do such a study in humans
- Whether a drug is a new chemical entity or part of a class of drugs that is known to have little to no potential for QT/QTc prolongation

If a thorough QT/QTc study is not done or the results of such a study are positive for QT/QTc prolongation, more extensive ECG and other cardiac evaluations are required during the later stages of clinical development. For maximal detection of QT prolongation, ECGs should be obtained during anticipated peak drug concentrations because QT/QTc changes may be dose related. If ECGs are obtained only during trough or low concentrations of the drug, a QT/QTc effect can be missed or underestimated.

Other Drug-Induced ECG Changes

Although QTc prolongation is of critical importance, other drug-related ECG changes can also indicate clinically important risks and must also be evaluated. Table 10-2 provides some examples.

AF is another clinically important arrhythmia that can be drug-induced. Figure 10-5 shows AF, the chaotic (fibrillatory) pattern that is often hard to see and not discernible in the figure is in contrast to the orderly and uniform appearance of the P waves seen in Figure 10-1. The intervals between one QRS complex and the next also vary in AF (Figure 10-5) compared to the regularity seen in Figure 10-1. Fibrillation of the atria increases the risk of formation and release of emboli (clots in the blood). This can result in stroke. AF can also occur at very rapid rates, and this can induce heart failure or precipitate myocardial ischemia (decreased blood flow to the heart) and angina (cardiac chest pain) in patients with heart disease.[12] For these reasons, drug-induced AF is an important finding.

References

1. Libby P, Bonow RO, Mann DL, Zipes DP. *Braunwald's Heart Disease: A Textbook of Cardiovascular Medicine.* 8th ed. Philadelphia, PA: Saunders 2007.

2. Wagner GS. *Marriott's Practical Electrocardiography.* 11th ed. Philadelphia, PA: Lippincott Williams & Wilkins; 2008.

3. eMedicine. http://emedicine.medscape.com/. Accessed March 15, 2010.

4. American Heart Association. http://www.americanheart.org/presenter.jhtml?identifier=10000052. Accessed March 15, 2010.

5. WebMD. http://www.webmd.com. Accessed March 15, 2010.

6. Mayo Clinic Diseases and Conditions. http://www.mayoclinic.com/health/DiseasesIndex/DiseasesIndex. Accessed March 15, 2010.

Table 10-2 Examples of Drug-Related ECG Abnormalities and Potential Clinical Consequences [1,11,12]

ECG Finding	Drugs[a]	Potential Clinical Consequences
Sinus bradycardia (a slowing of the heart rate to < 60 bpm)	Beta blockers, calcium channel blockers	Dizziness; hypotension; syncope
Sinus tachycardia (a speeding up of the heart rate above 100 bpm)	Sympathomimetics (stimulants)	Induce/worsen myocardial ischemia/angina
Complete heart block	Beta blockers, calcium channel blockers	Dizziness; hypotension; syncope; cardiac arrest
Prolonged QT/QTc	Class Ia and III antiarrhythmics; cisapride; long-acting antihistamines and concomitant use of other drugs affecting the P450 system	Syncope, TdP, VF, and sudden death
Atrial fibrillation	Sympathomimetics; cholinergics; anticholinergics, others	Risk of embolism and stroke; induce/worsen congestive heart failure/angina
Flattening or inversion of the T wave (negative T wave); increased prominence of the U wave; QTc prolongation; increased P wave; prolonged PR interval; premature ventricular contractions (extra, unexpected heart beats)/ventricular arrhythmias	Loop and thiazide diuretics causing hypokalemia (low potassium levels)	Risk of VT/VF and sudden death
Widened QRS complex ("Sine" wave), peaked T waves, prolongation of the PR interval and flattening/loss of the P wave	Potassium-sparing diuretics; ACE inhibitors causing hyperkalemia (high potassium values)	Increased risk of VF and cardiac arrest

[a] Partial list of drugs

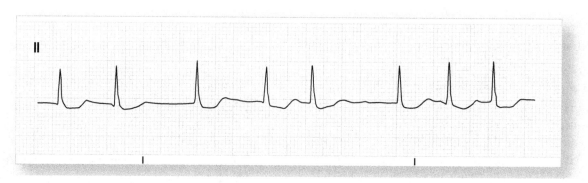

Figure 10-5 Atrial Fibrillation
Source: From Arrhythmia Recognition: The Art of Inter pretation, courtesy of Thomas B. Garcia, MD.

7. International Conference on Harmonisation of Technical Requirements for Registration of Pharmaceuticals for Human Use. *The Clinical Evaluation of QT/QTc Interval Prolongation and Proarrhythmic Potential for Non-Antiarrhythmic Drugs E14*. Geneva, Switzerland: ICH Secretariat; May 2005. http://www.ich.org/cache/compo/276-254-1.html. Accessed March 15, 2010.

8. Committee for Proprietary Medicinal Products. *Points to Consider: The Assessment of the Potential for QT Interval Prolongation by Non-Cardiovascular Medicinal Products*. vol. CPMP 986/96. London: The European Agency for the Evaluation of Medicinal Products; 1997.

9. Yap YG, Camm AJ. Drug-induced QT prolongation and torsades de pointes. *Heart*. 2003; 89:1363–1372.

10. International Conference on Harmonisation of Technical Requirements for Registration of Pharmaceuticals for Human Use. *The Non-Clinical Evaluation of the Potential for Delayed Ventricular Repolarization (QT Interval Prolongation) by Human Pharmaceuticals S7B*. Geneva, Switzerland: ICH Secretariat; May 2005. http://www.ich.org/cache/compo/276-254-1.html. Accessed March 15, 2010.

11. Zeltser D, Justo D, Halkin A, et al. Drug-induced atrioventricular block: prognosis after discontinuation of the culprit drug. *J Am Coll Cardiol*. 2004;44:105–108.

12. Van der Hooft CS, Heeringa J, Van Herpen G, Kors JA, Kingma JH, Stricker BH. Drug-induced atrial fibrillation. *J Am Coll Cardiol*. 2004; 44:2117–2124.

CHAPTER 11

Adverse Events That Should Be on Everyone's Radar Screen

In the world of risk determination, some adverse events (AEs) are "more equal" than others and should always be on everyone's radar screen. These events are historically linked to drug use and are associated with serious outcomes. Various regulatory agencies and pharmaceutical companies have prepared lists of such events. The majority of AEs presented in this chapter are from the Food and Drug Administration's (FDA) proposed list of always reportable AEs/reactions.[1] A word of caution: this group of AEs is not all encompassing but serves as a good start, providing a foundation upon which to build.

AEs are presented alphabetically by Medical Dictionary for Regulatory Activities system organ class.

➡ **NOTE:** This chapter is written for individuals with little or no clinical training. General

references are provided for those interested in learning more about the topic and are organized for those with [2–7] and without [8–11] clinical experience.

■ Blood and Lymphatic System Disorders

Agranulocytosis

Agranulocytosis is a condition in which there is a dangerously low level of white blood cells, referred to as granulocytes in the peripheral blood. These white blood cells have granules that contain substances that can kill bacteria when released. There are three types of granulocytes: neutrophils, basophils and eosinophils, which are discussed in Chapter 9. Technically, some would consider agranulocytosis to mean no granulocytes at all in the peripheral blood. This is unusual; in most cases there are some present. Some will define agranulocytosis as an absolute neutrophil count of fewer than 100 cells/mm^3.

Agranulocytosis is usually due to drugs including gold (used to treat arthritis but used less often now), some antiepileptics and antithyroid drugs (carbimazole and methimazole), penicillin, chloramphenicol, cotrimoxazole), some cancer drugs, indomethacin, naproxen, phenylbutazone, and clozapine. Many other drugs are suspected of rarely producing this condition. Other causes include rare genetic disorders, severe infections, and certain autoimmune diseases. Whenever agranulocytosis is seen, a drug etiology should be high on the list.

Agranulocytosis is diagnosed by doing a complete blood count test, which includes an automated count of the cells in the blood. This should be followed by a microscopic review of a stained (cell stains that are used to enhance the distinguishing features of the different white blood cells) blood smear by a trained medical person.

A low granulocyte count by itself usually does not produce symptoms. However, a low count predisposes the patient to infections, and the patient may present with a severe infection. Treatment usually involves removing the offending drug and allowing the cell count to rise. If an infection is present, it should be treated. Some high-risk patients should have prophylactic treatment for infections. Patients may also be treated with a granulocyte colony-stimulating factor to increase the production of granulocytes. White cell transfusions are rarely used.

Aplastic Anemia

Aplastic anemia is a very serious condition in which the bone marrow fails to produce blood cells, including red blood cells; white blood cells, primarily neutrophils; and platelets. Production in all 3 cell lines is decreased. This is usually manifested in the peripheral blood. A complete blood count (and smear) will show low counts of these 3 cell lines in most cases. Red blood cells are long lived (~90 days), so it will take some time before the production failure is seen in the blood count. Platelets and white cells, however, have much shorter lives and a low count will be seen quickly after onset of aplastic anemia. The definitive diagnosis requires a bone marrow biopsy to verify lack of production.

Although other causes are known, such as certain genetic and autoimmune diseases, toxins (benzene), malignancy and radiation, the most common cause of aplastic anemia is drug toxicity. Many drugs have been reported to do this including chloramphenicol (one of the first to do this), carbamazepine, gold, felbamate, phenytoin, quinine, and phenylbutazone.

The patient with aplastic anemia will present with 1 or more problems related to each cell line. For red blood cells, anemia will be seen (weakness, pallor, dyspnea, etc.). For low platelets, the patient may present with petechiae (minute hemorrhagic spots on the skin), ecchymosis (bruising), and bleeding. For low white cells, he or she might present with infection.

Treatment includes removing the offending agent in the hopes of a recovery, supportive care such as blood transfusions during the acute crisis, treatment of secondary infection, and if necessary immunosuppressive drugs and bone marrow transplantation.

■ Cardiac Disorders

Ventricular Fibrillation

Ventricular fibrillation (VF) is one of the most dangerous of the abnormal rhythms that can occur in the heart. It is characterized by the uncoordinated contraction of the muscle cells in the ventricles of the heart. This lack of coordinated muscle movement produces a situation in which the heart quivers (likened to a bowl of jelly) rather than contracting and pumping the blood out. Although there can be some nonspecific symptoms before VF actually occurs, such as dyspnea, fatigue, palpitations, and even syncope (fainting), once the fibrillation starts the patient rapidly becomes unconscious, stops breathing, and has no pulse. The electrocardiogram (ECG) shows a classic and usually diagnostic pattern. VF should not be confused with atrial fibrillation (AF), which is an entirely different rhythm disturbance (ECG tracings of VF and AF are shown in Chapter 10).

The immediate mechanism underlying VF usually relates to abnormalities in the ions (potassium, sodium, calcium) and/or the channels in the heart that bring them in and out of cells, which produce electrical abnormalities in the heart, preventing the appropriate signal to trigger coordinated pumping of the blood. The cardiac muscle (myocardial) cells are particularly sensitive to low oxygen levels and hypokalemia (low potassium). Causes of hypokalemia include the overzealous use of diuretics. Low oxygen levels in the heart can be secondary to respiratory failure, myocardial infarctions (heart attacks), and many other conditions. Low levels of potassium and/or oxygen make the myocardial cells very irritable, causing individual or groups of myocardial cells to start contracting on their own. This uncoordinated contraction of individual or groups of myocardial cells results in little to no blood being pumped from the heart.

There are many other causes of VF, including atherosclerosis, myocarditis (inflammation of the myocardium), cardiomyopathy (disease of the cardiac muscle), conduction diseases such as Wolff-Parkinson-White syndrome, metabolic problems, sepsis, electrical shock, lung disease, seizures, strokes, familial diseases (congenital long QT syndrome), and drugs. Drugs implicated in causing VF include various belladonna preparations, calcium products, and quinidine. In general, a heart that already has significant disease may be more prone to the development of VF compared to a normal heart.

VF is a medical emergency. Treatment is immediate defibrillation (electrical shock to the chest), as well as administration of certain antiarrhythmic medications, and correction of the underlying cause (e.g., metabolic problems). Cardiopulmonary resuscitation may be required. Immediate survival depends upon the ability to treat the patient on the spot. Communities with rapid emergency medical services and a trained general population have the most success. Even when a normal rhythm is reestablished quickly, long-term survival is often quite low due to the underlying problem that caused VF in the first place.

Ventricular Tachycardia and Torsades de Pointes

Ventricular tachycardia (VT) is a potentially life-threatening arrhythmia that starts in the ventricle. It is characterized by a rapid ventricular rate (> 100–120 beats per minute). Because the arrhythmia starts in the ventricles (lower heart chambers) and not in the atria (upper heart chambers), the ventricles do not receive blood from the atria in a coordinated way. The lack of blood from the atria and the rapid ventricular rate result in a significant decrease in the amount of blood the ventricle receives and can pump out. This results in lack of delivery of oxygen and other nutrients to the heart, brain, lungs, and other vital organs. If not treated, VT can deteriorate into VF and sudden death (see previous section). VT is divided into two types—*monomorphic* and *polymorphic*. Polymorphic VT is also referred to as *torsades de pointes* (*TdP*), French for *twisting of the points* because of its spiral-like appearance (an ECG tracing of TdP is shown in Chapter 10). Monomorphic VT (each ventricular waveform looks the same) usually occurs in patients with structurally abnormal hearts, e.g., scars that are left from previous myocardial infarctions. Scars in the myocardium cannot transmit electrical impulses, so the pathway of the impulse required for normal ventricular contraction is not taken, and the normal ventricular activation sequence is disrupted. In polymorphic VT (each ventricular waveform looks different), the problem is typically due to a prolonged QT interval (an ECG measurement discussed in Chapter 10). Prolonged QT intervals can be congenital (e.g., long QT syndrome) or acquired.

Causes of acquired QT are many and include metabolic problems (low magnesium, potassium, calcium), acidosis, hypoxia (low oxygen), heart failure, hypothermia (low temperature), and subarachnoid (brain) hemorrhage. Drugs are also a major precipitating factor or cause of TdP and include some antibiotics (certain macrolides and fluoroquinolones, but not all), especially if taken with certain other drugs, including methadone, lithium, tricyclics, phenothiazines, cisapride, and pimozide. A nonsedating antihistamine, terfenadine, quite surprisingly, produced prolonged QT intervals especially when it was taken along with other drugs (e.g., erythromycin, ketoconazole) that competed with the same enzymes necessary for terfenadine's metabolism. This resulted in higher terfenadine blood levels, greater QT prolongation, and a higher incidence of TdP and sudden death. These findings led to the removal of terfenadine and other similar drugs from the market. QT interval information is now a usual requirement for drug approval. TdP and prolonged QT intervals are a red flag that can represent a significant drug safety issue and must not be ignored.

VT is a medical emergency and requires cardioversion (an electric current to the heart) and intravenous antiarrhythmia treatment.

■ Congenital, Familial, and Genetic Disorders

Congenital Anomalies

Congenital anomalies are also called birth defects. The developing embryo/fetus is particularly susceptible to drugs and other toxic substances. According to the Centers for Disease Control and Prevention, about 3% of all babies born in the United States have a birth defect (though often minor).[12] The causes of many are unknown, though some known causes include familial transmission, smoking, alcohol use, and drugs (both legal and illicit). Most occur in the first 3 months (first trimester) of pregnancy, though they can occur in the later months, too. In the first trimester, organogenesis (formation of the various organ systems) is taking place. A defect during this time makes the baby particularly susceptible to significant anomalies. The birth defects associated with thalidomide are an unfortunate example of this. In the United States, European Union, and elsewhere, pregnancy registries are maintained by pharmaceutical companies and government agencies, some of which track all pregnancies (e.g., Sweden). Others track births or only abnormalities in births. Periodical examination of these registries looking for trends and clues to a possible previously unknown drug effect should be routine practice. If large numbers of pregnancies and/or anomalies are seen with a particular drug, a risk management plan should be put into place to minimize the risk of pregnancy during drug exposure.

Gastrointestinal Disorders

Pancreatitis

Pancreatitis is an inflammation of the pancreas. The pancreas is the organ that makes insulin and certain digestive enzymes. It can become inflamed due to various causes, including gallstones and other diseases of the bile ducts, excess alcohol ingestion, trauma, steroids, mumps, certain diseases of abnormal lipids, certain inherited diseases (e.g., porphyrias) and, in particular, drugs. By far the most common causes for pancreatitis include gallstones and alcohol. Many drugs implicated as causes of pancreatitis include, but are not limited to, the AIDS drugs didanosine and pentamidine; water pills (diuretics) including hydrochlorothiazide and furosemide given for high blood pressure; estrogen; steroids; and antibiotics such as sulfonamides and tetracycline. Drugs account for about 2% of all cases of pancreatitis.[13]

Pancreatitis may be acute, chronic, or in some classifications, subacute (in between chronic and acute) or relapsing. The major finding is abdominal pain radiating (shooting) to the back with nausea and vomiting. Other signs and symptoms may be surprisingly mild, such as abdominal tenderness, high or low blood pressure, and fever. If 1 of the severe complications, internal bleeding, occurs, then the clinical picture may turn into one of shock (low blood pressure, pallor, tachycardia, loss of consciousness, and even death). This is a medical emergency. Other complications include kidney failure (high blood urea nitrogen and creatinine), low blood count, low blood calcium and high blood glucose, infection of the pancreas, and, in chronic cases, pancreatic pseudocysts (balloon-like spheres filled with fluid). Diagnosis is made by the clinical picture as well as elevated serum amylase and/or lipase (2 enzymes made by the pancreas). Ultrasound or CT scan of the abdomen may also help confirm the diagnosis. Prognosis depends upon the severity of the disease on admission to the hospital and at 48 hours after treatment has begun.

Treatment is supportive and includes pain medications (usually morphine), fluids, electrolytes as needed, and no intake by mouth until the acute episode has subsided. Pancreatitis may recur or be chronic.

All cases of pancreatitis or elevated pancreatic enzymes (amylase and lipase) should raise the suspicions of a possible drug-related event.

General Disorders and Administration Site Conditions

Injection Site Reactions

Injection site reactions refer to pain, swelling, redness, and/or heat at the site of the injection of a medication. They can be seen with intravenous as well as intramuscular and subcutaneous (just below the skin) injections. These reactions are usually quite mild and resolve quickly. The presence of such reactions does not mean that the drug should be stopped, especially if it is for severe or chronic diseases (e.g., injections for hepatitis C or diabetes). In such cases, various maneuvers can be done to decrease the reaction, such as rotating the injection site, icing the area to be injected, and other techniques. If the reactions are severe, it may be necessary to switch to a different drug (e.g., a different insulin). Although the reaction is usually due to the drug product itself, it can also be due to the needle or tube (or lubricants, if any, on the needle or tube) or excipients ("theoretically" inert substances though some patients may actually have adverse reactions due to excipients) in the product. Although usually not severe, these injection site reactions should be noted and monitored.

Hepatobiliary Disorders

Acute Liver Failure

The liver is a large and complex organ with multiple functions in the body, including synthesis of various proteins (including those needed to make blood clot), production of bile for the digestion of fats, and the metabolism of various drugs into compounds that can be easily eliminated in the urine or stool. The liver can be harmed in multiple ways such as by drugs (including alcohol), viruses (hepatitis A, B, and C), bacteria, fungus, excessively high or low blood flow to it, cancer, and other diseases.

Acute liver failure is the rapid and often dramatic (days to a couple of weeks) deterioration of the liver's ability to function. The patient can very quickly develop progressive loss of appetite, weight loss, jaundice, abdominal swelling (due to the buildup of fluid called ascites), bleeding, confusion, coma, and death. The liver essentially ceases its functions, allowing toxins to build up in the body because they are no longer metabolized by the liver. Results of liver tests such as those for alanine aminotransferase (ALT), aspartate aminotransferase (AST), and total bilirubin levels are usually very abnormal. Results of coagulation (clotting) tests such as the activated partial thromboplastin time, prothrombin time, and the international normalized ratio are also likely to be abnormal, particularly in severe cases. Because the liver also produces protein, total protein and albumin values can also be abnormally low and, if so, may contribute to the development of ascites and edema elsewhere in the body. Scans may show a large (and later in the disease a shrinking and shriveling) liver. Physical examination may show pain and swelling of the abdomen and liver, bleeding in the skin or intestines, and confusion and stupor.

It is critically important to make a diagnosis of the cause of acute liver failure. Often it is not possible, but every effort should be made. Particular attention should be paid to drug history. This refers not only to prescribed (prescription) drugs but also to other drug products such as over-the-counter products, health foods, nutritional supplements, and herbals. Attention should also be paid to the sources of these products in order to get a clue as to whether there might be tampering, medication errors, counterfeiting, product quality issues, or other factors involved.

Liver Necrosis

Liver necrosis refers to the unnatural death of liver cells. Most cells in the body have natural life cycles and are programmed to die (apoptosis) and be replaced in the normal course of events. This is most visible in the skin, where the outer layer of skin cells flakes off (e.g., dandruff) and is replaced by new cells growing from the lower layers of the skin outward toward the surface. Necrosis is not natural death and is due to a cause that must be found. Acute liver failure always involves liver necrosis to some degree. However, liver necrosis may be minor in nature and does not necessarily lead to acute liver failure. Rather, it may be a self-limiting problem that resolves over time after the removal of the offending agent.

Actually, the liver has many different types of cells, but the ones referred to here are those called *hepatocytes*, which are the cells that metabolize the drugs and produce proteins and other chemicals needed for life.

The most direct way (the gold standard) to diagnose liver necrosis is obtaining actual tissue from the liver during surgery or by a biopsy. A pathologist then examines the cells microscopically, where necrosis can be seen. Because these are invasive, painful, and sometimes dangerous procedures in a diseased liver, they are not commonly done. Because coagulation factors can be abnormally low as a result of a diseased liver, a liver biopsy may lead to uncontrolled hemorrhage (bleeding) and death.

Instead, the usual methods to identify liver necrosis involve blood tests looking for elevations of bilirubin and certain enzymes; e.g., AST, ALT, alkaline phosphatase (ALP), and others, found in the liver and that escape into the blood from damaged liver cells. Not all elevations of enzymes are due to hepatocyte problems, because many of these enzymes are found in cells elsewhere (e.g., the heart, muscle, and bone). In addition, some elevations of these enzymes may be due to other liver problems not necessarily associated with hepatic necrosis, e.g., gallstones, (see Chapters 9 and 17).

RED HERRING ALERT: In drug-induced liver injury/liver necrosis, the hepatocyte, rather than other types of liver cells, is injured. ALT, AST, and bilirubin are typically elevated, but not ALP. If the ALP is elevated, it is usually only modestly elevated, e.g., $< 2 \times$ the upper limit of normal. If ALP, an enzyme found in both the liver and bone, is elevated $> 2 \times$ upper limit of normal, it usually points to a problem in the biliary (bile duct) system or bone. If ALP is elevated $> 2 \times$ upper limit of normal, think of something other than drug-induced liver injury/liver necrosis.

The drug safety message here is that whenever abnormal liver tests are seen in patients taking medications (again including over-the-counter drugs, health foods, nutritionals, etc.), a diagnosis of hepatic injury due to drug toxicity should always be considered.

Immune System Disorders

Anaphylaxis

Anaphylaxis is an acute, severe (sometimes fatal), immediate, usually allergic reaction to an external stimulus such as a food, drug, or bee sting. There are various types of anaphylaxis with somewhat different names (pseudoanaphylactic reaction, anaphylactoid reaction), which reflect the mechanism that produces the symptoms. However, the symptoms and treatments are largely identical no matter what the cause. Classically, this is a Type I hypersensitivity reaction, also referred to as an *immediate type hypersensitivity reaction*, which produces the rapid onset of symptoms due to the release of various immunologic products such as leukotrienes, histamine, and prostaglandins. These substances produce vasodilation (widening of blood vessels) and bronchoconstriction (narrowing of the breathing tubes). In classic anaphylaxis, the first exposure to the trigger (the offending agent) does not produce the reaction but rather sensitizes the individual. It is only on subsequent exposures that the anaphylactic reaction occurs. However, other mechanisms producing the variants of anaphylaxis may produce the reaction on first exposure. Major producers of anaphylaxis or variants of anaphylaxis include penicillin, cephalosporins, aspirin, nonsteroidal anti-inflammatory drugs (NSAIDs), polymyxins, fluorescein dye (used to examine the eye), X-ray contrast media, morphine, and others. Any drug can potentially produce this reaction either on a first or subsequent exposure. All routes of exposure (oral, intravenous, topical, eye, etc.) may also produce a reaction.

In anaphylaxis or its variants, blood pressure drops, fluid leaks out of the blood vessels into the tissues and produces tissue swelling, blood volume is lowered, and shock can follow if not treated. Major signs and symptoms include angioneurotic edema/angioedema (swelling of the face, eyes, lips, and tongue), laryngeal edema (swelling of the vocal cords), respiratory distress, hypotension, loss of consciousness, urticaria (hives), itching, flushing, diarrhea, and vomiting. Unless treatment is immediate, death can occur rapidly.

Anaphylaxis is a medical emergency. Treatment includes epinephrine (adrenaline), oxygen, antihistamines, corticosteroids, and supportive care (e.g., intravenous fluids) as required.

Sclerosing Syndromes

Sclerosing syndromes is an ill-defined category of terms (the FDA did not define it in its proposed reporting obligations of 2003)[1] and includes such diseases as scleroderma (an autoimmune disease that leads to the overproduction of collagen in connective tissue), progressive systemic sclerosis (a systemic connective tissue disease), CREST syndrome (calcinosis, Raynaud's phenomenon, esophageal dysmotility, sclerodactyly, and

telangiectasia) or limited scleroderma, peritoneal fibrosis, peritoneal sclerosis, sclerotic thickening of the peritoneal membrane, sclerotic obstructive peritonitis, calcific peritonitis, abdominal cocoon, sclerosing peritonitis, and sclerosing cholangitis. It does *not* refer to such diseases as multiple sclerosis or spinal sclerosis. These sclerosing diseases have common characteristics including inflammation and fibrosis of various tissues and organs, which interfere with the proper functioning of the involved organs. The diagnoses are complicated in many cases and the etiology often not found. The presence of one or more of these syndromes seen with a drug should trigger the possibility that the drug may have played a role in the disease.

■ Infections and Infestations

Confirmed or Suspected Endotoxin Shock

Shock is a medical emergency in which the oxygen delivery to the tissues is severely compromised, resulting in damage to organs. It is frequently fatal. There are several causes, e.g., heart problems, low blood volume, anaphylaxis (see "Anaphylaxis," previously discussed in this chapter) and septic shock (due to bacteria and the toxic substances they produce). Endotoxin shock is a type of septic shock in which gram-negative bacteria (often *Escherichia coli*) release toxic substances called endotoxins, which produce multiple effects. These include a drop in blood pressure due to negative effects on cardiac muscle and vasodilation of blood vessels, the formation of blood clots followed by bleeding, and organ failure (lungs, liver, kidneys).

The concern here is primarily one of the transmission of such an infectious agent in the drug product (see next section). Such cases should provoke consideration of product quality issues.

Confirmed or Suspected Transmission of Infectious Agent by a Study Drug or Marketed Product

Transmission of an infectious agent actually refers to a product quality problem, because the issue is not due to the drug or its excipients but rather a contamination or tampering of the drug during its manufacture, packaging, shipping, or dispensing. Pharmacovigilance workers play a key role in discovering this, because individual cases may not raise the suspicion of the treating nurse, physician, or pharmacist. Often it is only when there is a cluster of cases from the same geographic area or locale (e.g., one hospital) with a particular product having the same lot or batch number that there will be a suspicion of this problem. Contamination with an infectious agent can lead to severe infections, including endotoxin shock discussed previously.

Musculoskeletal and Connective Tissue Disorders

Rhabdomyolysis

Rhabdomyolysis refers to the rapid destruction and breakdown of muscle cells. When muscle cells are destroyed, they release their contents into the bloodstream. One of the released chemicals is myoglobin (one of the proteins in the muscle responsible for oxygen binding). In the circulation, however, myoglobin is very toxic to the kidneys and can produce acute kidney failure. There are multiple causes of rhabdomyolysis, including crush injury to muscles (usually large muscles such as in the leg or chest), trauma, keeping a part of the body in a fixed or awkward and immobile condition (e.g., as a result of confinement, torture, drunkenness, coma, and other causes) as well as seizures, excess exercise (in a dehydrated state), electric shock, artery obstruction (emboli and thrombi), infections, poisons, toxins, and muscle diseases. The reason there is a focus on rhabdomyolysis is that it may also be produced by medications. In particular, drugs that produce rhabdomyolysis include the widely used lipid-lowering HMG-CoA reductase inhibitors commonly referred to as *statins*, as well as certain anesthesia medications and some psychiatric drugs.

Rhabdomyolysis (also called *rhabdo*) usually presents with muscle pain (myalgia), weakness, and swelling. It may develop very rapidly and acutely, occurring over minutes to a couple of hours. The pain may get progressively worse and affect a large muscle or group of muscles. If the swelling (due to edema and the inrushing of fluid) is severe, this may produce a compartment syndrome in which the swelling muscle pushes against and damages the arteries, veins, and nerves nearby, producing further damage. As the products from the muscle breakdown enter the bloodstream, various other problems occur, producing nausea, vomiting, electrolyte problems that may lead to cardiac rhythm problems, kidney failure, a type of clotting disorder called disseminated intravascular coagulation, and even death.

Lab tests help in the diagnosis and include tests to detect elevations of the muscle enzyme called creatine kinase.

Cardiac troponin levels are also often elevated. Other lab abnormalities can occur if other organs are damaged; e.g., there might be elevated creatinine and blood urea nitrogen levels in patients with acute renal failure.

Rhabdomyolysis is a medical emergency. Treatment involves treating the cause (if known) plus immediate hydration, correction of abnormal electrolytes (e.g., potassium) and, if renal failure occurs, dialysis.

In the review of any safety data for drugs, a high level of suspicion should be maintained for any AEs or blood tests suggestive of muscle damage, muscle pain, and dysfunction.

Nervous System Disorders

Neuroleptic Malignant Syndrome

Neuroleptic malignant syndrome is a medical emergency that is usually due to an adverse drug reaction. It has almost exclusively been seen after taking antipsychotic medications (neuroleptics) and occasionally so-called dopaminergic drugs such as levodopa. It is believed to be due to the blockade of a particular receptor in cells to dopamine, though direct toxicity to muscle is also postulated.

The diagnosis is made clinically. Key features are muscle rigidity, very high fever, labile (variable) blood pressure, tachycardia (rapid heart rate), sweating, tremor, incontinence, gastrointestinal disturbances, abnormal behavior, altered consciousness including delirium, and in almost all cases, a history of taking a neuroleptic drug—particularly at high doses or after a dose increase. In severe cases, muscle breakdown and rhabdomyolysis may occur, leading to acute renal failure.

Lab tests are not specific for the disease but can show abnormal muscle enzymes (creatine kinase) elevations and possibly renal failure (elevated blood urea nitrogen and serum creatinine values), protein and myoglobin in the urine, and other derangements in the blood.

Treatment involves stopping the neuroleptic drug and supporting the patient with hydration, electrolytes, dialysis (if needed), cooling blankets, etc. Most patients recover if treatment is initiated rapidly. Recurrences are common, though most patients will be able to restart an antipsychotic drug at a later date if required. Obviously, this should be done under very careful medical supervision.

Because neuroleptic malignant syndrome is almost always due to a drug AE, even 1 case or suspected case should serve as an alert of an important safety issue.

Seizure

There are 2 categories of seizure: epileptic (due to abnormal brain activity) and nonepileptic (due to emotional stress or physiologic causes such as low blood sugar or fever in a child). Seizures can involve changes in mental state, clonus (muscles contract and relax many times producing a jerky, twitching-like movement), tonus (muscles contract and stay rigidly contracted), convulsions, or psychic symptoms (déjà vu). Seizures may be isolated or recurrent, in which case they are termed epilepsy or epileptic seizures.

Seizures are also classified depending upon whether they involve movement of all or parts or the body (motor), are associated with abnormal sensations or warnings (such as a specific smell or blinking lights that may herald a seizure), or abnormal body function such as abdominal pain, nausea, diarrhea, and bloating.[14] Seizures may be localized (focal, involving only a part of a body) or generalized. Generalized seizures are frequently associated with tonic/clonic or jerking movements and loss of consciousness and are often referred to as convulsions.

There are many causes of seizures, including fever (especially in children), diabetes mellitus, kidney failure, electrolyte and metabolic problems such as low sodium, brain injury, tumors of the brain, alcohol (and alcohol withdrawal), infections (AIDS, syphilis), and genetic/familial factors. Many drugs are implicated in causing seizures or *lowering the seizure threshold*—a vague and ill-defined concept that suggests that the drug will cause seizures in certain people who are prone to them. Other people with a higher seizure threshold would not have the seizure with the same particular stimulus. It is not actually possible to measure or quantitate a seizure threshold. Some drugs that are implicated include theophylline, bupropion, phenothiazines, meperidine, cyclosporine, chloroquine, ofloxacin, ceftazidime, camphor (inhaled), buspirone, indomethacin, antidepressants, oral contraceptives, and, somewhat paradoxically, certain antiseizure drugs given at high doses. Seizures, as mentioned previously, may be seen also upon drug withdrawal with some general anesthetics, alcohol, and some sleeping medications. Some illicit drugs such as cocaine are also believed to cause seizures, though other contributing factors such as the quality and purity of such street drugs makes such a judgment difficult. Toxins such as lead and strychnine may also produce seizures. Because seizures are common and seen with a fair number of medications, they should be thoroughly investigated when reported with drugs.

Diagnosis of seizures may be difficult. Electroencephalograms, which measure the brain's electrical activity, are the most useful laboratory tools. There are some reports of elevated serum prolactin (a hormone that stimulates milk secretion) levels associated with seizures, making this measurement a useful diagnostic tool in some cases.[15] The management of seizures varies depending upon the cause, acuteness, and severity of the seizure. Status epilepticus (a continuous seizure) is a medical emergency and requires medical intervention.

■ Renal and Urinary Disorders

Acute Renal Failure

Acute renal failure refers to the sudden loss of kidney function. There are multiple causes, and these are divided by anatomy into prerenal, renal, and postrenal causes.

Prerenal causes refer to blood volume problems such as low blood volume from shock or blood loss, excess use of diuretic drugs, infection, liver failure (see "Acute Liver Failure"), and obstruction of the blood vessels of the kidney.

Renal refers to direct damage to the kidney itself such as from drugs (e.g., aspirin, NSAIDs, aminoglycoside antibiotics, lithium). Other causes can include certain malignancies, systemic lupus erythematosus (an autoimmune disease that can attack the kidney and other organs), red blood cell damage (hemolysis), and massive muscle damage (rhabdomyolysis, discussed previously in this chapter).

Postrenal refers to problems in the urinary tract below the kidneys such as stones, bladder cancer, prostate problems, and drugs that obstruct bladder emptying.

Acute renal failure is associated with significant changes in laboratory values. The most important ones are increases in blood creatinine, blood urea nitrogen values, and potassium (hyperkalemia) values. Severe hyperkalemia (values > 7.0 mmol/L; normal range 3.5 to 5.5 mmol/L) is a medical emergency and can cause clinically important ECG changes and lead to cardiac arrest and sudden death. Metabolic acidosis can also occur because the kidney is unable to eliminate the acids that are formed during metabolism. Examination of the urine may reveal elevated protein levels, white and red blood cells (which are normally not found in any significant number in urine), and casts (which are tube shaped, and made up of red blood cells, white blood cells, or kidney cells). In some renal diseases (e.g., the nephrotic syndrome), the ability of the kidney to reabsorb protein is lost, and large amounts of protein are found in the urine (proteinuria), and correspondingly low levels of albumin and total protein are found in the blood. Protein in the blood acts like a sponge to keep fluid within the blood vessel. With the loss of protein, fluid leaks into the surrounding tissues, and edema (swelling) follows. Fluid retention and edema may also occur as a result of the inability of the failed kidneys to eliminate fluid. This results in decreased urine production (oliguria) or no urine production (anuria). It is possible to have acute renal failure while maintaining urine flow, but in such a situation the kidney is still not eliminating wastes. Other signs and symptoms of renal failure, largely due to the aforementioned biochemical changes, include loss of sensation, tremor, lethargy, seizures, agitation, foul breath (due to the buildup of urea), bleeding, and high blood pressure.

Diagnosis is generally straightforward and is based on the signs, symptoms, and laboratory findings discussed previously. Radiology examinations also help with the diagnosis, especially in postrenal failure. Determining the cause, however, may be much more difficult. Treatment must be urgent and includes removal of the cause as well as supportive therapy (fluid and electrolyte correction, treatment of acidosis, etc.) as well as dialysis if needed.

In terms of risk determination, a drug cause should always be suspected in acute renal failure (noting the possibility the offending agent can be an over-the-counter drug, nutraceutical, etc.).

■ Respiratory Thoracic and Mediastinal Disorders

Acute Respiratory Failure

Acute respiratory failure refers to the failure of the lungs to perform their oxygen exchange role (taking Carbon dioxide (CO_2) out of blood and putting O_2 in). Ventilation refers to the amount of air breathed in and out of the lungs. Perfusion is the amount of oxygen supplied to the various tissues of the body by the circulation of the blood. There are multiple causes for ventilation/perfusion problems, including some lung diseases as well as conditions resulting in decreased blood flow to the lungs (e.g., pulmonary embolism—a clot that blocks a pulmonary vessel). CO_2 levels can be high when the CO_2 produced by the body cannot be expelled from the lungs due to emphysema, asthma, or other diseases.

Acute respiratory failure may be directly due to lung disease. Conditions outside the lung can also cause respiratory failure. Examples of nonpulmonary causes include congestive heart failure resulting in pulmonary edema (fluid accumulation in the lungs), and conditions that adversely affect the respiratory center located in the brain, such as stroke and head trauma. Drugs can also play a causal role in acute respiratory failure either by their direct effect on the lungs or by having secondary effects such as precipitating heart failure or producing anemia (thus decreasing the ability to transport to the organs). Some drugs, such as morphine (or other narcotics) or benzodiazepines, can slow down respiration and play a role in acute pulmonary failure by depressing the brain's respiratory center. Drug overdoses can also induce the acute respiratory distress syndrome, a condition associated with damage to the alveoli (the air sacs where gas exchange occurs) and to the lung's capillaries.

Diagnosis of acute respiratory failure is made by a variety of means, including the physical exam noting rapid or very slow breathing, rales (a crackling sound) and other abnormal lung sounds, abnormal heart sounds (murmurs due to valve disease), abnormal chest X-ray, as well as measuring the amount of oxygen and CO_2 in arterial blood (blood gases) directly. Other tests may also be of use, including ECGs, lung scans, and lung biopsies.

Treatment is focused on treating the underlying condition, e.g., treatment with the antidote naloxone used to reverse respiratory depression caused by a narcotic overdose, while ensuring adequate oxygenation and removal of excess CO_2. Patients may have to use a respirator until the underlying condition resolves.

Pulmonary Fibrosis

Pulmonary fibrosis is a disease (or diseases) in which normal lung tissue becomes scarred over (with fibrous or connective tissue) and is no longer able to function in the exchange of oxygen (O_2) and CO_2. Causes include radiation therapy, scleroderma and similar diseases, cigarette smoking and certain environmental pollutants (asbestos, silica) as well as drugs (methotrexate, cyclophosphamide, amiodarone, propranolol, aspirin, gold, penicillamine, nitrofurantoin, sulfasalazine, and others). Drug administration does not have to be by inhalation. Patients typically complain of dyspnea (shortness of breath), dry cough, fatigue, and rapid weight loss. Tachypnea (increased respiratory rate) and hypoxia (low blood oxygen levels) may also be evident. Pulmonary fibrosis may progress to pulmonary hypertension and respiratory failure.

Pulmonary fibrosis should always be investigated for a possible drug cause.

Pulmonary Hypertension

Pulmonary hypertension is a condition characterized by high blood pressure in the vessels of the lung including the pulmonary arteries, veins, and capillaries. Normally the pressures in the pulmonary vessels are low. The right ventricle, unlike the left ventricle, is not designed to pump against a high resistance system. With this extra workload, right-sided heart failure can ensue. There are multiple causes for pulmonary hypertension, including familial (genetic) as well as lung diseases such as emphysema (often due to smoking), liver cirrhosis, scleroderma, sickle cell disease, and heart disease. Many times the actual cause is not found and the condition is labeled as *idiopathic*. Pulmonary hypertension is a different disease from the usual high blood pressure found in many patients when their systemic blood pressure (measured in the arm) is elevated. Drugs implicated include cocaine, methamphetamines, and alcohol. If pulmonary hypertension is seen at a greater frequency than expected, be suspicious of a drug-related cause.

■ Skin and Subcutaneous Tissue Disorders

Erythema Multiforme, Stevens-Johnson Syndrome, and Toxic Epidermal Necrolysis

These skin reactions represent a range of conditions that share certain characteristics but differ in severity. Erythema multiforme (EM) is the mildest form and toxic epidermal necrolysis, also called Lyell syndrome, is the severest. Stevens-Johnson syndrome (SJS) is intermediate between these two. In these disorders, the epidermis (the upper layer of skin) detaches from the layers underneath. Nikolsky's sign, which is separation of the upper and lower layers of the skin when rubbed, is often present. It may involve small areas of skin or the whole body. It can be due to viral infections, cancer, and very often, drugs. The drugs most often implicated include sulfa, phenytoin, penicillin, chloramphenicol, quinolones, NSAIDs (including phenylbutazone, piroxicam, ibuprofen, indomethacin, sulindac, and tolmetin), phenobarbital, carbamazepine, and valproic acid, with sporadic reports for many other drugs seen. The mechanism is thought in some cases to be immunologic. In many cases, a cause is never found. It presents with various skin manifestations including erythema (redness), vesicles (blisters), plaques (solid, raised, flat-topped lesions), and bullae (very large fluid-filled blisters).

Target lesions are concentric layers of redness and paleness, which look like a bull's-eye, and are characteristic of EM. When bullae form, significant amounts of fluid can be lost from the body and result in shock. When these bullae rupture, large amounts of skin are lost, resembling a bad burn to some degree. A superimposed infection may also be present, which will produce other symptoms, depending upon the location of the infection.

Diagnosis is made definitively by a skin biopsy. In addition to discontinuing the offending drug, treatment is similar to the treatment for severe burns, which is primarily fluid replacement, supportive care, and treatment of any secondary infection. Mortality can approach 30% in some SJS series if extensive areas of the skin are involved and slough (fall off).[16]

Whenever the diagnosis of EM, SJS, or toxic epidermal necrolysis is made, a drug cause should be considered.

Fixed Drug Reactions

Fixed drug reactions are skin reactions, sometimes in one place on the skin, sometimes at multiple sites, which are due to a drug. They are usually mild and may recur each time the offending drug is used. The lesion itself is usually red, round, and well defined, and it may have a blister. What typically distinguishes fixed drug reactions from EM are the relatively mild nature of the skin reactions and the fixed location of the lesions when they recur. They may occur from minutes to hours after the drug is taken. Drugs implicated include acetaminophen; tetracyclines; sulfa drugs including cotrimoxazole, and sulfasalazine; aspirin; NSAIDs (including ibuprofen); benzodiazepines; and quinine. Other drugs have also been sporadically implicated. Treatment is discontinuation of the drug.

■ Vascular Disorders

Malignant Hypertension

Malignant hypertension refers to very high blood pressure associated with organ damage. Systolic pressure is usually > 220 mm Hg and diastolic pressure > 120 mm Hg.[17] The term *malignant* as used here has nothing whatsoever to do with cancer, and it is an unfortunate use of the word. Nonetheless, this is the term that has been used for many years and remains in use.

Malignant hypertension is associated with nausea, vomiting, and organ damage to the eye (papilledema or swelling of the optic disk), the heart (chest pain, myocardial infarction, congestive heart failure), the kidneys (acute renal failure), and nervous system (stroke, headache, visual problems, encephalopathy or brain dysfunction). It is usually seen in patients with a history of (benign) hypertension.

Malignant hypertension can be drug induced (e.g., the use of cocaine, amphetamines, steroids, monoamine oxidase inhibitors, and certain oral contraceptives). It can also occur with the sudden withdrawal of certain drugs including beta-adrenergic blockers, clonidine, and alcohol.

Malignant hypertension is a medical emergency and must be treated immediately.

References

1. Food and Drug Administration. "Safety Reporting Requirements for Human Drug and Biological Products." Federal Register/Vol. 68, No. 50/Friday, March 14, 2003/Proposed Rules. 12406–12497. http://edochet.access.gpo.gov/2003/03-5204.htm. Accessed February 28, 2010.

2. Goldman L, Ausiello DA, Arend W, et al. *Cecil Medicine: Expert Consult-Online and Print (Cecil Textbook of Medicine)*. Philadelphia, PA: Saunders; 2008.

3. Fauci AS, Kasper DL, Longo DL, et al. *Harrison's Principles of Internal Medicine*. 17th ed. New York, NY: McGraw-Hill Professional; 2008.

4. McPhee SJ, Papadakis MA. *Current Medical Diagnosis and Treatment*. 49th ed. New York, NY (LANGE CURRENT Series) McGraw-Hill Medical; 2010.

5. Warrell DA, Cox TM, Firth JD, Berz ED. *Oxford Textbook of Medicine*. 4th ed. Oxford University Press; 2003.

6. Brenton LL, Lazo JS, Parker KL. *Goodman & Gilman's The Pharmacological Basis of Therapeutics*. 11th ed. New York, NY: McGraw-Hill Professional; 2005.

7. eMedicine. http://emedicine.medscape.com/. Accessed February 28, 2010.

8. WebMD. http://www.webmd.com. Accessed February 28, 2010.

9. Mayo Clinic Diseases and Conditions http://www.mayoclinic.com/health/DiseasesIndex/DiseasesIndex. Accessed March 23, 2010.

10. NIH Medline Plus. http://www.nlm.nih.gov/medlineplus/druginformation.html. Accessed February 28, 2010.

11. FDA http://www.fda.gov. Accessed February 28, 2010.

12. Department of Health and Human Services. Center for Disease Control and Prevention. Birth Defects. http://cdc.gov/ncbddd/bd/. Accessed February 28, 2010.

13. Wilmink T, Frick TW. Drug-induced pancreatitis. *Drug Saf*. 1996 Jun;14(6):406–423.

14. Peppercorn MA, Herzog AG, Dichter MA, Mayman CI. Abdominal epilepsy: A cause of abdominal pain in adults. *JAMA*. 1978;40:2450–2451.

15. Chen DK, Yuen TS, Fisher RS. Use of serum prolactin in diagnosing epileptic seizures: Report of the Therapeutics and Technology Assessment Subcommittee of the American Academy of Neurology. 2005;65:668–675.

16. Bastuji-Garin S, Fouchard N, Bertocchi M, Roujeau J, Revuz J, Wolkenstein P. SCORTEN: A severity-of-illness score for toxic epidermal necrolysis Bastuji-Garin, Nathalie Fouchard[*], M Bertocchi[*], Jean-Claude Roujeau[*], Jean Revuz[*] and Pierre Wolkenstein. *J Invest Dermatol*. 2000; 115: 149–153.

17. JD Bisognano. Hypertension, Malignant, September 2009. http://emedicine.medscape.com/article/24160-overview. Accessed February 28, 2010.

Approaches to the Analysis, Summary, and Interpretation of Safety Data

Exposure

NOTE: In an integrated analysis of safety (IAS) demographics and disposition of subjects are discussed in the exposure section of the report;[1,2] in clinical study reports these topics are discussed in separate sections of the study report.[3] In Chapters 13 and 14 demographics and disposition are respectively discussed.

Exposure information provides an essential framework for understanding and interpreting safety data. It serves a number of purposes in both the premarketing and postmarketing settings. These include:

Premarketing

- Determining the adequacy of the safety database in support of drug approval. Exposure information provides answers to the following questions:
  - Have enough patients been exposed at recommended doses for long enough periods to support approval of the drug?
  - Does the profile of the subjects who participated in the clinical development program represent the patient population that will receive the marketed drug in the real world?
  - If not, what is missing? Too few Blacks, Asians, and other races? Too few elderly or pediatric patients?
- Providing the denominator for the calculation of rates of safety findings, e.g., adverse event (AE) rates, as discussed in Chapter 6.

Postmarketing

- Determining the extent of use of the drug once marketed.
- Providing the denominator for the calculation of AE reporting rates discussed in Chapter 6.

■ Adequacy of the Safety Database

For long-term treatment of non–life-threatening conditions, a minimum of 1500 patients exposed to the investigational drug during clinical development is recommended. Of these subjects, at least 300 should be exposed for 6 months, and

100 exposed for 12 months at doses recommended for clinical use.[4] Even though recommended, it should be understood these numbers are still too small to identify and characterize rare events during clinical development (see Chapter 2). In addition to the number of patients exposed and the duration of exposure, the types of patients treated are also evaluated. Are the patients who participated in the clinical development program representative of the patients who will be using the drug once marketed? The answer is usually no. For instance, Blacks, Asians, other racial groups, the elderly, the pediatric population, and patients with a variety of different concomitant diseases, e.g., hepatic disease, are often underrepresented at the time of drug approval. Exposure deficiencies in terms of the number of patients, length of exposure, or the types of patients exposed can result in nonapproval of the drug or a requirement for additional studies postapproval.

Estimated Exposure

Estimates of exposure are required primarily in 2 situations—for ongoing clinical trials that are blinded and for the Periodic Safety Update Report for Marketed Drugs (PSUR).

Blinded Trials

Exposure estimates from blinded trials are required for periodic reports (usually submitted annually) during clinical development and for the IAS. Examples of periodic reports include the Development Safety Update Report the investigational new drug Annual Report (United States), and the Annual Safety Report (European Union).[5–7] This information is part of the annual overview of safety and aids in the identification of any adverse findings/trends that can represent a new risk while trials are still ongoing. In the IAS, all subjects exposed to study medication must be included in summarizing exposure. For blinded studies that are ongoing at the time of the data cutoff date, an estimate of the number of subjects exposed to study medication should be provided. How to arrive at this estimate is described later in the chapter.

The Periodic Safety Update Report for Marketed Drugs

Estimated exposure is a requirement of the PSUR.[8,9] This is determined in a number of different ways (e.g., prescriptions written, bottles of drug distributed, tablets sold or manufactured), but this is only an estimate for 2 main reasons. The first is that the number of prescriptions written and sales data are usually not accurate or complete and are often only a sampling of the complete universe of prescriptions written or tablets sold. The second is there is no certainty as to how much of the drug that was sold was actually taken and for how long it was used. There are many bottles of half-used drugs sitting in patients' medicine cabinets.

How to Summarize Exposure—Clinical Trials

This section explains how to summarize exposure during clinical trials. Appendix II, "The Integrated Analysis of Safety for Mepro," provides examples of how exposure data can be summarized.

1. Prepare a table that lists all the studies included in the IAS. This provides the reviewer with a snapshot view of the types of studies included, number of subjects exposed per trial, doses given, and duration of treatment. The *Common Technical Document for the Registration of Pharmaceuticals for Human Use—Efficacy—M4E (R1): Clinical Overview and Clinical Summary of Module 2 Module 5: Clinical Study Reports* and *Guideline for the Format and Content of the Clinical and Statistical Sections of an Application* provide specific information of what should be included in this table.[1,2] Some of the more general information provided in this type of table includes:

   ■ Study number
   ■ Location of where the study was conducted and date the study was completed
   ■ Study design
   ■ The treatment groups and the doses received
   ■ The number of patients in each treatment group
   ■ The duration of the study

2. Include a brief narrative description of each study in the IAS, providing the reviewer with an overview of the types of studies that were done, the numbers of subjects exposed to the various treatments, and the duration of treatment.

3. Account for *every* subject who received one or more doses of study medication—this includes investigational drug, placebo and active control.

   Table 12-1 is an example of a tabular display of the number of subjects who participated in the studies

| Table 12-1 | Enumeration of Subjects in Completed Studies |

Study Number	Placebo	Investigational Drug	Active Control	Other[#]
		Phase 2/3 Studies		
Placebo-controlled studies				
MP2001	25	50		
MP2002	25	75		
MP2004	150	450		
MP3002	2000	2000		
Active-controlled studies				
MP2003		450	150	
MP3001		2000	2000	
MP3003		150	75	
Total controlled Phase 2/3 studies	2200	5175	2225	
Uncontrolled (open) studies				
MP2003X		125[a]		
MP2004X		110[b]		
Total all Phase 2/3	2200	5410[a,b]	2225	
		Phase 1 Studies		
Single-dose studies				
MP1001	6	18		
MP1002	6	36		
MP1005		12[c,d]		
MP1006		24		
MP1007	6	36		
MP1009		24		
MP1011		12		
MP1012		12		
MP1015		12[d]		12[d]
MP1016		12[d]		12[d]
MP1019	6	36		
Multiple-dose studies				
MP1003	6	24		
MP1004	6	24		
MP1008		12		
MP1010	35	35		35
MP1013		12[d]		12[d]
MP1014		12[d]		12[d]
MP1017		12[d]		12[d]
MP1018		8[c]		
Total phase 1	71	373[c,d]		95
Grand total	2271	5783[a,b,c,d]	2225	95[d]

[#] Other includes moxifloxacin, digoxin, lithium, fluconazole, methotrexate, and warfarin.

[a] 25 and 100 patients who received active control and investigational drug, respectively, in study MP 2003 received investigational drug in study MP 2003X.

[b] 10 and 100 patients who received placebo and investigational drug, respectively, in study MP 2004 received investigational drug in study MP 2004.

[c] In these crossover studies subjects received investigational drug in more than one period in the study.

[d] Subjects received digoxin, lithium, fluconazole, methotrexate, or warfarin alone and in combination with investigational drug.

included in an IAS, organized by study, treatment group, study design, and phase of study.

This is a complicated table with lots of footnotes. The footnotes are necessary because exposure data do not typically fall into nice discrete categories and explanations are necessary. In this example, the footnotes explain what drugs are included in the other category; that some subjects participated in more than one trial and therefore are counted more than once in the denominator in the same or different treatment groups; subjects in crossover studies received investigational drug in more than one period in the study; and for some of the Phase 1 studies, subjects received both the investigational drug and another drug concomitantly.

4. Indicate the number of *unique* subjects. In an IAS where data are pooled (combined) across studies, it is not unusual to find subjects who participated in more than one study. This is shown in the footnote in Table 12-1 that describes subjects who received placebo and active control in a short-term study, who then went on to receive investigational drug in a long-term extension study. The footnotes also indicate that some subjects who received investigational drug in a short-term study also continued to receive investigational drug in a long-term extension study and were counted in the denominators for both the short-term and long-term studies. Because the same subjects can be counted more than once in the same treatment group or be counted in different treatment groups, it is useful to show the actual number of *unique* subjects who participated in the clinical trials.

In the example given in Table 12-1, 25 and 10 subjects (for a total of 35 subjects) received placebo, and active control, respectively, in a short-term study and then went on to receive the investigational drug in a long-term study. These respective subjects were counted in the placebo, active control, and investigational groups. Two hundred subjects received the investigational drug in a short-term study and then went on to receive investigational drug in a long-term study and were counted in the denominators of both the short-term and long-term studies. The grand total of subjects who received investigational drug in Table 12-1 is 5783, which includes the 235 subjects who participated in more than 1 study. The number of unique subjects who received the investigational drug, however, is 5583, because the 200 subjects who received the investigational drug more than once (i.e., in both short-term and long-term studies) are counted only once in the calculation of unique patients who received investigational drug.

5. Show the number of subjects included in each data set summarized in the IAS. In an IAS studies are grouped in different ways or different data sets. These groupings provide different views of the data. Examples of data sets include: controlled Phase 2/3 studies, all Phase 2/3 studies, and Phase 1 studies (see Chapters 3 and 15). To understand the rates of AEs and other safety findings summarized for each data set, the number of subjects included in each data set (N–denominator) must be specified.

Table 12-2 is an example of a summary of the number of subjects included in 3 different data sets. The numbers shown are based on the information from Table 12-1.

The controlled Phase 2/3 studies data set is similar to the all-Phase 2/3 studies data set, except that the open long-term studies (MP2003X and MP2004X) are not included.

6. Provide exposure information by dose and duration. This information is often combined and can be displayed in different ways. One example is illustrated in Table 12-3.

In this example the number of subjects who were exposed to investigational drug for ≥ 36 weeks and ≥ 52 weeks is 704 and 116, respectively.

Table 12-2   **Summary of the Number of Subjects by Data Sets**

Data Sets	Placebo	Investigational Drug	Active Control
Controlled Phase 2/3 studies	2200	5175	2225
All Phase 2/3 studies	2200	5410	2225
Phase 1 studies	71	373	0

Table 12-3 **Summary of Exposure by Dose and Duration**

Duration of Exposure (Weeks)	Placebo N = 2200	ID = 5 mg N = 2450	ID = 10 mg N = 2400	ID = 15 mg N = 325	Total ID N = 5175
0 to < 1	38 (1.7%)	34 (1.4%)	36 (1.5%)	6 (1.8%)	76 (1.5%)
≥ 1 to < 4	275 (12.5%)	257 (10.5%)	204 (8.5%)	43 (13.2%)	504 (9.5%)
≥ 4 to < 12	550 (25.0%)	473 (19.3%)	400 (16.7%)	87 (26.8%)	960 (18.6%)
≥ 12 to < 24	792 (36.0%)	562 (22.9%)	581 (24.2%)	189 (58.2%)	1332 (25.7%)
≥ 24 to < 36	545 (24.8%)	729 (29.8%)	754 (31.4%)	0	1483 (28.7%)
≥ 36 to < 52	0	340 (13.9%)	364 (15.2%)	0	704 (13.6%)
52	0	55 (2.2%)	61 (2.5%)	0	116 (2.2%)

ID = investigational drug.

Calculation of duration and dose can be confusing and challenging to do in 2 situations. Situation 1 involves calculating exposure for subjects who first participated in a short-term study (i.e., a study of < 6 months) and then continued in a long-term extension of the short-term study. Situation 2 involves calculating the dose for subjects who participated in dose-titration studies where a fixed dose was not used but the dose was increased based on how efficacious the drug was (e.g., blood pressure control in a hypertension study) or how well the dose was tolerated. How are these situations handled?

Approach for Situation 1: For subjects who received placebo or an active control in a short-term study and then went on to receive the investigational drug in a long-term extension study, exposure to the investigational drug is calculated from the time the subject received the first and last dose of investigational drug in the long-term extension study. For subjects who received the investigational drug in the short-term study and continued to receive investigational drug in a long-term extension study, exposure is calculated from the first dose of investigational drug received in the short-term study to the last dose received in the long-term extension study.

Approach for Situation 2: For studies where the dose was titrated, a decision needs to be made regarding what dose group to select and the rationale for the dose group selected should be provided. For instance, the mean (average), modal dose (i.e., the most frequent dose given), or dose used for the longest duration are all options that can be used.

Which method is used should be clearly noted and the same methodology should be used across studies.

7. Calculate person-years exposure (PYE) indicating duration of exposure. PYE is calculated by adding up the actual days each subject received treatment and dividing this number by 365 days.

8. Estimate exposure for ongoing, blinded studies by: (1) determining the number of subjects randomized as of the data cutoff date; and (2) using the randomization ratio of investigational drug to placebo or active comparator. For example, if 300 subjects were randomized as of the data cutoff date, and the randomization ratio of investigational drug to placebo is 2:1, the estimated exposure is assumed to be 200 subjects for the investigational treatment group and 100 placebo subjects.

■ How to Determine Exposure Postmarketing

Postmarketing exposure estimates are a requirement of each PSUR.[8,9] As mentioned previously, it can be determined in a number of different ways. Examples include but are not limited to prescriptions written, bottles of drug distributed, and tablets sold or manufactured.

1. Clearly document the method used to calculate the exposure.

2. Calculate exposure estimates using the same method from report to report; this allows comparison of results from one reporting period to the next.

References

1. International Conference on Harmonisation of Technical Requirements for Registration of Pharmaceuticals for Human Use. *The Common Technical Document for the Registration of Pharmaceuticals for Human Use—Efficacy—M4E (R1): Clinical Overview and Clinical Summary of Module 2 Module 5: Clinical Study Reports*. Geneva, Switzerland: ICH Secretariat; September 2002. http://www.ich.org/cache/compo/276-254-1.html. Accessed March 23, 2010.

2. Center for Drug Evaluation and Research, Food and Drug Administration, Department of Health and Human Services. *Guideline for the Format and Content of the Clinical and Statistical Sections of an Application*. July 1988. http://www.fda.gov/downloads/Drugs/GuidanceComplianceRegulatoryInformation/Guidances/UCM071665.pdf. Accessed March 23, 2010.

3. International Conference on Harmonisation of Technical Requirements for Registration of Pharmaceuticals for Human Use. *Structure and Content of Clinical Study Reports E3 ICH*. Geneva, Switzerland: ICH Secretariat; November 1995. http://www.ich.org/cache/compo/276-254-1.html. Accessed March 23, 2010.

4. International Conference on Harmonisation of Technical Requirements for Registration of Pharmaceutical for Human Use. *The Extent of Population Exposure to Access Clinical Safety for Drugs Intended for Long-Term Treatment of Non-life-threatening Conditions E1*. Geneva, Switzerland: ICH Secretariat; October 1994. http://www.ich.org/cache/compo/276-254-1.html. Accessed March 23, 2010.

5. International Conference on Harmonisation of Technical Requirements for Registration of Pharmaceuticals for Human Use. *Development Safety Update Report E2F*. Geneva, Switzerland: ICH Secretariat; June 2008. http://www.ich.org/cache/compo/276-254-1.html. Accessed March 23, 2010.

6. Code of Federal Regulations. PART 312—INVESTIGATIONAL NEW DRUG APPLICATION, Subpart B—Investigational New Drug Application, Sec. 312.33 "Annual reports." April 2009. http://www.accessdata.fda.gov/scripts/cdrh/cfdocs/cfcfr/CFRSearch.cfm?fr=312.33. Accessed March 23, 2010.

7. "Detailed guidance on the collection, verification and presentation of adverse reaction reports arising from clinical trials on medicinal products for human use." April 2006. http://ec.europa.eu/enterprise/pharmaceuticals/eudralex/vol-10/21_susar_rev2_2006_04_11.pdf. Accessed March 23, 2010.

8. International Conference on Harmonisation of Technical Requirements for Registration of Pharmaceuticals for Human Use. *Clinical Safety Data Management: Periodic Safety Update Reports for Marketed Drugs E2C (R1)*. Geneva, Switzerland: ICH Secretariat; November 2005. http://www.ich.org/cache/compo/276-254-1.html. Accessed March 23, 2010.

9. Volume 9A of The Rules Governing Medicinal Products in the European Union—Guidelines on Pharmacovigilance for Medicinal Products for Human Use. September 2008. http://ec.europa.eu/enterprise/sectors/pharmaceuticals/documents/eudralex/vol-9/index_en.htm. Accessed March 23, 2010.

Demographics and Other Baseline Characteristics

Demographics, as the term is used in the pharmacology and medical world, refer to the characteristics of a population with respect to age, gender, race, and other baseline factors such as weight, renal status, concomitant diseases, coexistent illnesses, and tobacco and alcohol use. Demographics and other population characteristics are used in several different ways. For the individual case safety report, the patient's demographics, concomitant medications, and coexistent diseases can be important contributing factors to the reported event. For these reasons, this information is collected and included in the narrative of the event. Demographic factors can also impact a drug's risk profile. For example, the risk of developing Stevens-Johnson syndrome—a serious and potentially life-threatening skin condition—is increased in Asians taking the anticonvulsant drugs carbamazepine and

phenytoin.[1] The primary focus of this chapter is to understand how this information is used in clinical study reports and in the integrated analysis of safety (IAS).

Demographics and other baseline characteristics are used to determine:

- If there are any differences among treatment groups at baseline.
- If the study population is representative of the real world population that will be receiving the drug once marketed. This is one of the factors considered in the drug approval process.

■ Baseline Considerations

The basis of aggregate analysis (the analysis of data by treatment groups) is to look for differences between the investigational drug and the control group (placebo and/or an active control) as discussed in Chapter 6. If the treatment groups are similar (balanced) at baseline, then any differences found in the study suggest a potential drug effect. If baseline differences exist, this can be a reason or at least a contributing factor explaining why there is a difference in results between treatment groups. If no drug effect is seen, baseline difference could be a factor in masking, hiding, or even counteracting a drug effect. Baseline imbalances confound (confuse) the interpretation of safety findings. For instance, the results of a study show a baseline difference between treatment groups—the investigational drug group has more male patients compared to the placebo group. The rate of myocardial infarctions is also higher in the investigational group than in the placebo group. Is this due to the gender difference alone, a drug effect, or an interaction between the drug and males? In this example, gender differences confound the interpretation of the myocardial infarction findings. For this reason, it is important to determine whether at baseline the different treatment groups are demographically similar (balanced) or different (an imbalance is seen). In randomized, controlled clinical trials, the gold standard type study design, demographics and other baseline characteristics across treatment groups are typically balanced. This is because treatment assignment is based on a computer-generated list where allocation to different treatment groups is randomly (by chance alone) determined.

TIP: Be suspicious if baseline differences are found in a randomized, controlled trial—it may mean the randomization schedule was not followed.

TIP: In an IAS, as discussed in Chapter 3, studies are allocated and pooled (combined) to different data sets; e.g., a controlled Phase 2/3 studies data set, an all-Phase 2/3 studies data set, etc. If demographics and other baseline characteristics are not balanced, this may be a *clue* the allocation of some of the studies selected for the data set are not appropriate for inclusion.

The Study Population Versus the Real World

The characteristics of the study population must also be compared to the real world population that will be taking the drug once it is marketed (presuming one knows the demographics of the real world). If there is not a good match between the study population and the real world population, this can result in nonapproval of the drug or a postapproval requirement to evaluate more patients of a certain demographic group. Health agencies can also limit the approved labeling to only patients with the demographics from the study population. For example, if only 1% of all the study patients are Black, but it is estimated that 24% of those likely to use the marketed drug are Black, the prescribing information might state that the safety and efficacy of the drug in Blacks have not been adequately studied and also prompt a regulatory agency request for more safety information as a postapproval requirement.

How to Summarize Demographics and Other Baseline Characteristics

This section explains how summarizing demographic's and other baseline characteristics by treatment group as required for clinical study reports and the IAS. Appendix II, "The Integrated Analysis of Safety for Mepro," provides an example of how this information can be summarized in the IAS.

1. Prepare a summary table by treatment group that includes:
   a. Age
   b. Gender
   c. Race
   d. Other characteristics of the study population, including:
      i. Ethnicity (e.g., Hispanic, non-Hispanic)
      ii. Weight, body mass index (BMI)
      iii. Smoking and alcohol use
      iv. Renal status
2. For continuous variables (a continuous variable is one that can have any value within a range), e.g., age, weight, BMI, provide:
   a. Mean—the average
   b. Standard deviation (measures the statistical dispersion of the data). If the data points are close to the mean, the standard deviation is small; if many of the data points are far from the mean, the standard deviation is large.
   c. Median—arranging all the values in order and selecting the value in the middle.
   d. Range of values—shows the upper and lower bounds of the sample.

Table 13–1 is an example of how demographic's and other baseline characteristics can be displayed.

Table 13-1 **Summary of Demographic's and Other Baseline Characteristics—Controlled Phase 2/3 Studies**

Demographic Variable	Placebo N = 2200	Investigational Drug N = 5175	Active Control N = 2225
Gender			
Male	752 (34%)	1597 (31%)	756 (34%)
Female	1448 (66%)	3578 (69%)	1469 (66%)
Race			
Caucasian	1628 (74%)	3788 (73%)	1691 (76%)
Black	396 (18%)	1073 (21%)	423 (19%)
Asian	110 (5%)	201 (4%)	89 (4%)
Other[a]	66 (3%)	113 (2%)	22 (1%)
Age (years)			
Mean	43.8	45.4	45.1
SD	11.0	9.8	11.1
Median	44	45	45
Range	18–79	18–81	18–80
Age category			
< 40 years	770 (35%)	1708 (33%)	801 (36%)
40–64 years	968 (44%)	2432 (47%)	1001 (45%)
≥ 65 years	462 (21%)	1035 (20%)	423 (19%)
Weight (kg)			
Mean	81.3	79.1	79.9
SD	19.2	18.6	18.8
Median	79.0	78.5	78.1
Range	47–137.1	46.5–140.3	49–141.4
BMI (kg/m^2)			
Mean	27.8	27.7	26.8
SD	6.0	6.0	5.9
Median	27.1	27.3	26.1
Range	18.8–40.1	18.5–40.8	18.5–40.3

[a] Includes Native Americans and Pacific Islanders.

This table shows the treatment groups are well balanced with respect to demographics and other baseline characteristics. The table also shows there are more females than males, Caucasians are the predominant racial group, and the majority of patients are > 40 years of age.

3. Provide summary tables by treatment group for coexistent diseases and concomitant medication to determine if there are any baseline differences across treatment groups.

4. Document the method used to determine baseline differences. This can range from looking at simple descriptive statistics such as means for treatment group differences by *eyeballing* the data (making a judgment call) as discussed in Chapter 6, or doing a statistical test or analysis to determine whether an observed difference is statistically significant. A statistician should be consulted to determine the best approach to take. Of course, randomization serves as the best defense against baseline imbalances.

Reference

1. Locharernkul C, Loplumlert J, Limotai C, et al. Carbamazepine and phenytoin induced Stevens-Johnson syndrome is associated with HLA-B*1502 allele in Thai population. *Epilepsia*. 2008;49: 2087–2091.

Disposition

Disposition is the determination of what happened to each subject who participated in a clinical trial. Did the subject complete treatment or was treatment stopped prematurely (other terms include premature withdrawal, premature termination, premature discontinuation, and dropout)? If treatment was stopped prematurely, it is important to know why—was it due to lack of efficacy, a safety concern, or another reason?

The reasons for not completing treatment usually fall into 4 main categories:

1. Lack of efficacy
2. Adverse event (AE) (which also includes death)
3. Lost to follow-up
4. Other. This category is a catch-all category and includes but is not limited to the following examples: the subject no longer wanted to participate in the study, poor compliance, the subject moved away, the subject became pregnant, the investigator

no longer wanted to participate in the study, the sponsor stopped the study because of slow enrollment.

TIP: Be suspicious of all subjects who were lost to follow-up or were put into the *other* category. Death can be a reason for being lost to follow-up. It can also mean the investigator was not diligent enough in tracking down the subjects who didn't return to the study. Also, in the rare instances when fraud occurs, subjects sometimes fall into the lost to follow-up category.

■ How to Summarize Disposition Data—Clinical Trials

This section outlines how to summarize disposition data, including advising readers of a number of potential pitfalls that can occur in determining disposition. Appendix II, "The Integrated Analysis of Safety for Mepro," provides an example of how disposition data can be summarized in an integrated analysis of safety.

1. Establish *standard* categories for reasons for premature termination. Data collected from individual studies will eventually have to be pooled with other studies for the integrated analysis of safety (IAS). This reality underscores the importance of establishing at the beginning of the clinical development program the standard categories for premature termination to be used across all studies. If plans for data integration are not put into place at the beginning of the clinical development program and the reasons for discontinuation are not standardized (i.e., are not the same) across all studies, this must be done at the time of preparation of the IAS, which can be problematic and a drain on resources (see Chapters 2 and 3).

2. Check the rate of AEs that led to discontinuation in the disposition section of the clinical study report or IAS and the rate shown for AEs that led to discontinuation that are in the AE section of the report. These rates should match. Sometimes mismatches occur because AEs that led to premature discontinuation are captured on 2 different (electronic or paper) case report form (CRF) pages—the End of Study and Adverse Events pages. The End of Study CRF page indicates if the subject completed or prematurely discontinued treatment, and if discontinued, the reason why (e.g., lack of efficacy, AE, etc.). The Adverse Event CRF page provides details of all reported AEs (e.g., the description of the event, whether it was mild, moderate, or severe; whether it was related to study medication, whether the event resulted in discontinuation of treatment, whether it was serious, and whether it resolved or not). The summary tables of disposition data are usually programmed from the End of Study CRF page, while AEs leading to discontinuation are programmed from the Adverse Event CRF page. Any AE mismatches between these two 2 data sets will result in different AE discontinuation rates. Although this data collection and programming convention violates one of the first laws of good data practices—"never collect the same data in two 2 different places"—this is a commonplace and unfortunate method of data collection and programming. Because of this known inherent weakness in the way these data are collected and handled, as part of good planning, it is important to set up routine checks of the data to ensure that the subjects who

discontinued treatment due to AEs captured on the End of Study CRF match those captured on the Adverse Event CRF.

> **CAUTION:** If routine consistency checks are not planned or done, any data mismatches resulting in rate differences can have significant negative consequences. Adding missed AEs to already programmed tables requires reprogramming and reanalysis of the AE tables. In an IAS where there are typically scores of AE tables, this translates into significant wasted time/resources and increased costs. *Bottom line*: if these mismatches are first identified at the IAS stage, it is simply too late.

3. Determine and document the convention to be used for categorizing *disease progression* (also referred to as *worsening, aggravation,* or *exacerbation* of the condition being evaluated). Disease progression is often handled inconsistently. In some cases, investigators will list disease progression as lack of efficacy, while others will list disease progression as an AE. This situation arises for treatment of diseases such as cancer, congestive heart failure, and stroke, where hospitalizations and deaths are expected. When hospitalization or death results, disease progression is handled as a serious AE. In some situations, the investigator suspects the study medication is actually making the condition being treated worse and lists the event as an AE, and this can be true. Historically, some drugs initially prescribed for treatment of specific diseases were subsequently shown to cause worsening of the disease being treated. Examples include (1) flecainide and encainide, which are antiarrhythmic drugs that increase the risk of arrhythmic deaths in patients with acute myocardial infarctions and ventricular arrhythmias; and (2) increased hepatotoxicity in patients given fialuridine for the treatment of hepatitis B.[1–3]

> **TIP:** A way to make it clear to the reviewer how these inconsistencies are handled is to add "Disease Progression" as an AE subcategory and include in this subcategory all disease progression events listed on the AE page that led to discontinuation. A footnote explaining what is included in this subcategory is useful. This approach is shown in Table 14-1.

Table 14-1	**Disposition**	
Patient Disposition	Placebo N = 100	Investigational Drug N = 100
Completed	65 (65%)	80 (80%)
Discontinued	35 (35%)	20 (20%)
Lack of efficacy	28 (28%)	10 (10%)
Adverse event	4 (4%)	7 (7%)
Adverse event[a]	*2 (2%)*	*6 (6%)*
Disease progression[b]	*2 (2%)*	*1 (1%)*
Lost to follow-up	1 (1%)	2 (2%)
Other[c]	2 (2%)	1 (1%)

[a] Includes AEs not related to disease progression.
[b] Includes disease progression, worsening disease, disease aggravated, disease exacerbated, which were listed on the Adverse Event CRF and led to premature discontinuation.
[c] Includes withdrew informed consent, poor compliance, subject moved away.

This table also shows that more subjects completed treatment and more discontinued due to AEs in the investigational drug group compared to placebo.

4. If both lack of efficacy and AE are listed, state the convention used to count such patients; e.g., the patient was counted in both the lack of efficacy and AE categories or was counted only in the AE category.

TIP: The Food and Drugs Administration recommends that patients who discontinue for both lack of efficacy and AE be counted in the AE category.[4]

---

5. Summarize only those subjects who prematurely discontinued *treatment*, not those who prematurely discontinued the *study*. In some studies, the clinical study protocol states subjects must

CAUTION: If this convention is not followed, subjects can erroneously be counted as premature discontinuations even though treatment was completed. Of course, it is possible that a patient who completed treatment developed a latent (late-occurring) adverse drug reaction to the investigational drug resulting in discontinuation from the study before the study was completed. This information is also important but is addressed in the "Withdrawal and Rebound" section of the IAS where posttreatment AEs are summarized and discussed.

be followed for a prespecified period after the last dose of study medication (e.g., 3 months, 1 year, etc.) regardless of whether or not the subject completed treatment. This can lead to confusion regarding what should be analyzed. For the analysis of safety, premature discontinuation of *treatment* should be summarized, *not* premature withdrawal from the *study*.

References

1. Pratt CM, Moye LA. The Cardiac Arrhythmia Suppression Trial: background, interim results and implications [review]. *Am J Cardiol.* 1990;65(4): 20B–29B.

2. McKenzie R, Fried MW, Sallie R, et al. Hepatic failure and lactic acidosis due to fialuridine (FIAU), an investigational nucleoside analogue for chronic hepatitis. *N Engl J Med.* 1995;333(17):1099–1105.

3. Committee to Review the Fialuridine (FIAU/FIAC) Clinical Trials, Division of Health Sciences Policy, Institute of Medicine, Manning FJ, Swartz M, eds. *Review of the Fialuridine (FIAU) Clinical Trials.* Washington, DC: National Academies Press; 1995.

4. Center for Drug Evaluation and Research, Food and Drug Administration, Department of Health and Human Services. *Guideline for Conducting a Clinical Safety Review of a New Product Application and Preparing a Report on the Review.* February 2005. http://www.fda.gov/downloads/Drugs/GuidanceComplianceRegulatoryInformation/Guidances/ucm072974.pdf. Accessed March 23, 2010.

Adverse Events Part 1: Common Adverse Events

The analysis of adverse event (AE) data plays the largest role in determining a drug's risk profile. In this chapter, the analysis of common AEs is covered. The next chapter discusses deaths, other serious adverse events (SAEs), other significant AEs, and the analysis of AEs by organ system or syndrome.

The emphasis of this chapter and the next is on the integrated analysis of safety (IAS) and the Periodic Safety Update Report for Marketed Products (PSUR), for investigational and marketed drugs, respectively. The information provided in these chapters, however, can also be applied to other reports. Reference should be made to the regulations and guidance documents regarding content and format for specific requirements for clinical study reports (CSRs), the Summary of Clinical Safety (SCS), the Integrated Summary of Safety (ISS), the Periodic Adverse Drug Experience Report (PADER), and the PSUR for Marketed Drugs.[1–7] There are many different ways to apply the information provided in these

regulation and guidance documents. Appendix II and Appendix IV provide an abbreviated IAS and PSUR, respectively, for the fictitious nonsteroidal anti-inflammatory drug (NSAID) meproamine dihydroacetate (Mepro). These examples will show how the approaches discussed in these chapters can be applied.

■ Defining *Common*

In discussing common AE rates for clinical studies, or the IAS, it is useful to start by defining *common*. Unfortunately there is no set number to use, because *common* is dependent on the number of subjects exposed. For instance, in small studies with 50 subjects per treatment group, common might be defined as $\geq 10\%$. However, for an IAS where overall exposure is 1500 or more patients, common might be a rate of $\geq 1\%$. The definition of *common* is therefore a judgment call. Because common is not a specific number, the chosen threshold that is used for common AEs should be clearly defined or specified in the report, e.g., "For adverse events in this study report, common is defined as $\geq 5\%$."

Once a drug is marketed, the definitions for *common*, *uncommon*, and *rare* used in prescribing information are as follows[8]:

Common (frequent): ≥ 1/100 and < 1/10 (≥ 1% and < 10%)

Uncommon (infrequent): ≥ 1/1000 and < 1/100 (≥ 0.1% and < 1.0%)

Rare: ≥ 1/10,000 and < 1/1000 (≥ 0.01% and < 0.1%)

■ The Collection of Adverse Event Information

Clinical Trials

In clinical trials, there is a specific AE case report form (CRF) designed for the collection of AE information that includes:

- The AE—this should be listed as a diagnosis or syndrome whenever possible rather than individual signs and symptoms if the diagnosis or syndrome is clear and reasonably well known. For example, *influenza* should be listed rather than *pyrexia, myalgia, headache, malaise, cough, pharyngitis,* and *rhinitis.*
- Onset date
- Resolution date (if resolved)
- Intensity—mild, moderate, or severe
- Relationship to treatment—e.g., none, remote, unlikely, possible, probable, and definite (or some other standardized grading system)
- Action taken—none, adjusted dose, temporarily held dose, permanently discontinued
- Serious—whether the outcome of the event met one or more criteria for seriousness, e.g., death, hospitalization, etc.
- Outcome—recovered, recovered with sequelae, ongoing, death

Postmarketing

For postmarketing, AE information is captured on an intake form (paper or electronic) that includes data fields required for completion of regulatory reporting forms (e.g., the CIOMS I form in Europe and elsewhere and the MedWatch 3500A form in the United States).[9–11] The content of these forms was discussed in Chapter 5.

■ The Analysis of Common Adverse Events—Clinical Trials

Data Conventions Used in the Aggregate Analysis of Adverse Events Data From Clinical Trials

Before an aggregate analysis of AEs from clinical trials is done, there are certain data conventions that are followed. Conventions are specific rules applied to the data regarding how the data are counted and analyzed. Data conventions are needed so any reviewer knows what rules were used and can use these rules to replicate the results, if desired. If a reviewer does not agree with the results of the analysis and feels the conventions utilized were not correct, the reviewer can choose to use other conventions and redo the analysis based on the conventions the reviewer thinks valid. Data conventions should be documented in the report and should be transparent to the reviewer. Conventions used in the analysis of common AEs include:

- A definition of a treatment-emergent AE.
- A determination of causality, i.e., whether the AE was considered not related or related to the study drug as judged by the investigator.
- A rule for handling missing data.
- A rule for counting AEs.
- A determination of which data should or should not be pooled (combined), if dealing with an integrated analysis (i.e., the analysis of more than one study).
- A statement of the method(s) (see "Adverse Events Versus Adverse Drug Reactions") used to determine common adverse drug reactions (i.e., treatment related AEs).

Definition of a Treatment-Emergent Adverse Event

In clinical trials, treatment-emergent AEs and posttreatment AEs are analyzed. The latter are analyzed to determine if there is a withdrawal/rebound effect or a late-occurring event. The definition of a treatment-emergent AE includes one of the following:

- Any AE that occurred during the treatment period or within the period of *residual effect* posttreatment.
- Any AE present at baseline that worsened in intensity during the treatment period or within the *residual effect period* of the drug.

The residual effect period refers to the period of time after the last dose of medication when measurable drug levels are still likely to be present. Many drugs have negligible residual effects following the last dose; while others have noticeable residual effects. A number of factors determine the length of this period; 2 include the drug's half-life and whether the drug is protein bound. For example, if an AE occurred 8 days after treatment with a drug with a half-life of 20 days, the AE should be counted as a treatment-emergent (and not a posttreatment) AE. A clinical pharmacologist should be consulted in determining a drug's residual effect period.

> **NOTE:** There are rare instances of AEs produced long after treatment and long after the drug has left the body. Various mechanisms are possible, including immediate effects that are not manifested until much later; this was seen with diethylstilbestrol,[12] which was given to pregnant women and in whom a serious and severe AE (vaginal cancer) was seen in the offspring when they attained puberty years later. Another example is the cumulative toxicity that can build up over time but may not manifest itself until a stressor occurs much later. An example of this is doxorubicin (Adriamycin), which may produce cardiac toxicity years later.[13]

How to Count Adverse Events and Calculate Adverse Event Rates

The simple or crude AE rate is calculated (as discussed in Chapter 6) using the following formula:

$$\text{Adverse event rate (\%)} = (n/N) \times 100$$

where n is the number of subjects who reported an AE, and N is the number of subjects who were exposed to treatment.

This calculation does not include duration of exposure or number of episodes of the AE. If a subject reported the same AE more than once, it should be coded to the same Medical Dictionary for Regulatory Activities (MedDRA) preferred term (PT), but the subject is counted only once. For example, if the same subject reported 5 different episodes of headache, the subject is counted only once in the rate calculation for headache rather than 5 times. If a subject reports different AEs coded to different PTs but within the same system organ class (SOC), the subject

is counted only once in the rate calculated for that SOC. For example, if a subject reported both nausea and constipation, the subject would be counted only once in the calculation of the rate for the SOC *Gastrointestinal disorders*. If the same AE is reported more than once by the same patient, and a causal assessment of not related is assigned to one event, and related to the other, counting the AE as a related event is recommended. If the same AE is listed more than once, and different intensities are assigned (e.g., moderate and severe), assigning the worst intensity (i.e., severe) is recommended.

As previously noted, this is the simple or crude AE rate, and it doesn't take into account differences in exposure. In the crude rate, a patient exposed to the drug for 1 day and another exposed for 365 days are counted, and both have equal weight in the calculation. Exposure, however, is an important consideration. The longer the exposure, the more at risk a subject is of having an AE, even for events that are not drug related. For instance, the risk of developing malaria is greater if you stay in Africa for 1 year rather than if you stay for 1 day. To account for exposure differences, rates based on person-years exposure (PYE) are used.

PYE is calculated by adding up the actual days each person received treatment and dividing this number by 365 days. For example, if 100 persons were treated for 180 days, the PYE = 49.3, based on the following equation:

$$\text{PYE} = (100 \text{ persons} \times 180 \text{ days exposed})/365 \text{ days}$$
$$\text{per year} = 49.3 \text{ person-years exposed}$$

Because these numbers can be small, the results are multiplied by 100, 1000, or more, and expressed as 100 PYEs, 1000 PYEs, and so on.

> **NOTE:** In the calculation of rate using PYEs, it is assumed that the risk of the AE remains constant over time.

Let's look at an example of how the crude rate and the rate based on exposure can show different things.

Example—Crude Rate Versus Rate Based on Person-Years Exposure

All placebo-controlled studies were pooled in the calculation of the rate of myocardial infarction. Five hundred subjects were exposed to placebo, and 1000 subjects were exposed to the investigational drug. All subjects in the placebo group received placebo for 90 days. In the investigational drug group, 500 patients were treated for 90 days, and 500 subjects for 1 year. In the placebo group 10 patients had myocardial infarctions compared to 50 in the investigational drug group. Table 15-1 summarizes the crude rate for myocardial infarction and the rate per 100 PYE.

In this example, exposure to the investigational group is approximately 5 times that of placebo. If this exposure difference is not taken into account, one might conclude based on the crude rate alone, the risk for myocardial infarction is more than twice placebo, a finding that would be quite worrisome. When exposure is factored in, the rates are found to be essentially the same. This example should underscore the importance of calculating rates based on PYE if exposure differences between treatment groups exist.

Defining *Not Related* and *Related* as Judged by the Investigator

One of the aggregate AE analyses routinely done is looking at the relationship to treatment as judged by the investigator. The information captured on the AE CRF as discussed previously includes several choices, e.g., none, remote, unlikely, possible, probable, and definite. For analysis, these terms are usually collapsed into 2 categories. A common convention is to include the terms *none*, *remote*, and *unlikely* into the not related category, and *possible*, *probable*, and *definite* into the related category.

➡ **NOTE:** There is a controversy in the AE world regarding the words *remote* and *unlikely*. Some argue that both of these terms still imply that a drug cause is possible and thus should be included in the related group. This argument says that *not related* means just that— no possibility of being related and that any possibility of a causal relationship, however remote, should not be included in this category. Until this issue is resolved, whatever convention is used should be clearly documented.

An example of how this information can be displayed is shown in Table 15-2.

➡ **NOTE:** Although this type of analysis is routinely done for common AEs, its usefulness is limited because inconsistencies across investigator assessments are routinely seen. Causality is better determined by the

---

Table 15-1 **The Rate of Myocardial Infarction**

Treatment Group	No. of Patients	No. of Myocardial Infarctions	Crude Rate	Person-Years Exposure (PYEs)	Myocardial Infarctions per 100 PYE
Placebo	500	10	2%	123.3	8.1
Investigational drug	1000	50	5%	623.3	8.0

Table 15-2 **Summary of Adverse Events by Relationship to Treatment (as Judged by the Investigator)**

Adverse event MedDRA PT	Placebo N = 100			Investigational Drug N = 100		
	NR	R	Total	NR	R	Total
Headache	6 (6%)	3 (3%)	9 (9%)	9 (9%)	1 (1%)	10 (10%)

NR = not related; R = related.

Table 15-3	Missing Data—Value Selected for Analysis
Missing Information	**Value Selected for Analysis**
Start date of adverse event	Date of first dose of study medication
End date of adverse event	Event is considered ongoing
Intensity	Severe
Relationship to treatment (as judged by the investigator)	Related

difference in AE rates observed between treatment groups rather than the causality assessment provided by the investigator. Investigator causality assessments are more useful in the assessment of individual case safety reports (ICSRs).

How to Handle Missing Data

For missing AE data, 1 of 2 approaches should be considered:

1. Exclude missing data from the analysis. For example, if there are 1000 subjects who received an investigational drug, and 100 of the subjects have missing information regarding the intensity of the AE, these 100 subjects are excluded from the AE by intensity analysis. If this approach is followed, the denominator used in the rate calculation is 900 rather than 1000.

2. Assign the *worst* value for the missing information according to Table 15-3.

This is an important decision to make in safety analyses. Excluding patients is sometimes considered suspect, because some reviewers might conclude that the analysis is attempting to hide or minimize bad or unfavorable data. Whatever approach is used should be clearly documented in the methods section of the report.

■ Adverse Events Versus Adverse Drug Reactions

For an IAS, it is especially important to identify common *adverse drug reactions* (i.e., AEs that are related to the drug) from AEs (all *bad* things whether believed to be related to the drug or not). This will allow the medical writer and reviewer to focus on adverse drug reactions and the factors that can increase or minimize them. In aggregate analyses (as opposed to an ICSR), the determination of whether a common AE is in reality an adverse drug reaction is based on various methods including whether or not there is a *meaningful difference* in the AE rates observed across treatment groups. The methodologies used to determine this meaningful difference are:

- *Statistical* method—Testing hypotheses; e.g., utilizing *p*-values of ≤ 0.05, to test the null hypothesis of no difference in the rate of a safety finding for the investigational drug versus placebo is not advised, especially if the study is not powered adequately to detect important safety differences. However, using 95% confidence intervals around the difference between the rate in the investigational drug group and the placebo group can be informative. The 95% confidence interval provides a best estimate of the difference between the investigational drug and placebo for the safety parameter along with an interval estimate that displays the precision of the estimate. As with any statistical assessment, the use of confidence intervals must be interpreted using clinical judgment because there may be real differences identified through statistical methodology that are not of clinical importance.

- *Rule of thumb* **method**—Specifying the rate of change in the investigational group *and* the magnitude of difference that is observed between the investigational group and control group. For instance, a rate of $\geq 5\%$ in the investigational group and $\geq 2 \times$ the rate in the placebo group.[4]

- *Eyeballing the data* **method**—Looking at the difference in rates between treatment groups and making a clinical judgment call whether these differences are clinically meaningful even if the rates do not reach statistical significance (*Statistical* method) or meet specified criteria (*Rule of thumb* method). The pattern of the data can also suggest a potential drug effect, e.g., a dose response is seen.

All these methods have their own pros and cons as discussed previously in Chapter 6. Regardless of which method is chosen, clinical judgment is typically used in combination with either the statistical or rule of thumb method.

To illustrate, the following is a summary of AEs for an investigational drug with vasodilator properties. Table 15-4 summarizes those AEs with rates of ≥ 1% and shows the rates for the same events in the placebo group.

The shaded terms are those events considered potential adverse drug reactions based, with one exception, on the rule of thumb method previously described; i.e., a rate of ≥ 5% in the investigational group and ≥ 2 times the rate in the placebo group. Although the AE *Blood pressure decreased* is < 5% and < 2 times the rate of placebo, it is included anyway based on the following rationale:

- The event is consistent with the mechanism of action of a vasodilator (a drop in blood pressure is expected when blood vessels dilate).
- The rate in the investigational drug group is almost 2 times greater than the rate in placebo.

Based on this, a drug effect cannot be ruled out and *Blood pressure decreased* is included as a potential adverse drug reaction. So we see in this example that *both* the rule of thumb method and clinical judgment are often used together in the identification of potential adverse drug reactions.

> ➡ **NOTE:** The word *potential* is included for several reasons. The majority of safety analyses are retrospective rather than prospective; therefore, a causal relationship to drug is not

proven but inferred. Causality determination is not always straightforward as illustrated in the example just discussed regarding blood pressure decreases. Moreover, safety results are not always consistent from study to study. For these reasons, *potential* is used until there is more evidence gathered to support a firm conclusion of a causal relationship.

Table 15-4 also illustrates another important concept in the determination of common adverse drug reactions—the need, from time-to-time to use combined terms. Because MedDRA has so many terms that are medically related, similar PTs may have to be combined and counted to avoid underreporting a rate. In the example shown in Table 15-4, a combined term was created for *Blood pressure decreased*.

The AE rate for *Blood pressure decreased* would be underestimated if this was not done, as illustrated in Table 15-5. In this table, the rates of medically similar AEs with different names are shown for each treatment group. Combining these terms and rates into a combined term provides a more accurate picture of the true rate of events related to the reduction of blood pressure (placebo = 2.3%, investigational drug = 4.3%) than if these events were presented separately.

■ Characterization of Common Adverse Drug Reactions

Once an AE is identified as an adverse reaction, it needs to be fully characterized; i.e., more information is needed

Table 15-4	Summary of Adverse Events With a Rate ≥ 1%	
Adverse Events **MedDRA Preferred Term**	**Placebo** **N = 1000**	**Investigational Drug** **N = 1000**
Headache	104 (10.4%)	233 (23.3%)
Dizziness	55 (5.5%)	124 (12.4%)
Pharyngitis	76 (7.6%)	50 (5.0%)
Blood pressure decreased[a,b]	23 (2.3%)	43 (4.3%)
Fatigue	20 (2.0%)	30 (3.0%)
Nausea	10 (1.0%)	10 (1.0%)

[a] Blood pressure decreased includes the MedDRA PTs: Blood pressure ambulatory decreased, Blood pressure decreased, Blood pressure diastolic decreased, Blood pressure orthostatic decreased, Blood pressure systolic decreased, Diastolic hypotension, Hypotension, and Orthostatic hypotension.

[b] This event is considered a potential adverse drug reaction based on clinical judgment.

| Table 15-5 | Summary of Medically Similar Adverse Events Related to Decreased Blood Pressure |

Adverse Event MedDRA Preferred Term	Placebo N = 1000	Investigational Drug N = 1000
Blood pressure decreased	18 (1.8%)	30 (3.0%)
Blood pressure systolic decreased	5 (0.5%)	8 (0.8%)
Hypotension	0	5 (0.5%)
Blood pressure ambulatory decreased	0	0
Blood pressure diastolic decreased	0	0
Blood pressure orthostatic decreased	0	0
Diastolic hypotension	0	0
Orthostatic hypotension	0	0

to better understand the event and any factors that might influence the adverse reaction rate. These include:

- The information captured on the AE CRF, e.g., intensity, relatedness, any interventions, discontinuation from treatment, and whether the event had a serious outcome
- Dose and dose-related factors such as dosing regimen, dose and weight (mg/kg or mg/m^2), total dose, and drug concentration
- Onset of the event
- Duration of the event (the time it took for the event to resolve)

Other factors that also should be explored include:

- Potential interactions with the drug including the following:
  - Drug–demographic interactions
  - Drug–drug interactions
  - Drug–disease interactions
- Geographic regional differences

What Data to Pool

Individual clinical studies are often too small in terms of both the numbers of subjects exposed to treatment and the length of exposure. This limits the ability to identify and characterize drug-related safety findings. For these reasons, an IAS is done across all studies to enhance the ability to determine drug-related safety findings and to identify the factors that can increase or mitigate the risk.

The decision to pool certain studies and present others separately is data driven. It is important not to pool data that can confound the results. Important factors that can preclude pooling include:

- Different study designs—e.g., a parallel study versus a crossover study (where a subject first receives placebo and then is crossed over and receives the investigational product, and vice versa)
- Different doses—e.g., doses considerably lower (10 mg) than the recommended doses (100 mg and 200 mg)
- Different formulations—e.g., topical application—where little systemic absorption is expected versus intravenous administration
- Different study durations—e.g., a 1-day study versus a 1-year study
- Different study populations—e.g., an investigational antibiotic being evaluated in subjects with mild superficial infections versus subjects with life-threatening infections

The data for an IAS are usually divided into the following 3 major pooled data sets:

- Controlled Phase 2/3 studies—This is the best data set to use for across treatment group comparisons.
- All Phase 2/3 studies—This data set includes *all* subjects who participated in Phase 2/3 studies, including uncontrolled studies. Many long-term studies are uncontrolled therefore, and this important information is captured in this data

set. This data set also includes *all* deaths, SAEs, and other significant AEs that occurred in any Phase 2/3 (controlled or uncontrolled) study.

- Phase 1 studies—This data set is of limited value because these studies are typically of short duration; use doses below or above the recommended dose's and include subjects (usually healthy males) that often do not reflect the Phase 2/3 study population. Nevertheless, an important AE or other safety finding can occur in a Phase 1 subject, and all subjects, exposed to one or more dose's of study drug have to be accounted for.

Other data sets can be used, such as by indication (e.g., hypertension and angina) and formulation (oral and topical).

What studies to pool and not to pool, and what data sets should be used, can be quite complicated. Input from different disciplines, such as clinical pharmacology, biostatistics, clinical research, and drug safety, is sometimes needed.

■ Time to Onset—Time to Resolution

Time to onset and time to resolution provide useful information to both the health professional and patient in terms of when an adverse drug reaction is likely to occur and when it is likely to resolve.

Time to Onset

In general, most AEs reported in clinical trials occur early, i.e., within the first several weeks of treatment. Because most clinical studies are short term and cover a period of only a few months (e.g., ≤ 3 months) or less, information about long-term effects is usually limited. Long-term studies, especially for indications for chronic use, e.g., treatment of diabetes, rheumatoid arthritis, and osteoporosis, are necessary in the identification of important safety findings that are late in onset. The effect on bone mineralization and the risk of fractures with long-term antiepileptic treatment is an example of the development of an important adverse drug reaction after long-term exposure.[14]

Analyzing time to onset helps in the determination of whether an adverse drug reaction occurs early or is late in onset. This information can be presented in a number of different ways and includes:

- Evaluating the onset of AEs based on specified time intervals, e.g., 0 to < 2 weeks, ≥ 2 to < 4 weeks, ≥ 4 weeks to < 3 months, etc.

- Calculating the mean or median time to onset
- Doing a Kaplan-Meier analysis, a type of statistical analysis that provides a graphic representation by treatment group of the actual time to onset of the event

---

CAUTION: Mistakes are sometimes made when sponsors incorrectly compare the rate of AEs from short-term studies to those of long-term studies and ignore when the onset of these events occurred. This is illustrated in Table 15-6. In this example, a short-term study is defined as a study with a duration of less than 6 months, and a long-term study as a study with a duration of 6 months or longer. The rates shown in this table do not take into consideration the time to onset of the AE. If a patient from a long-term study had an event after 1 day of treatment and another patient had an AE after 1 year of treatment, these 2 events would get counted the same way. From this table, it is impossible to identify those events that occurred after longer-term treatment.

In this table, it is noted that 4000 patients participated in short-term studies, while 200 patients participated in long-term studies. No difference in AE rates is seen in short-term versus long-term studies. These results are misleading.

To get a better understanding of the effects after long-term exposure, the data should be analyzed by time to onset of the AE as illustrated in Table 15-7.

In this table both types of studies are pooled and the number of patients exposed (*N*) in each column represents how many patients received treatment during the time periods shown. It should be noted that subjects counted in the Ns of one interval are also counted in the Ns of the *preceding* interval(s). For example, patients who were exposed to the drug for ≥ 12 months are also included in the N in each column, because they received the drug during the time periods of < 3 months, ≥ 3months to < 6 months, ≥ 6 months to < 12 months, and ≥ 12 months. In other words, each interval represents a *snapshot* of time when the patient was receiving the drug. The rates are then calculated based on the number of patients reporting the *first* onset of an event at each time interval. If, for example, the onset of rash occurred during the ≤ 3–< 6 months time interval, the patient is counted only in the rate in that column (even if the rash persisted into the next time interval). When the table is structured this way, different results are seen. This table shows that nausea and vomiting occur early

Table 15-6   *Incorrect:* **Comparison of Adverse Event Rates from Short-Term Versus Long-Term Studies**

Adverse Events MedDRA Preferred Term	Patients from Short-term Studies N = 4000	Patients from Long-term Studies N = 200
Nausea	600 (15%)	28 (14%)
Vomiting	480 (12%)	28 (14%)
Rash	400 (10%)	18 (9%)
Dyspnea	360 (9%)	20 (10%)

Table 15-7   *Correct:* **Summary of Adverse Events—Time to Onset**

Adverse Events MedDRA Preferred Term	< 3 months N = 4200	≥ 3–< 6 months N = 4000	≥ 6–< 12 months N = 200	≥ 12 months N = 100
Nausea	620 (14.8%)	2 (< 0.1%)	4 (2.0%)	2 (2.0%)
Vomiting	504 (12.0%)	4 (0.1%)	0	0
Rash	252 (6.0%)	153 (3.8%)	8 (4.0%)	5 (5.0%)
Dyspnea	361 (8.6%)	1 (< 0.1%)	0	18 (18.0%)

with the rate for these events diminishing over time. Rash appears to be relatively constant over time. For dyspnea, a biphasic distribution is seen, both early on and again after 12 months' exposure, with the higher rate observed after longer-term exposure. This should alert the reviewer that dyspnea needs further review and exploration, because this finding can be a signal of a latent effect of the drug.

Keep in mind that the longer a study runs, the higher the number and rate of AEs. That is, a study that runs several years will often show that all patients have had at least 1 AE and that the AEs that are common in the population as a whole (e.g., headache, nausea) may be seen in 80% or more of the patients. This makes comparisons with short-term studies even more difficult. To put it another way, if you take a placebo for long enough, you'll still die someday!

Time to Resolution

The methods used to calculate the time to resolution are similar to the methods described for time to onset. It is likely, however, that some events will be ongoing by the time the treatment period is over. Adverse reactions with long resolution times or those that do not resolve are of particular clinical concern. Every effort should be made to follow patients until their AEs resolve.

■ Reviewer-Friendly Data Displays

Whenever possible, in-text "dashboard" displays of data should be used. The word *dashboard* is used in a similar context to the dashboard of a car, where all the key information regarding the status and operation of a car can be seen at a glance. Dashboard data displays are reviewer friendly, and if done properly can provide an overview of all the relevant information in 1 place. This makes the reviewer's job easier by avoiding or reducing the need to go to many different appendices looking for information that can be buried in stacks of data that provide very little useful or important information. These in-text data displays can take a bit more time to create but are worth the investment for the clarity and usefulness that are provided. Examples of dashboard and other reviewer-friendly data displays are given in this chapter as well as throughout the book.

The Analysis of Common Adverse Events—Postmarketing

The purpose of analyzing common postmarketing AEs is to determine if the types, frequency, and severity of AEs have changed over time, resulting in a change in a drug's benefit–risk profile. The methods used to do this, however, are very different than the methods used for the analysis of AEs from clinical trials. Unlike clinical trials, where AE rates can be calculated and compared across treatment groups, this cannot be done for spontaneously reported AEs. The reasons for this are largely due to under-reporting of AEs'[15] uncertainty regarding the extent of exposure, and lack of a control group (see Chapter 2). The methods used to determine increased frequency are discussed in Chapter 6. AEs from *postmarketing studies*, however, are analyzed the same way as AEs from clinical trials.

How to Summarize Common Adverse Events—Clinical Trials

This section explains how to summarize common AEs. Appendix II, "The Integrated Analysis of Safety Mepro," provides examples of how common AE data can be summarized for an IAS.

1. Read these chapters:
   - Chapter 3: The Dynamic Integrated Safety Database—Something You Shouldn't Live Without
   - Chapter 4: Coding Basics
   - Chapter 5: Determining Causality—The Individual Case Safety Report
   - Chapter 6: Determining Causality— Aggregate Data
   - Chapter 7: Determining the Weight of Evidence—Patterns and Links
   - Chapter 8: Determining Clinical Significance. . . and Then What?

2. Review the Investigator's Brochure. Animal toxicological findings and the drug's pharmacokinetic and pharmacodynamic profiles can provide insight into potential adverse drug effects. For example, you should be on the lookout for the following potential adverse reactions: cataracts in humans if there is a high rate of cataracts observed in dogs exposed to the investigational drug; potential *renal injury* if the drug accumulates in the kidney;

and potential hypotension if the drug causes vasodilatation.

3. If the investigational drug is a member of a drug class, be alert for similar types of adverse drug reactions described for the drug class, e.g., gastric hemorrhage if the investigational drug is an NSAID.

4. Collect complete and accurate AE information.

5. In the methodology section of the report, define *treatment-emergent AEs* and indicate the conventions used for calculating rates as described earlier in the chapter.

6. Remember to calculate AEs by PYE if exposure is different across treatment groups.

7. Do the following AE analyses (other analyses may be required depending on what the results of these analyses show):

➡ **NOTE:** The results of these various different and voluminous AE analyses will be placed in appendices, and most of these data will not be discussed in the text of the report. Only a subset of relevant informant is typically included for in-text discussion. Examples are included in this chapter and the IAS in Appendix II.

- Overview of AEs—this provides a *snapshot* summary of relevant AE information across treatment groups and includes:
  - Overall rate of AEs; i.e., any subject who reported 1 or more AE
  - Related AEs (as judged by the investigator)
  - Severe AEs
  - Serious AEs
  - Deaths
  - AEs leading to discontinuation
- AEs by PT and SOC
- AEs by decreasing frequency
- AEs by dose
- AEs that led to discontinuation of treatment
- AEs by relationship to drug (as judged by the investigator)
- AEs by intensity
- AEs by time to onset
- AEs by time to resolution
- AEs—short term versus long term
- AEs by concomitant medication

- AEs by demographics and baseline characteristics
  - Age
  - Gender
  - Race
  - Weight
  - Renal status (as measured by baseline creatinine values)

➡ **NOTE:** The renal of subgroup analysis is often omitted if there are too few subjects with abnormal baseline creatinine values to analyze.

- AEs by geographic location

These analyses are usually done for each data set included in the IAS, e.g., controlled Phase 2/3 studies, all Phase 2/3 studies, Phase 1 studies, etc. As you can imagine, all these different cuts of the data can result in hundreds of tables and volumes of appendices.

8. Avoid unnecessary programming.

9. Create user-friendly table formats.

TIP: For in-text tables, the format used for Table 15-9 is recommended. This particular format includes placebo, investigational drug by dose and total (i.e., all dose groups in the investigational group combined), as well as the active control. This type of format allows easy comparison across treatment groups and also allows easier identification of dose-related findings.

➡ **NOTE:** Table 15-9 is another example of data displays that aid in the identification of potential adverse drug reactions. The table summarizes the results of a fictitious investigational NSAID and a fictitious marketed NSAID (active control) compared to placebo. The gray shaded terms, with the exception of PUBs (GI perforations, ulcers, and bleeds) all meet the criteria for adverse drug reactions using the rule of thumb method discussed previously. The decision to include PUBs in the list of potential adverse drug reactions is a clinical judgment call based on the following reasons:

- PUBs are a known class effect of NSAIDs
- The rate of PUBs in the total investigational drug group is ≥ 2 times the rate in placebo
- A dose effect is seen

TIP: Sponsors will often include a totals column in tables, representing the sum of results from the different treatment groups as illustrated in Table 15-8. This makes absolutely no sense from a review perspective, because the goal is to identify treatment differences, and this is achieved by comparing results *across* treatment groups. Including this type of totals column requires additional programming, wastes time and space, increases costs, and only serves as a distraction. The proper way to use a totals column is to total all the patients *within* a treatment group as shown in Table 15-9.

Table 15-8	*Incorrect*: Summary of Adverse Events		
Adverse Events MedDRA Preferred Term	**Placebo N = 100**	**Investigational Drug N = 100**	**Total N = 200**
Headache	51 (51%)	48 (48%)	99 (50%)
Dizziness	22 (22%)	45 (45%)	67 (34%)
Pharyngitis	8 (8%)	6 (6%)	14 (7%)

Table 15-9	**Summary of Adverse Events With a Rate of $\geq 1\%$[a]–Controlled Phase 2/3 Studies**					
Adverse Events MedDRA Preferred Term	Placebo N = 2220	ID = 5 mg N = 2450	ID = 10 mg N = 2400	ID = 15 mg N = 325	Total ID N = 5175	Active control N = 2225
Any adverse event	1376 (62.0%)	1853 (75.6%)	1883 (78.5%)	268 (82.5%)	4004 (77.4%)	1802 (81.0%)
Dizziness	333 (15.0%)	360 (14.7%)	377 (15.7%)	44 (13.5%)	781 (15.1%)	334 (15.0%)
Epigastric discomfort	24 (1.1%)	174 (7.1%)	188 (7.8%)	30 (9.2%)	392 (7.6%)	200 (9.0%)
Nausea	69 (3.1%)	142 (5.8%)	170 (7.1%)	29 (8.9%)	341 (6.6%)	276 (12.4%)
Headache	533 (24.0%)	183 (7.5%)	126 (5.3%)	13 (4.0%)	322 (6.2%)	267 (12.0%)
Nasopharyngitis	144 (6.5%)	152 (6.2%)	110 (4.6%)	24 (7.4%)	286 (5.5%)	122 (5.5%)
Abdominal pain upper	67 (3.0%)	123 (5.0%)	180 (7.5%)	30 (9.2%)	333 (6.4%)	185 (8.3%)
Dyspepsia	44 (2.0%)	100 (4.1%)	142 (5.9%)	21 (6.5%)	263 (5.1%)	232 (10.4%)
Vomiting	64 (2.9%)	105 (4.3%)	132 (5.5%)	21 (6.5%)	258 (5.0%)	174 (7.8%)
PUBs	1 (0.05%)	17 (0.7%)	40 (1.7%)	10 (3.1%)	67 (1.3%)	97 (4.4%)

[a] $\geq 1\%$ greater in the total investigational group.

ID = investigational drug; PUBs = gastrointestinal perforations, ulcers, and bleeds.

The shaded areas are considered to be potential adverse drug reactions.

The table also shows the same adverse drug reactions for both the investigational and active control group. The rates, however, appear consistently greater in the active control group, especially when compared to the investigational drug's two lower dose groups. This, however, does not prove the investigational drug is safer than the active control [see Chapter 6]. Of note, a lower rate of headache is also observed in both the investigational drug and active control groups compared to the placebo—this finding is expected and is consistent with the analgesic property of NSAIDs.

10. Decide what data set(s) will be the primary one(s) discussed in the text. Although these decisions are data driven, a focus on the controlled Phase 2/3 studies for comparison of common AE rates is recommended. This is the most objective type of presentation and the best way to identify common adverse drug reactions. The potential for confounding (confusing) results is also minimized.

Although the main focus of the text should be on the controlled Phase 2/3 studies data set, some mention in the text should be made stating whether the results from the all Phase 2/3 studies data set substantially differed from the results from the controlled Phase 2/3 studies data set, and if so, what these differences were. Any important findings from the Phase 1 studies data set should also be mentioned in the text.

⮕ **NOTE:** For deaths, other SAEs, and other significant AEs, a shift in focus to the all Phase 2/3 studies data set is recommended. In this way no important event is excluded, e.g., a death in an uncontrolled Phase 3 study. This is discussed further in the next chapter. Regardless of what data sets are used, indicate in the text in which appendices the complete results of each data set can be found. This way, if the reviewer wants to review the data not highlighted in the text, the information can easily be found. (This will make more sense when you read the sample IAS in Appendix II.)

TIP: In Table 15-9, the gray shaded areas represent the common potential adverse reactions. Once the common potential adverse drug reactions are

Table 15-10 Summary of Potential Adverse Drug Reactions by Dose-Controlled Phase 2/3 Studies

Adverse Events MedDRA Preferred Term	Placebo N = 2220	ID = 5 mg N = 2450	ID = 10 mg N = 2400	ID = 15 mg N = 325	Total ID N = 5175	Active control N = 2225
Any adverse event	1376 (62.0%)	1853 (75.6%)	1883 (78.5%)	268 (82.5%)	4004 (77.4%)	1802 (81.0%)
Epigastric discomfort	24 (1.1%)	174 (7.1%)	188 (7.8%)	30 (9.2%)	392 (7.6%)	200 (9.0%)
Nausea	69 (3.1%)	142 (5.8%)	170 (7.1%)	29 (8.9%)	341 (6.6%)	276 (12.4%)
Abdominal pain upper	67 (3.0%)	123 (5.0%)	180 (7.5%)	30 (9.2%)	333 (6.4%)	185 (8.3%)
Dyspepsia	44 (2.0%)	100 (4.1%)	142 (5.9%)	21 (6.5%)	263 (5.1%)	232 (10.4%)
Vomiting	64 (2.9%)	105 (4.3%)	132 (5.5%)	21 (6.5%)	258 (5.0%)	174 (7.8%)
PUBs	1 (0.05%)	17 (0.7%)	40 (1.7%)	10 (3.1%)	67 (1.3%)	97 (4.4%)

ID = investigational drug; PUBs = gastrointestinal perforations, ulcers, and bleeds.

identified, these events should be the focus of in-text tables and discussion in the text. Discussion of common events that are not related to treatment is distracting and provides little insight into the drug's risk profile.

11. Provide in-text tables summarizing only the potential adverse drugs reactions by:
    - Dose
    - Relationship to drug (as judged by the investigator)
    - Intensity
    - Time to onset
    - Time to resolution
    - Short-term versus long-term
    - Concomitant medication
    - Demographic and baseline characteristics
    - Geographic region
    - AEs leading to discontinuation (see next chapter).

Table 15-10 is an example of data display looking at the effect of dose on the rate of potential adverse reactions. This table looks similar to Table 15-9, but it includes only those events identified as potential adverse drug reactions. More examples of data displays for the other required analyses listed previously are shown in the sample IAS in Appendix II.

In this table, the first row of results summarizes the rates of patients with *any* AE. Including this information provides the reviewer with an overview of all events (AEs and potential adverse reactions combined). The remainder of the table focuses on only the potential adverse reactions. When the data are displayed in this dashboard fashion, the reviewer can easily compare the results across treatment groups and determine if there is a dose effect—which is seen in Table 15-10.

12. Do not be afraid of overlooking a potential adverse reaction(s). As long as you are diligent and objective in your review, and the methods for identification of potential adverse reactions are documented and transparent, the reviewer can decide which terms he or she feels are adverse drug reactions. If you have done an honest, thorough, and comprehensive review, it is unlikely the reviewer will discover something major that you missed. *The opposite of this is also true!*

13. Look at the most common concomitant medications (i.e., used during the treatment period). This analysis provides more evidence of a drug-related effect. For instance, the results in Table 15-10 show GI-related adverse reactions in both the investigational and active control groups. If a higher rate of the concomitant use of proton pump inhibitors, antacids, and other GI remedies is seen, this finding increases the weight of evidence that the GI-related events are drug related.

14. Keep an open mind—AEs are not always *adverse* (see Chapter 6).

How to Summarize Common Adverse Events—Postmarketing Data

This section explains how to summarize common AEs. Appendix IV, "6-Month Periodic Safety Update Report—Mepro," shows how this information can be displayed and summarized in the PSUR.

1. Read the chapters mentioned in the previous section.

2. Provide a tabular summary of all the AEs reported during the PSUR's reporting period, as shown in Table 15-11 (this is a duplicate of Table 6-2 from Chapter 6). The format and content of this type of summary table can vary somewhat as noted in the International Conference on Harmonisation guidance document *E2C (R1): Clinical Safety Data Management: Periodic Safety Update Reports for Marketed Products*.[6] Unless a health authority specifically requests a particular format, the format shown in Table 15-11 is recommended because

it provides a dashboard display of all events across all sources of information and includes serious and nonserious events.

➡ **NOTE:** This table shows the most common AEs reported during the reporting period were *Ecchymosis, Palpitations, and Anemia*. It also shows the majority of the events were nonserious. Although serious events carry more clinical weight, it is also important to look at nonserious events. The same AE, regardless of seriousness, can be telling the same story, even if the magnitude and severity of the event are different. For instance, one person can have a nonserious case of thrombocytopenia [low platelet count]; i.e., a value of $100 \times 10^3/mm^3$ [normal platelet count = $140–400 \times 10^3/mm^3$] and be asymptomatic, while another patient may have a platelet count of $20 \times 10^3/mm^3$, be actively bleeding, and require hospitalization (a serious event). Even though the degree of thrombocytopenia is very different in these 2 cases, both signal a potential platelet effect. A high volume of similar cases is a clue to a potential drug effect but

Table 15-11 Summary of Postmarketing Reports by Adverse Event Term[a]				
Adverse Event Term by MedDRA SOC/PT	Spontaneous/ Regulatory Bodies	Postmarketing Studies	Literature	Total
Blood and lymphatic system disorders				
Ecchymosis	98 (5)	15	5 (2)	118 (7)
Anaemia	47 (3)	4	5 (2)	56 (5)
Leukocytosis	19 (2)	10 (1)	0	29 (3)
Neutropenia	1	1	0	2
Thrombocytopenia	1 (1)	0	0	1 (1)
Cardiac disorders				
Palpitations	40	27	10	77
Hypertension	10 (2)	1 (1)	5 (2)	16 (5)
Tachycardia	9	7	4 (1)	20 (1)
Myocardial infarction	3 (3)	0	1 (1)	4 (4)
Nervous system disorders				
Insomnia	20	16	1	37
Depression	5 (1)	2 (1)	1	8 (2)
Anxiety	3	3	0	6

[a] The number in ( ) represents the number of terms considered serious. The *italicized* events are unlisted AEs.

can be a red herring [false signal]. Other determinations [as discussed in Chapters 5–8] have to be done to weigh the evidence for or against a causal relationship.

3. Refer to Chapter 6 for suggested approaches for determining increased frequency.

CAUTION: How to calculate increased frequency is not specified by regulatory agencies. In 1997, the Food and Drug Administration (FDA) actually revoked the requirement to report increased frequency of events on an expedited basis.[16] Prior to dropping this requirement, the FDA provided a formula to use; however, this method did not contribute to the timely identification of safety problems, and expedited reporting for increased frequency based on this formula was dropped.[17] Because there are no standard approved formulas currently available, the method that is used should be clearly described in the PSUR, and the same method should be used from one reporting period to the next.

In addition to the issues discussed previously regarding underreporting, lack of accurate exposure information, and absence of an appropriate method to calculate increased frequency, many other factors can lead to false conclusions. **Bottom line:** Frequency calculations for marketed drugs are at best hypothesis generating. But it at least forces us to look at the data where there may be an undiscovered clue waiting to be found.

References

1. International Conference on Harmonisation of Technical Requirements for Registration of Pharmaceuticals for Human Use. *Structure and Content of Clinical Study Reports E3.* Geneva, Switzerland: ICH Secretariat; November 1995. http://www.ich.org/cache/compo/276-254-1.html. Accessed February 18, 2010.

2. International Conference on Harmonisation of Technical Requirements for Registration of Pharmaceuticals for Human Use. *The Common Technical Document for the Registration of Pharmaceuticals for Human Use—Efficacy—M4E (R1) Clinical Overview and Clinical Summary of Module 2 Module 5: Clinical Study Reports.* Geneva, Switzerland: ICH Secretariat; September 2002.

http://www.ich.org/cache/compo/276-254-1.html. Accessed February 18, 2010.

3. "Guideline for the Format and Content of the Clinical and Statistical Sections of an Application." July 1988. www.fda.gov/downloads/Drugs/GuidanceComplianceRegulatoryInformation/Guidances/UCM071665.pdf. Accessed March 26, 2010.

4. Center for Drug Evaluation and Research, Food and Drug Administration, Department of Health and Human Services. *Guideline for Conducting a Clinical Safety Review of a New Product Application and Preparing a Report on the Review.* February 2005. http://www.fda.gov/downloads/Drugs/GuidanceComplianceRegulatoryInformation/Guidances/ucm072974.pdf. Accessed March 26, 2010.

5. Code of Federal Regulations. PART 314—APPLICATION FOR FDA APPROVAL TO MARKET A NEW DRUG, Subpart B—Applications, Sec. 314.80 Postmarketing reporting of adverse drug experiences. April 2009. http://www.accessdata.fda.gov/scripts/cdrh/cfdocs/cfcfr/CFRSearch.cfm?fr=314.80. Accessed March 26, 2010.

6. International Conference on Harmonisation of Technical Requirements for Registration of Pharmaceuticals for Human Use. *Clinical Safety Data Management: Periodic Safety Update Reports for Marketed Drugs E2C (R1).* Geneva, Switzerland: ICH Secretariat; November 2005. http://www.ich.org/cache/compo/276-254-1.html. Accessed March 26, 2010.

7. Volume 9A of The Rules Governing Medicinal Products in the European Union—Guidelines on Pharmacovigilance for Medicinal Products for Human Use. September 2008. http://ec.europa.eu/enterprise/sectors/pharmaceuticals/documents/eudralex/vol-9/index_en.htm. Accessed March 26, 2010.

8. A Guideline on summary of product characteristics (SMPC). September 2009. http://ec.ewopa.eu/enterprise/sectors/pharmaceuticals/documents/eudralex/vol-2/index_en.htm h2-volume-2c—regulatory-guidelines. Accessed March 26, 2010.

9. US Department of Health and Human Services, Food and Drug Administration. *Voluntary reporting* [Form FDA 3500]. http://www.fda.gov/Safety/MedWatch/HowToReport/DownloadForms/default.htm. Accessed March 26, 2010.

10. US Department of Health and Human Services, Food and Drug Administration *Mandatory reporting*

[Form FDA 3500A]. http://www.fda.gov/Safety/MedWatch/HowToReport/DownloadForms/default.htm. Accessed March 26, 2010.

11. Council for International Organizations of Medical Sciences. *Suspect adverse reaction* report. http://www.cioms.ch/cioms.pdf. Accessed March 26, 2010.

12. Giusti RM, Iwamoto K, Hatch KE. Diethylstilbestrol revisited: A review of the long-term health effects. *Ann Intern Med.* 1995; 122(10): 778–788.

13. Saltiel E, McGuire W. Doxorubicin (Adriamycin) Cardiomyopathy—A critical review. *West J Med.* 1983; 139(3): 332–341.

14. Epstein S, Tannirandorn P. Drug-induced bone loss. *Osteoporos Int.* 2000; 11:637–659.

15. Hazell L, Shakir SA. Under-reporting of adverse drug reactions: a systematic review. Drug Safety. 2006;29: 385–396.

16. Department of Health and Human Services. Postmarketing Expedited Adverse Experience Reporting for Human Drug and Licensed Biological Products; Increased Frequency Reports. Federal Register. 62 FR 34166, June 25, 1997.

17. Center for Drug Evaluation and Research, Food and Drug Administration, Department of Health and Human Services. *Guideline for Postmarketing Reporting of Adverse Drug Experiences.* March 1992. http://www.fda.gov/downloads/Drugs/fda.gov/Guidances/ucm071987.pdf. Accessed March 26, 2010.

Adverse Events Part 2: Deaths, Other Serious Adverse Events, Other Significant Adverse Events, and Analysis of Adverse Events by Organ System or Syndrome

In the previous chapter, common adverse events (AEs) were discussed. The objective of this chapter is to focus on less common but nevertheless clinically important events—deaths, other serious adverse events (SAEs), and other significant AEs. Adverse drug reactions (treatment-related AEs), even if uncommon, can significantly affect a drug's risk profile and tilt the benefit–risk profile to unfavorable. The ability to detect uncommon and rare AEs is limited during clinical development because too few patients are exposed to the investigational drug for too short a time. The uncertainty of the number of reports and the number of patients exposed, the lack of a comparator, as well as incomplete and poor quality information, underscore the challenges of identifying less common but important AEs once the drug is marketed. For these reasons, finding an uncommon/rare AE and

determining whether the event is drug related may be as difficult as finding a needle in a haystack. In attempting to find a needle in a haystack, the first step is to identify the haystacks. As far as drug safety is concerned, these "haystacks" are deaths, other SAEs, and other significant AEs.

Other Significant Adverse Events

Guidance documents define *other significant adverse events* as:[1–4]

- Any event that led to an *intervention*, including withdrawal of treatment of the investigational drug, dose reduction, or significant additional concomitant medication
- Marked hematological or other lab abnormalities not meeting the definition of serious
- Potentially important abnormalities that are not serious but nevertheless clinically important, e.g., a single seizure, a syncopal episode, orthostatic symptoms

The events in the first category are objective and the easiest to identify, while the events in the other 2 categories are subjective and require clinical judgment to identify. The events in these last 2 categories are referred to in this chapter as *adverse events of interest*. AEs of interest can at first appear nonserious, clinically unimportant, and easily overlooked if viewed in isolation. If, however, these isolated events are grouped together with other medically similar events and other related safety findings, a different picture can emerge. For this reason, in the Summary of Clinical Safety (SCS), there is a section entitled "Analysis of Adverse Events by Organ System or Syndrome."[2] An analysis of AEs by system organ class (SOC) should also be used in the Periodic Safety Update Report for Marketed Drugs (PSUR).[5,6] This type of review improves the odds of finding that needle in the haystack. What this analysis is, and how to do it, are explained in this chapter.

An Integrated Review

To increase the chance of identifying an uncommon finding, all possible *clues* must be searched for. These clues may be similar AEs with different names, e.g., syncope and loss of consciousness. These clues may appear in different places; e.g., AEs and laboratory tests—hypertension reported as an AE, and an increased trend in blood pressure seen with measurement of blood pressure. All available evidence needs to be presented and integrated together to get the full picture. In Chapter 7, *Determining the Weight of Evidence—Patterns and Links*—ways to look for these clues are discussed.

A Top–Down Approach

A systematic top–down approach should be taken in the analysis and review of deaths, other SAEs, and other significant events. The data should be reviewed going from the more general (group or aggregate information) to the specific (information on individual patients) in the order that follows:

- AE rates by treatment group. Rates should also be calculated using person-years exposure (PYE) if there is an exposure imbalance among the various treatment groups as discussed in Chapter 15.
- Listings or patient profiles (see specifics later in this chapter).
- Narratives.

Complete information should be provided in the appropriate appendices of the report. Selected information, e.g., listings and narratives of treatment-related AEs, should be discussed in the text of the report. What is selected for presentation in the text of the report are data driven with the understanding that one size doesn't fit all. Remember, you are writing a story about the risk of the drug. All the *evidence* supporting the risk assessment should be presented in a user-friendly way that allows the reviewer to reach the same conclusions as you did. So you have to decide which data are best to present. How this is done is illustrated in the sample integrated analysis of safety and PSUR in Appendices II and IV, respectively.

TIP: Deaths, other SAEs, and other significant AEs that are considered treatment related (as judged by the investigator or the sponsor) should be briefly described in the text unless the volume of events is too large to make this feasible (e.g., certain cancer drugs where most or all patients succumb). This gives the reviewer a better understanding of the event. Have a look also at the deaths and other significant AEs that are not considered to be treatment related to be sure that nothing is lurking in there that might, in fact, be treatment related.

What Is an Analysis of Adverse Events by Organ System or Syndrome, and How Does One Do It?

Let's begin by first understanding the meaning of the word *syndrome*. A syndrome is a constellation of signs and symptoms that are associated with a specific disease or syndrome (such as Hermansky Pudlak syndrome) or diseases with the same name but with different causes (such as nephrotic syndrome). A symptom as described in Chapter 7 is a *subjective* abnormal feeling or disturbance of the body experienced and recounted by the patient. Examples include headache, abdominal pain, and dizziness. In contrast, a sign is *objective* evidence of an abnormality that is observed by someone other than the patient. Examples include fast heart rate, elevated blood pressure, hepatomegaly (enlarged liver), an elevated glucose value, and the number, size, and the location of cancer metastases seen with magnetic resonance imaging.

Some syndromes include *syndrome* in the name of the condition; e.g., *neuroleptic malignant syndrome*, a life-threatening condition associated with the use of antipsychotic medication, while others do not, e.g., rhabdomyolysis—a condition associated with severe muscle damage (see Chapter 11 for a description of these events). The use of the word *syndrome* can be misleading because every disease is associated with a constellation of signs and symptoms. For instance, an acute myocardial infarction (heart attack) is associated with chest pain (symptom), elevated cardiac enzymes (sign), and a specific ECG finding (sign). Whether an AE is a specific syndrome or a specific disease is really unimportant. What is important, though, is whether the reported AE represents a *diagnosis* rather than an individual sign or symptom. Signs and symptoms can be nonspecific, and the same ones can be found in many different conditions. Furthermore, signs and symptoms for a specific disease/syndrome can be scattered across many different SOCs, significantly limiting the reviewer's ability to identify discrete medical conditions/syndromes when reviewing AE summary tables grouped by SOCs. The purpose of looking at AEs by organ system or syndrome is to proactively look and identify specific diseases/syndromes from the many individual AE terms found in many different SOCs. In addition to AEs, laboratory test values, vital signs, ECGs, and physical examinations may also reveal findings consistent with a particular syndrome or disease. All these different safety findings should be integrated, i.e., presented together, to determine the weight of evidence for or against a drug-related finding.

These concepts are illustrated by rhabdomyolysis. Rhabdomyolysis as previously mentioned is a condition where muscle tissue is severely damaged. The muscle enzyme *creatine phosphokinase* leaks out of the muscle cell, resulting in elevated blood levels. In some severe cases, *myoglobin* (a protein similar to hemoglobin that binds O_2) also leaks out of the muscle cell. Myoglobin can damage the kidney and cause renal failure. The symptoms of rhabdomyolysis include muscle pain (myalgia) and muscle weakness. The signs of the disease include elevated creatine kinase levels and may also include myoglobin in the blood (myoglobinemia), myoglobin in the urine (myoglobinuria), and evidence of renal impairment, e.g., elevated blood creatinine levels (creatinine is a laboratory measure of kidney function), oliguria (decreased urine output), or even acute renal failure.

Standardised MedDRA Queries (SMQs), if available, provide the AE search terms that best help to identify specific diseases/syndromes, especially if the AEs associated with the disease/syndrome are found in different SOCs. The AE terms included in the SMQ for rhabdomyolysis/myopathy are shown in Table 16-1. There are 45 preferred terms (PTs) found in 6 different SOCs. The PTs that are more specific to rhabdomyolysis are designated as narrow terms; those terms that are less specific (i.e., can be found in other conditions) are referred to as *broad* terms.

Because rhabdomyolysis is associated with muscle damage, creatine kinase (the values obtained from the lab test) should also be evaluated. This is an example of using an integrated approach (i.e., looking at both AEs and relevant laboratory data).

TIP: All relevant safety information including AEs, labs, vitals signs, and ECGs (if applicable) can be displayed in a dashboard fashion to give the medical reviewer a quick and user-friendly overview of the relevant findings in 1 snapshot view as shown in Table 16-2. This type of display helps the reviewer identify data trends and patterns that, if present, add to the weight of evidence of a drug-related finding.

The results from this table show a higher rate of AEs in the investigational drug and active control groups compared to placebo, as well as a corresponding trend toward increases in creatine kinase levels (the types of laboratory analyses shown in this table are discussed in Chapter 17). All these findings increase the weight of evidence that both the investigational drug and active control groups have an adverse effect on muscle.

In the next section, the methods recommended for such searches are described in greater detail.

MedDRA SMQs are not available for all diseases/syndromes; for example there is currently no SMQ for *cytokine release syndrome*; i.e., signs and symptoms that occur within 24 hours of the infusion of monoclonal antibodies (immunotherapy). In these situations, search criteria have to be defined/specified by medical and coding experts. This type of search criteria or query is referred to as an *ad hoc query* (AHQ).

The selection of AE terms to be included in the AHQ requires medical knowledge and sometimes review of the medical literature. The following AEs (based on

Table 16-1 Preferred Terms Included in Standardised MedDRA Query for *Rhabdomyolysis/Myopathy* [a,b]

Injury, Poisoning, and Procedural Complications	Investigations	Metabolism and Nutrition Disorders	Musculoskeletal and Connective Tissue Disorders	Renal and Urinary Disorders	Respiratory, Thoracic, and Mediastinal Disorders
Muscle rupture	*Myoglobin blood increased; Myoglobin blood present; Myoglobin urine present;* Biopsy muscle abnormal; Blood calcium decreased; Blood creatine phosphokinase abnormal; Blood creatine phosphokinase increased; Blood creatinine phosphokinase MM increased; Blood creatinine abnormal; Blood creatinine increased; Creatinine renal clearance abnormal; Creatinine renal clearance decreased; electromyogram abnormal; glomerular filtration rate abnormal; glomerular filtration rate decreased; muscle enzyme increased	Hypercreatinemia; Hypocalcemia	*Muscle necrosis; Myoglobinemia; Myopathy; Myopathy toxic; Rhabdomyolysis;* Compartment syndrome; Muscle disorder; Muscle fatigue; Muscle hemorrhage; Muscular weakness; Musculoskeletal discomfort; Musculoskeletal disorder; Musculoskeletal pain; Myalgia; Myalgia intercostal; Myositis	*Myoglobinuria;* anuria; Chromaturia; oliguria; Renal failure; Renal failure acute; Renal failure chronic; Renal impairment; Renal tubular necrosis	Diaphragm muscle weakness

Italicized terms = narrow terms.
[a] MedDRA version 12.0.
[b] PTs shown in primary system organ class.

a publication in the *Oncologist*) were selected as part of the search criteria for identification of possible cases of cytokine release syndrome.[7]

Because the natural history of the cytokine release syndrome is rapid onset after an infusion, another search criterion should be the time of the event. For cytokine release syndrome, a reasonable time frame would be ≤ 24 hours. So the search criteria established for cytokine release syndrome would be (1) the AEs shown in Table 16-3 and (2) those that occurred within 24 hours of infusion.

Table 16-2 **Dashboard Summary of Changes in Creatine Kinase and Adverse Events Related to Rhabdomyolysis**

	Placebo	ID = 5 mg	ID = 10 mg	ID = 15 mg	Total ID	Active Control
CK (U/L)						
N	2100	2315	2290	300	4905	2095
Baseline mean	144.3	144.7	144.3	145.2	144.5	144.4
Mean change	−0.1	−0.5	−0.8	−1.5	−0.7	2.4
N	2100	2315	2290	300	4905	2095
Categorical shifts[a] L/N to H	109 (5.2%)	167 (7.2%)	202 (8.8%)	30(10.0%)	399 (8.1%)	465 (22.2%)
N	1987	2183	2145	287	4615	1906
Clinically significant increases[b]	10 (0.5%)	17 (0.8%)	25 (1.2%)	5 (1.7%)	47 (1.0%)	63 (3.3%)
Rhabdomyolysis-Related Adverse Events						
N	**2200**	**2450**	**2400**	**325**	**5175**	**2225**
Rhabdomyolysis/ myopathy (SMQ)	11 (0.5%)	37 (1.5%)	50 (2.1%)	9 (2.8%)	96 (1.9%)	129 (5.8%)

[a] Subjects who shifted from a below normal (L) or normal (N) baseline value to a value above normal range (H) during treatment.
[b] Clinically significant change = normal value at baseline and > 3 × upper limit of normal during treatment.

Table 16-3 **Adverse Events Associated With the Cytokine Release Syndrome[3]**

Symptoms	Signs
Pruritus/itching	Allergic reaction/hypersensitivity (including drug fever)
Rigors/chills	Rash/desquamation
Headache	Urticaria (hives, welts, wheals)
Arthralgia/myalgia	Sweating
Tumor pain	Cough
Fatigue (asthenia, lethargy, malaise)	Bronchospasm
Dizziness	Hypotension/hypertension
Nausea/vomiting	Tachycardia
Dyspnea	

Source: Adapted from Lenz HJ. Management and preparedness for infusion and hypersensitivity reactions. *The Oncologist.* 2007;12:601–609.

Based on the results of the search, the original search criteria may need to be broadened or narrowed and the search redone.

For all cases that meet prespecified search criteria, a listing or patient profile (i.e., a more comprehensive listing) for each patient should be provided. This information helps identify common findings across patients and should include the following:

- Patient ID, study number
- Age, gender, race
- Study medication including dose and route of administration
- AE—both the verbatim term and the MedDRA preferred term
- Onset and resolution dates of AE. The study day the event started and ended should also be included
- Whether the AE was serious or not
- Whether the AE led to premature discontinuation
- The intensity of the AE
- Relationship to treatment (as judged by the investigator)
- Outcome of the event
- All concomitant medication that the patient was taking at the time the event of interest occurred. This should include the dates and study days the subject was taking the concomitant medication

■ All other AEs (i.e., AEs other than the event of interest) reported for the patient including AE onset and resolution dates, as well as study days

A summary of your review of the listings (even if nothing of importance was seen) should be provided. For example, "The majority of cases were nonserious, considered unrelated to treatment, did not lead to premature termination, and occurred only in patients taking an HMG-CoA reductase inhibitor (a statin) concomitantly." From this review, further investigation should be done if any unusual findings are seen. In this example, further investigation should be done to determine if the statin was the culprit or there was an interaction between the investigational drug and the statin.

Narratives of deaths, SAEs, AEs leading to discontinuation, and any other significant finding should be provided and put in the appendix of the report. The ones that are considered drug related (as judged by either the investigator or the sponsor) should be briefly described in text or hyperlinked if the report is electronic. The approaches to writing a good narrative are discussed in Chapter 5.

■ How to Summarize Deaths, Other Serious Adverse Events, Other Significant Adverse Events, and Analysis of Adverse Events by Organ System or Syndrome—Clinical Trials

This section explains how to summarize deaths, other SAEs, and other significant advents and how to do an analysis of adverse events by organ system or syndrome. Appendix II, "The Integrated Safety Analysis for Mepro," provides examples of how this is done.

1. Obtain *complete* information in *real time* for *all* SAEs including deaths. Even though SAEs that are unexpected and treatment related are the highest priorities, SAEs initially considered expected and/or unrelated can turn out to be serious adverse drug reactions, which becomes apparent only when all the cases are analyzed together. That is, only after multiple cases or a particular pattern is observed does one realize that seemingly unrelated AEs are really due to the study drug (and are adverse drug reactions). In particular, investigators who see only 1 case of an SAE may not realize that other similar cases may have been reported and the AE judged unrelated is in reality drug-related.

> **CAUTION:** Incomplete case information is all too often found during preparation of an IAS. It is not always feasible to get additional information later on, because the investigator site may no longer be active, or there is insufficient time due to submission deadlines. Discovery of insufficient SAE information at time of the preparation of the IAS is simply too late!

2. Read the following chapters:
   ■ Chapter 4: Coding Basics
   ■ Chapter 5: Determining Causality—The Individual Case Safety Report
   ■ Chapter 6: Determining Causality—Aggregate Data
   ■ Chapter 7: Determining the Weight of Evidence—Patterns and Links
   ■ Chapter 8: Determining Clinical Significance … and Then What?
   ■ Chapter 11: Adverse Events That Should be on Everyone's Radar Screen

3. Present the data for deaths, other SAEs, and AEs leading to discontinuation in a top–down fashion. Start from the general and drill down to the most specific information.
   ■ Provide the rates of these events across treatment groups.
   ■ Provide a separate line listing of all the patients who died, had an SAE, or discontinued study medication due to an AE.
   ■ Provide narratives for all deaths, other SAEs, AEs leading to discontinuation, and any other significant events.

4. For events where there are exposure differences across treatment groups, calculate rates using PYE as illustrated in Table 16-4 summarizing deaths from Phase 2/3 studies. A similar table should also be used for other SAEs and AEs leading to discontinuation. All deaths, other SAEs, and AEs leading to discontinuation must be accounted for. If any occurred in Phase 1 studies, this should also be mentioned in the text of the report.

➡**NOTE:** This table shows the rates of death calculated by crude rate and rate by 100 PYE are similar between the investigational group and placebo and somewhat higher in the active control group).

➡️**NOTE:** Deaths that occur during treatment and within 30 days posttreatment should be included. For posttreatment deaths, the table and listing should be footnoted to indicate the number of posttreatment deaths and when they occurred posttreatment. The 30-day rule is a means of capturing important adverse reactions that are late occurring (*latent*), i.e., that are due to the investigational drug but did not appear until sometime after treatment ended. For drugs with long elimination half-lives, a longer post-treatment follow-up period may be needed.

If a disease process starts during the treatment period or during the period of residual effect post-treatment (i.e., when drug levels are still detectable) and results in death, the death should be captured even if it occurred more than 30 days posttreatment.[1-4] Also note that the 30-day posttreatment period (although stated in guidance documents) is somewhat arbitrary and is used more by tradition than by a clear scientific reason for such a time frame.

5. Refer to guidance documents for the format and content of the listings for deaths, other SAEs, and AEs leading to discontinuation.[1-4] Although similar, the listings for the SCS and and the Integrated Summary of Safety have some minor differences.

6. Place listings and narratives in the appropriate appendices and number them according to the specific regulations/guidances for that report.[1-3]

7. Provide brief in-text narratives of deaths, other SAEs, AEs leading to discontinuation, and other significant AEs that are considered treatment related (by either the investigator or the sponsor), unless the volume of events precludes doing so. If there are too many events, just summarize the rates in the text and/or present a few cases of those that differ substantially from the rest.

8. Provide the patient number and study number whenever mentioning an individual patient in the text; the reviewer can then search for more patient information if warranted.

9. Select the events to be included in the Analysis of Adverse Events by Organ System or Syndrome. Selection criteria are based on a number of factors that include:

   ■ **The pharmacology of the drug**—The mechanism of action, the way the drug is metabolized, excreted etc., provides some direction as to what AEs to include. For example, the mechanism of action for any immunosuppressant is to modify the immune response in some way. Due to this action, there is at least a theoretical risk for infections, autoimmune disease, and malignancies. For a drug with this property, the rates of infections, autoimmune disease, and malignancies should be selected for summary in this section of the report. If nothing is found, this too should be stated in the text.

   ■ **Drug class**—If the investigational drug belongs to a drug class with drugs that are already approved for market, the significant

| Table 16-4 | **Summary of Deaths—All Phase 2/3 Studies** | | | | |

Treatment Group	Total Number of Patients	Total Number of Deaths	Crude Mortality Rate	Person-Years Exposure (PYE)	Mortality per 100 PYE
Placebo	2200	2	0.10%	947.8	0.21
Investigational drug	5410	4[a]	0.07%	3433.8	0.12
Active control	2225	7[b]	0.31%	1221.6	0.57

[a] One death occurred 17 days posttreatment.
[b] One death occurred 23 days posttreatment.

risks known for the drug class should be discussed. For example, if the investigational drug is a member of the nonsteroidal anti-inflammatory drug class of drugs, the AEs that should be discussed include:

- Gastrointestinal perforations, ulcers, and bleeds
- Cardiovascular and cerebrovascular disease
- Hematologic effects (anemia, platelet function)
- Hepatic effects
- Renal effects
- Hepatic effects
- Congestive heart failure and edema
- Hypertension
- Anaphylaxis
- Skin reactions
- Preexisting asthma

- Include any of the AEs discussed in Chapter 11 "Adverse Events That Should Be on Everyone's Radar Screen," e.g., seizures, hepatotoxicity, renal toxicity, severe skin reactions, torsades, etc., if reported, even if the investigator considered these events to be nonserious and/or unrelated to treatment.

- Include other *adverse events of interest*—The selection of these events is based on the safety data findings and clinical judgment. What specific approach to take cannot be precisely defined.

TIP: Put your detective hat on and be alert for anything that catches your eye (anything unusual or unexpected). Keep digging for answers until you feel you have explored the data to your satisfaction. Once you complete your investigation, make a decision whether this event qualifies in your opinion as an AE of interest.

TIP: One suggestion is to start by looking at those AEs that are reported in 3 or more subjects in the investigational group and none in the placebo group. Note, however, that even if you identify cases it may mean nothing, especially if exposure is 3 times greater in the investigational group compared to placebo. Depending on exposure

differences, you may want to start at 4, 5, or more subjects rather than at 3—what number to pick is totally arbitrary. This approach is not scientific by any means—it is just a starting point—a way to provide some focus and organization to your review.

---

10. Consider the following methodology for searching, counting, and reviewing cases included in the Analysis of Adverse Events by Organ System or Syndrome:

- State the SMQ used for the event of interest (if one is available) and whether the search is limited to only narrow terms or all terms. Sometimes the SMQ may not be just right, and you may want to modify the SMQ is some way; i.e., use a modified SMQ (mSMQ). If you decide to modify the SMQ, describe the terms that were added or deleted from the original SMQ.

- If there is no SMQ for the event of interest, do a literature search or establish your own AHQ, and state the specific terms included in the AHQ. Make sure one or more experts knowledgeable in the disease(s) in question and in MedDRA are involved in the selection of terms to be sure the right terms in the AHQ are correct.

- Calculate the rate for any subject with at least 1 event included in the SMQ, mSMQ, or AHQ. If the subject reports the same event more than once or reports more than 1 event within the SMQ, mSMQ, or AHQ, the subject should be counted only once in the rate calculation. Rates should be calculated for all

---

CAUTION: Not all AE terms in a query are equal. For example, in the SMQ *Anaphylactic reactions*, Anaphylaxis is included, as are *Cough and Sneezing*. Anaphylaxis is a life-threatening condition, while cough and sneezing are nonspecific events that are typically nonserious. For this reason, it is important to review a listing/patient profile of all subjects who were identified in the search and were included in the rate calculation. It is also important to specify how many events were serious, led to discontinuation, and were considered treatment related.

treatment groups and compared for treatment differences as shown in Table 16-2.

■ Specify a time frame as part of the search criteria. For example, for events that are acute in onset, e.g., immediate-type hypersensitivity reactions, you may want to limit the search to only those events that occurred within ≤ 24 hours; for events with no known specific time to onset, you may want to use a broader search criterion, e.g., AEs that occurred anytime during the treatment period or within the residual effect of the drug.

■ If there is an imbalance in exposure across treatment groups, rates should also be calculated using 100 PYE.

■ A listing for all subjects identified in the search should be provided. The listing should include information shown in the previous section of this chapter.

■ Summarize the methodology used in the text (including the AE terms selected). If the methodology is too long, put it in an appendix and reference the location in the text.

■ Summarize in the text the relevant findings of the search.

TIP: Remember to make preemptive strikes in interpreting the data. If you think the data will raise any concerns, discuss the issue *before* you get a regulatory request for more information. State whether you think the finding is real, a red herring (false finding), or that you simply do not know what to make of the data at this time, and provide the *evidence* supporting your conclusion. Remember, if you have a question regarding the data, the health authority is likely to have the same question.

■ How to Summarize Deaths, Other Serious Adverse Events, Other Significant Adverse Events, and Analysis of Adverse Events by Organ System or Syndrome—Postmarketing

This section explains how to summarize postmarketing deaths, other SAEs, other significant AEs, and do

an analysis of AEs by organ system or syndrome. Appendix IV, "6-Month Periodic Safety Update Report—Mepro," provides examples of how the data can be summarized.

1. Review the chapters recommended in the previous section.

2. Develop a detailed questionnaire for all AEs discussed in Chapter 11. Add AEs of interest to this list based on the known or theoretical risks of the drug. Drug safety associates or call center personnel responsible who collect postmarketing reports should be trained on these questionnaires so that maximum case information is collected when talking with the reporter.

3. Focus your review to determine if the benefit–risk profile has changed, based on the following:

   ■ A new safety finding is identified

   ■ The characteristics of a known risk have changed; e.g., the risk is more frequent, more severe, more specific (drug-induced nephrotic syndrome rather than drug-induced renal failure)

4. In the PSUR, give priority attention to unlisted AEs, especially serious unlisted events. *Unlisted* means that the AE is not found in the *company's core safety information* in effect during the reporting period of the PSUR. An unlisted event can signal a new or previously unidentified safety finding. If the unlisted event is also serious, this can indi-

---

CAUTION: Realize that the same AE term can be categorized as both serious and nonserious, e.g., anemia. One case of anemia may have required hospitalization (serious), while another was not severe enough to cause hospitalization (nonserious) but had similar characteristics to the first case. AEs that fall into the medically important category where some degree of clinical judgment is required can also lead to different classifications of the same event. This issue is further compounded in large multinational companies where handling of postmarketing reports is done locally rather than centrally. For this reason, it is important to evaluate all similar AE terms regardless of whether they are serious or nonserious events. It is also important not to dismiss or ignore listed events because increased frequency and/or severity of listed events can also signal an important change in the risk profile as discussed in Chapters 6 and 15.

cate a clinically important finding that can potentially affect the benefit–risk profile. For these reasons, brief narratives of serious unlisted events should be included in the text of the PSUR.

5. Include all serious unlisted AEs (and any other events you consider relevant) organized by SOC in the "Overall Safety Evaluation" of the PSUR.[5,6] If already mentioned in a different section(s) of the report, cross-reference to this section.

6. Follow the methods described in the previous sections for Analysis of Adverse Events by Organ System or Syndrome to identify AEs of interest that should be included in the Overall Safety Evaluation of the PSUR.

7. Include brief narratives of serious and significant unlisted AEs in the text of the PSUR.

References

1. International Conference on Harmonisation of Technical Requirements for Registration of Pharmaceuticals for Human Use. *Structure and Content of Clinical Study Reports E3.* Geneva, Switzerland; ICH Secretariat: November 1995. http://www.ich.org/cache/compo/276-254-1.html. Accessed March 26, 2010.

2. International Conference on Harmonisation of Technical Requirements for Registration of Pharmaceuticals for Human Use. *The Common Technical Document for the Registration of Pharmaceuticals For Human Use—Efficacy—M4E (R1) Clinical Overview and Clinical Summary of Module 2 Module 5: Clinical Study Reports.* Geneva, Switzerland; ICH Secretariat: September 2002. http://www.ich.org/cache/compo/276-254-1.html. Accessed March 26, 2010.

3. Center for Drug Evaluation and Research, Food and Drug Administration, Department of Health and Human Services. *Guideline for the Format and Content of the Clinical and Statistical Sections of an Application.* 1988. http://www.fda.gov/downloads/Drugs/Guidance ComplianceRegulatoryInformation/Guidances/ UCM071665.pdf. Accessed March 26, 2010.

4. Center for Drug Evaluation and Research, Food and Drug Administration, Department of Health and Human Services. *Guideline for Conducting a Clinical Safety Review of a New Product Application and Preparing a Report on the Review.* 2005. http://www.fda.gov/downloads/Drugs/Guidance ComplianceRegulatoryInformation/Guidances/ ucm072974.pdf. Accessed March 26, 2010.

5. International Conference on Harmonisation of Technical Requirements for Registration of Pharmaceuticals for Human Use. *Clinical Safety Data Management: Periodic Safety Update Reports for Marketed Drugs E2C(R1).* Geneva, Switzerland; ICH Secretariat: November 2005. http://www .ich.org/cache/compo/276-254-1.html. Accessed March 23, 2010.

6. Volume 9A of The Rules Governing Medicinal Products in the European Union—Guidelines on Pharmacovigilance for Medicinal Products for Human Use. September 2008. http://ec .europa.eu/enterprise/sectors/pharmaceuticals/ documents/euralex/vol-9/index_en.htm. Accessed March 23, 2010.

7. Lenz HJ. Management and preparedness for infusion and hypersensitivity reactions. *Oncologist.* 2007;12:601–609.

The Analysis of Laboratory Data

In Chapter 9, clinical laboratory tests, and what the tests mean, were discussed. The objective of this chapter is to provide approaches for the analysis of laboratory data. Although the primary focus is on the integrated analysis of safety (IAS), the information presented in this chapter should also be relevant for clinical study reports.

Laboratory evaluations play an integral part in the determination of the risk profile of a drug. Drug-related changes in laboratory tests provide important insights into a drug's toxicity. The findings may be predictable based on the mechanism of action of the drug such as electrolyte abnormalities associated with diuretic use, or they may be idiosyncratic and unpredictable. How a drug is metabolized and eliminated can result in hepatic and renal abnormalities, respectively. Changes in laboratory tests can also signal an allergic or immunologic problem, for instance the development of hemolytic anemia (destruction of red blood cells) with penicillin use. Which laboratory value is affected and whether it is associated with other safety findings provide important *clues* in understanding the risk profile of a drug.

There are no absolute standards across clinical development programs regarding what laboratory tests should be done. The ones discussed in this chapter reflect the more common tests. Based on the profile of your drug, some additional lab tests may be warranted.

■ Pooling Laboratory Data Across Studies

With the knowledge that lab data will eventually have to be pooled for the IAS, plans should be put into place early in the clinical development program to collect data in a way that will facilitate data pooling. Two factors to consider are:

1. The selection of laboratory units that will be used in the analysis of laboratory data
2. The use of central versus local labs

Conventional Versus International System of Units

Laboratory values can be expressed in 2 ways—the conventional or classic units used in the United States and the international system of units (SI units) used in Europe and other countries. Researchers in the United States tend to use a mix of English (e.g., Fahrenheit, feet, and inches) and metric units (e.g., mmol/L), whereas outside the United States, metric units are used almost exclusively. Laboratory values collected from different studies and from different study sites must be in the same units to be analyzed together. For this reason, it should be decided early on what the *standard unit* for all studies should be. Once this decision is made, all laboratory values should be recorded using this standard. If this is not done, the data will have to be converted to the standard unit used for analysis in the IAS. Data conversion increases the risk for errors and takes up valuable time and resources. This can be avoided by using the same standard unit throughout the clinical development program.

Central Versus Local Labs

Central laboratories should be used whenever possible. This reduces the need to deal with many different normal ranges. When data are pooled and different normal ranges are used, data need to be *normalized* to one *standard normal range*. Normalization of the data is the process of converting laboratory values obtained in different studies/sites with different normal ranges, to values based on the standard normal range established for data analysis.[1] This is illustrated in Table 17-1. Because laboratory 1 and laboratory 2 have different normal ranges, the alanine aminotransferase (ALT) values from these 2 labs have to be normalized or converted to the standard normal range used for analysis in the IAS.

Table 17-1 Conversion of ALT Values to Normalized ALT Values			
IAS Standard Normal Range = 0–20 U/L[a]			
	Normal Range	Actual Value	Normalized Value
Laboratory 1	10–60 U/L	60 U/L	20 U/L
	10–60 U/L	110 U/L	40 U/L
Laboratory 2	0–40 U/L	40 U/L	20 U/L

IAS = integrated analysis of safety.
[a] Standard normal range used in the IAS.

Normalization of the data can be complex, error prone, and time consuming. On occasion, the normalization process can result in negative values or have other problems. For a further discussion of these issues and suggestions for resolving them, see Chuang-Stein.[2]

The Types of Laboratory Analyses and Conventions Used

Analysis of laboratory data includes the following:[3–6]

- Determining the *central tendency*; i.e., mean or median changes from baseline
- *Categorical shifts*; i.e., the rate of shifts from a category (below normal, normal, above normal) at baseline to another category during the treatment period (e.g., shifts from normal to below normal values, below normal to above normal values, etc).
- The rate of *clinically significant or markedly abnormal laboratory changes*
- The rate of *laboratory-related adverse events* (AEs)

Mean or Median Change From Baseline

In a mean or median change from baseline analysis, the change from baseline to a treatment visit is calculated for all patients who have a baseline value and a treatment visit. The mean/median change from baseline value is then calculated as the mean (arithmetic average)/median (mid-point) of these changes.

➡ **NOTE:** The mean change from baseline will equal the mean value at a visit minus the mean baseline value, but this property does not hold for the median.

This calculation is done for each treatment visit and at the end point (i.e., the last treatment value obtained). For the IAS, the mean change from baseline to the *worst* (ie., the most extreme) treatment value is also recommended.[6] Mean/median changes from baseline are then compared across treatment groups to determine if there are any differences. Any *meaningful difference* (as discussed in Chapter 6) suggests a potential drug effect.

Categorical Shifts

In a categorical shift analysis, the rate of subjects with lab values that shifted from one category at baseline to

Table 17-2	Categorical Shifts		
Baseline	**On Treatment**		
Low (L)	Low (L)	Normal (N)	High (H)
Normal (N)	Low (L)	Normal (N)	High (H)
High (H)	Low (L)	Normal (N)	High (H)
Low (L) = below normal values; high (H) = above normal values.			

a different category during the treatment period is calculated. All of the possible shifts are shown in Table 17-2. The shaded boxes indicate the categories that show no shifts from baseline to the treatment period. The rates are then compared across treatment groups.

TIP: To simplify this type of analysis, a *modified* categorical shift table is recommended. In the modified shift analysis, the baseline normal (N) categories are combined with the below normal (L) and the above normal (H) baseline categories. Rates are then calculated for subjects who had:

- A high (H) *or* normal (N) baseline value that shifted to a low (L) value during treatment (H/N to L).

- A low (L) *or* normal (N) baseline value that shifted to a high (H) value during treatment (L/N to H).

For this type of analysis, one of the following 2 options needs to be selected:

- **Option 1**: Calculating rates based on change in categories from baseline to end point (i.e., last treatment measurement obtained).

- **Option 2**: Calculating rates based on change in categories from baseline to *any* on-treatment measurement. If option 2 is selected, these additional conventions should be followed:

  - For categorical shifts from L/N to H, the subject is counted only once if the subject has more than 1 high treatment value.

  - For categorical shifts from H/N to L, the subject is counted only once if the subject has more than 1 low treatment value.

- If a subject has both a shift of H/N to L and a shift of L/N to H, the subject is counted in the rates for both types of shifts.

Option 2 is more conservative, and it is the one recommended. Whatever convention is used should be stated in the methods section of the report.

Clinically Significant or Markedly Abnormal Changes

➡ **NOTE:** Throughout the book *clinically significant and markedly abnormal* are used interchangeably.

Important outliers can go unnoticed in the mean change or categorical shift analyses. For example, treatment group mean changes can be small, e.g., a +2 unit mean increase in ALT values, but included in the mean value may be a patient with a very abnormal value, i.e., an ALT value > 20 times the upper limit of normal (ULN). In the categorical shift analysis, any patient with a value above normal, whether it is 1 unit (not clinically significant) or 1000 units (clinically significant) above normal, would fall in the high category. For this reason it is important to identify subjects who have clinically significant/markedly abnormal changes and then determine if the observed rates are different across treatment groups. To do this, criteria defining what a clinically significant/markedly abnormal change is need to be specified. These criteria contain 2 parts: (1) defining at what level a laboratory value is considered clinically significant; and (2) specifying the degree of change from the baseline value. Two approaches can be used—both require clinical judgment. As with most things in medicine and drug safety, once you pick 1 method, stick with it and don't change in the middle of the study or program unless there are compelling reasons to do so.

- **Approach 1:** Include only subjects with normal values at baseline that shifted to a clinically significant value during the treatment period.

  ➡ **NOTE:** If this method is chosen, a listing of all subjects with abnormal baseline values who had clinically significant values during the treatment period should be reviewed. This will ensure that no subjects with preexisting abnormal values that worsened to a clinically significant extent during the treatment period are overlooked.

■ **Approach 2:** For subjects with abnormal values at baseline, specify the degree of change that will be considered clinically significant, e.g., ALT > 3 times the baseline value. To determine the magnitude of change considered clinically significant for each laboratory parameter, clinical judgment is required. For instance, a 25% increase/decrease may be a clinically significant change for potassium but not necessarily for ALT.

For values that meet clinically significant criteria, the next step is to determine how these patients are to be counted. The same options/conventions used for the categorical shift analysis discussed previously should be considered:

■ **Option 1:** Calculate the rate based on the number of patients with clinically significant changes at end point.

■ **Option 2:** Calculate the rate based on the number of patients with clinically significant changes during *any* on-treatment visit. If this option, which is the recommended option, is chosen, these additional conventions should also be followed:

  ▫ If a subject has more than 1 clinically significant change for a given laboratory parameter, the subject is counted only once if the changes are in the same direction, e.g., both increased.

  ▫ If a subject has both a clinically significant increased change and a clinically significant decreased change, the subject is counted in the rates for both types of clinically significant changes.

Laboratory-Related Adverse Events

Laboratory-related AEs should also be evaluated because any real trends in mean changes, categorical shifts, and clinically significant values are also likely to show increased rates of related laboratory AEs. Because of the MedDRA dictionary's convention of having different preferred terms (PTs) for laboratory signs (such as *Blood sodium decreased*) versus laboratory diagnoses (such as *Hyponatraemia*), it is possible to underestimate the true rate of a laboratory-related event if the rates of these terms are calculated separately, because these terms are often used interchangeably. For instance, if the rate of *Hyponatraemia* is 3% and the rate of *Blood sodium decreased* is 1%, the rate for low sodium events is actually 4%. For this reason, for in-text table displays similar lab terms should be combined and

rates should be calculated on these combined terms as discussed in Chapters 4 and 15.

In some cases, using high-level terms, high-level group terms, a Standardised MedDRA query (SMQ), a modified SMQ (mSMQ), or an ad hoc query (AHQ) rather than an individual PT are better options to use and more comprehensive than using a single PT (see Chapter 4 for discussion of SMQs, mSMQs, and AHQs).

Once the AE terms are selected, the conventions used in calculating AE rates described in Chapter 15 should be followed.

Laboratory-related AEs that are serious or lead to premature discontinuation and considered treatment related (as judged by either the investigator or the company) should be discussed in the text of the report.

➡ **NOTE:** The FDA guidance document *Cancer Drug and Biological Products—Clinical Data in Marketing Applications* should be reviewed for cancer studies or other indications where preexisting clinically significant abnormal laboratory values, especially hematology values, are expected. This guidance provides information on the collection and evaluation of laboratory data in these types of studies.[7]

■ An Integrated Approach to Laboratory Analyses

An integrated approach should be used in the analysis of laboratory data. Findings in more than 1 of these analyses strengthen the *weight of evidence* for a drug-related laboratory effect. For this reason, when feasible, a "dashboard" display of all the relevant data should be presented in a way that will aid in the identification of similar trends and patterns. Table 17-3 is a summary of the hemoglobin (Hb) changes and associated AEs for placebo, a fictitious investigational nonsteroidal anti-inflammatory drug (NSAID) that is supposed to have a lower risk of bleeding events than other NSAIDs, and an active control (a fictitious marketed NSAID). Because hematocrit and red blood cell values trend in a similar fashion to Hb, only Hb is shown in the table.

➡ **NOTE:** Notice the denominators [*Ns*] are different for some of these analyses. This difference represents the number of subjects

Table 17-3 Dashboard Summary of Hemoglobin and Related Adverse Events

		Placebo	ID = 5 mg	ID = 10 mg	ID = 15 mg	Total ID	Active Control
Hb (g/L)							
	N	2100	2315	2290	300	4905	2095
Baseline		144.3	144.7	144.3	145.2	144.5	144.4
mean		−0.1	−0.5	−0.8	−1.5	−0.7	−2.4
Mean change[a]							
	N	2100	2315	2290	300	4905	2095
H/N to L		109 (5.2%)	167 (7.2%)	202 (8.8%)	30 (10.0%)	399 (8.1%)	465 (22.2%)
	N	1987	2183	2145	287	4615	1906
Clinically significant decreases[b]		10 (0.5%)	17 (0.8%)	25 (1.2%)	5 (1.7%)	47 (1.0%)	63 (3.3%)
Anemia-related Adverse Events							
	N	2200	2450	2400	325	5175	2225
Erythropenia (SMQ)		11 (0.5%)	37 (1.5%)	50 (2.1%)	9 (2.8%)	96 (1.9%)	129 (5.8%)
Haemolytic disorders (SMQ)		1 (< 0.1%)	0	1 (< 0.1%)	0	1 (< 0.1%)	0
Haemorrhages (SMQ)		5 (0.2%)	24 (1.0%)	52 (2.2%)	11 (3.4%)	87 (1.7%)	103 (4.6%)

[a] Normal baseline value and a clinically significant treatment value.

ID = investigational drug; H = above normal range, N = normal range, L = below normal range.

included in the specific analyses. For the AE analysis, all subjects who received 1 or more doses of study drug were included, whereas for the clinically significant change analysis, only subjects who had a normal baseline value and at least 1 on-treatment lab test were analyzed; consequently the Ns are smaller.

The table shows a decrease in Hb in the mean change, categorical, and clinically significant change analyses in both the investigational drug and active control groups compared to placebo. The changes in the investigational drug group are dose related. Consistent with these findings is a trend toward higher rates for AEs related to erythropenia and hemorrhages (but not hemolytic anemia). Changes in the active control group appear to be consistently greater than those seen in the investigational group. In real life, it is unlikely the data will show this type of consistency across all analyses. Nevertheless, dashboard data displays providing a snapshot view of all relevant data at one glance are reviewer friendly and improve the chances of identifying data patterns and trends.

Further Detective Work

When a laboratory safety signal is identified, further investigation at the individual patient level is warranted because aggregate analyses can hide important information. For instance, the SMQ *Acute renal failure* includes the PT *Proteinuria* that can be a clinically unimportant finding if mild, and *Acute renal failure*, which is always serious and clinically important. Therefore, identifying the specific AEs reported in the SMQ is essential. Similarly, for subjects with markedly abnormal laboratory changes, a transient isolated finding does not carry the same weight as progressive and sustained changes. Temporal association with other information such as other AEs and concomitant medications provide additional insight into whether the finding is treatment related. Examples of this detective work are shown in the information summarized from individual patient listings illustrated in Tables 17-4 and 17-5.

In both examples, each patient has the same clinically significant blood, urea, nitrogen (BUN) value on the same study day. The other information in the listings provides very different pictures of what might be going on. For Subject 1 (Table 17-4), in addition to the markedly abnormal BUN value, the subject also has increased

Table 17-4 **Listing for Subject 1**

Study Day	Creatinine µmol/L	BUN mmol/L	Albumin g/L	Urinalysis	Adverse Events	Concomitant Medications
0 (baseline)	62	2.8	42	Normal	None	None
28	75	2.9	38	Normal	None	None
56	104 (H)	11.1 (H, CS)	51 (H)	SG: 1.030 (H)	Diarrhea, dehydration	None
84 (final visit)	73	3.0	39	Normal	None	None
98 (14 days posttreatment)	72	3.0	45	Normal	None	None

L = value below normal range; H = value above normal range; CS = clinically significant change; SG = specific gravity.

Table 17-5 **Listing for Subject 2**

Study Day	Creatinine µmol/L	BUN mmol/L	Albumin g/L	Urinalysis	Adverse Events	Concomitant Medications
0 (baseline)	62	2.8	42	Normal	None	None
28	170 (H)	10.8 (H, CS)	23 (L, CS)	Protein: 1+	None	None
56 (PT)	185 (H, CS)	11.1 (H, CS)	20 (L, CS)	Protein: 3+	Edema, weight increased, proteinuria	None
70 (14 days posttreatment)	73	3.0	30 (L)	Protein: Trace	None	None

PT = premature termination; L = value below normal range; H = value above normal range; CS = clinically significant.

creatinine, albumin, and specific gravity values. Diarrhea and dehydration are also reported. These results when reviewed in total suggest the changes in renal function tests are due to dehydration secondary to diarrhea (a non-renal cause), rather than due to a direct toxic effect on the kidney. Furthermore, all abnormal values return to normal after resolution of the diarrhea and dehydration while the subject remains on treatment. Table 17-5 shows something very different. In this case there is progressive and markedly abnormal creatinine and BUN values. Albumin values decrease to clinically significant low values, and increasing amounts of protein are seen in the urine. At the same time, edema (fluid in the tissue that is likely due to the loss of albumin), weight gain (presumably due to the increased fluid), and proteinuria are reported as AEs and the subject is prematurely discontinued from treatment. These abnormalities are consistent with the nephrotic syndrome (see Chapters 9 and 11). No concomitant medications or coexistent conditions that might explain these findings are reported. Moreover,

the abnormal findings improve or return to normal after the drug is prematurely discontinued, indicating a *positive dechallenge* (the condition resolves/improves when the drug is stopped). Based on the *weight of evidence* of all these findings, drug-related renal toxicity cannot be ruled out. Because of the magnitude of the laboratory changes, the concomitant AEs, and the need to discontinue treatment prematurely, these findings are also clinically significant (see Chapter 8). These two examples underscore the need to dig deeper into the data when a potential safety signal is identified.

Drug-Induced Liver Injury

Drug-induced liver injury (DILI) is the most frequent cause of safety-related drug withdrawals reported in the past 50 years.[8] The type of DILI of predominant concern is severe hepatocellular damage (damage to the liver cells) as was discussed in Chapters 9 and 11. Enzymes referred to as aminotransferases (ATs) leak out of injured liver cells into the blood. These enzymes, ALT and aspartate aminotransferase (AST), are easily measured by a blood test and are elevated with hepatocellular injury. Generally, elevated ALT or AST values are not uncommon in clinical trials, and are usually not significant or associated with permanent liver injury if mild and transient. The association of clinically significant ALT/AST elevations in association with elevated total bilirubin levels (TBLs), however, is an ominous sign. The liver has a great capacity to clear bilirubin. The presence of elevated bilirubin values in the absence of gallbladder and bile duct disease suggests severe liver damage. Regulatory reviewers are especially on the alert for any evidence of DILI that meets the criteria for *Hy's Law*.[8] Hy's Law was named after Dr. Hyman Zimmerman, a hepatologist, who observed that drug-induced hepatocellular injury (i.e., AT elevation) accompanied by jaundice (a yellowish discoloration of the skin and white part of the eye) due to elevated TBLs had a poor prognosis, with a 10–50% mortality from acute liver failure (in pretransplantation days).[9,10] From this observation, Hy's Law evolved. Cases identified as Hy's Law usually include the following findings:[8]

1. The drug causes hepatocellular (liver cell) injury, generally shown by a higher incidence of threefold or greater elevations above ULN of ALT or AST than the (nonhepatotoxic) control drug or placebo.

2. Among trial subjects showing such AT elevations, often with ATs much greater than 3 times ULN, one or more also show elevation of serum TBL > 2 times ULN, without initial findings of *cholestasis*. Cholestasis refers to the block of bile flow in the bile tract. An example of cholestasis is gallstones in the biliary tract blocking bile flow. The enzyme alkaline phosphatase is usually elevated in biliary tract disease, but not in hepatocellular disease.

3. No other reason can be found to explain the combination of increased AT and TBL, such as viral hepatitis A, B, or C; preexisting or acute liver disease; or another drug capable of causing the observed injury.

According to the FDA, finding 1 Hy's Law case in the clinical trial database is worrisome. Finding 2 is considered highly predictive that the drug has the potential to cause severe DILI when given to a larger population.[4]

Due to the importance of DILI, the FDA issued a guidance indicating the specific analyses that should be done. These are discussed in the next section.

➡ **NOTE:** Any potential Hy's Law case should be considered serious and unexpected and submitted to the FDA as an expedited report.

■ How to Summarize Clinical Laboratory Data—Clinical Trials

This section explains how to summarize clinical laboratory data from clinical trials. Appendix II, "The Integrated Analysis of Safety for Mepro," provides examples of how laboratory data can be summarized for an IAS.

➡ **NOTE:** There are a number of available software tools that can assist in creating user-friendly graphic data displays and help the reviewer drill down to individual or subsets of data of interest. The approaches and conventions recommended in the following steps provide the framework and focus of how clinical laboratory data should be handled regardless of how the data are displayed and should be relevant whether tables, graphs, or figures are used.

1. Review the pharmacokinetic profile of the drug to determine the potential for laboratory abnormalities. For instance, abnormalities in liver function tests and renal parameters are more likely to be seen with drugs that are metabolized by the liver and excreted by the kidney, respectively.

2. If the investigational drug is a member of a drug class with known drug-related lab effects, summarize and discuss these specific lab tests in the text of the report. For instance, nephrotoxicity (kidney injury) is associated with treatment with the class of drugs known as aminoglycosides—antibiotics used to treat serious infections. Consequently, for such drugs the analysis of the renal-related parameters, creatinine, BUN, etc., should be comprehensively summarized in the text rather than sending the reviewer to the appendix for the results of these tests.

3. In the methodology section of the report, describe the conventions used in the analysis of mean/median change, categorical shifts, clinically

significant change analyses, and laboratory-related AEs. The conventions summarized under "The Types of Laboratory Analyses and Conventions Used" are the ones recommended.

TIP: Appendix V provides suggested criteria for clinically significant/markedly abnormal laboratory changes. Some of the criteria shown in Appendix V are based on published recommendations while others are based on clinical judgment; i.e., subjective criteria. Because there is no 1 standard, there may be disagreements among various reviewers as to what constitutes a clinically significant change. Until standard criteria are established, the best that can be done is to clearly show what criteria were used. If a reviewer disagrees, the data can be reanalyzed based on the reviewer's preferred criteria.

TIP: It is both useful and reviewer friendly to group and display laboratory parameters that measure the same organ system or similar physiologic functions together rather than in alphabetical order. This helps in the identification of data trends and patterns. Recommended (but arbitrary) groupings were described in Chapter 9.

TIP: Liver function tests, lipids (excluding high-density lipoproteins), uric acid, creatine kinase, and creatinine values that shift to below normal values are usually of little or no clinical importance.

---

4. Whenever possible in the text, use dashboard displays of the data as illustrated in Table 17-3 and Table 17-6.

5. Prepare and review a listing or patient profile for *each* subject who had one or more clinically significant values (even those subjects with baseline abnormal values). At a minimum, the listing should include values for all visits including baseline and posttreatment, medical history, AEs, and concomitant medications. If the lab parameter is associated with other lab parameters within the same lab grouping (e.g., creatinine, BUN, and albumin), the values for these other lab tests should also be shown in the listing/patient profile. These types of listings provide valuable information as shown in Tables 17-4 and 17-5.

6. Provide a brief description or narrative in the text of the report for any lab-related AE that was serious or led to premature discontinuation and was considered treatment related (as judged by either the investigator or the sponsor). Include the patient number and study number so the reviewer can search for additional information not included in the narrative if warranted. For electronic reports, a hyperlink can be used.

7. If an SMQ, mSMQ, or AHQ is used, review a listing of the subjects identified in the query. Because these queries can include a range of events from nonspecific and nonserious signs and symptoms, e.g., *Blood glucose increased*, to clinically important diagnoses such as *Diabetic coma*, it is important to see the details of the reported events, e.g., actual AE(s), whether the event was serious, severe, considered treatment related, led to discontinuation, etc.

8. To determine DILI, the following conventions and analyses based on the FDA guidance document, are recommended:[8]

   - The rate of subjects with a *normal* baseline ALT value and *any* treatment value $\geq 3 \times$ ULN, $\geq 5 \times$ ULN, $\geq 10 \times$ ULN, and $\geq 20 \times$ ULN*

   - The rate of subjects with a *normal* baseline AST value and *any* treatment value $\geq 3 \times$ ULN, $\geq 5 \times$ ULN, $\geq 10 \times$ ULN, and $\geq 20 \times$ ULN*

   - The rate of subjects with *normal* baseline ALT and AST values with *any* treatment values $\geq 3 \times$ ULN, $\geq 5 \times$ ULN, $\geq 10 \times$ ULN, and $\geq 20 \times$ ULN* for *both* ALT and AST

     * A subject should be counted in only 1 category, e.g., if a subject has an ALT value $\geq 10 \times$ ULN, the subject should be counted only in the $\geq 10 \times$ ULN category and not in the $\geq 3 \times$ ULN or $\geq 5 \times$ ULN categories.

   - The rate of subjects with a *normal* baseline TBL and *any* treatment value above normal value (H).

Table 17-6 **Dashboard Summary of Liver Function Tests and Liver-Related Adverse Events—Controlled Phase 2/3 Studies**

		Placebo	ID = 5 mg	ID = 10 mg	ID = 15 mg	Total ID	Active Control
				Liver Function Tests			
ALT							
	N	1915	2208	2187	261	4656	1988
≥ 3 × ULN		21 (1.1%)	66 (3.0%)	92 (4.2%)	14 (5.4%)	172 (3.7%)	157 (7.9%)
≥ 5 × ULN		2 (0.1%)	7 (0.3%)	7 (0.3%)	2 (0.8%)	16 (0.3%)	12 (0.6%)
≥ 10 × ULN		0	1 (< 0.1%)	0	0	1 (< 0.1%)	0
≥ 20 × ULN		0	0	0	0	0	0
AST							
	N	1898	2190	2165	252	4607	1963
≥ 3 × ULN		28 (1.5%)	61 (2.8%)	95 (4.4%)	13 (5.2%)	169 (3.7%)	167 (8.5%)
≥ 5 × ULN		4 (0.2%)	11 (0.5%)	6 (0.3%)	2 (0.8%)	19 (0.4%)	10 (0.5%)
≥ 10 × ULN		0	1 (< 0.1%)	0	0	1 (<0.1%)	0
≥ 20 × ULN		0	0	0	0	0	0
ALT and AST							
	N	1898	2190	2165	252	4607	1963
≥ 3 × ULN		18 (0.9%)	50 (2.3%)	73 (3.4%)	3 (1.2%)	126 (2.7%)	120 (6.1%)
≥ 5 × ULN		1 (<0.1%)	2 (0.1%)	1 (<0.1%)	0	3 (< 0.1%)	3 (0.2%)
≥ 10 × ULN		0	1 (< 0.1%)	0	0	1 (<0.1%)	0
≥ 20 × ULN		0	0	0	0	0	0
Total bilirubin							
	N	2100	2315	2290	300	4905	2095
N to H		23 (1.1%)	23 (1.0%)	18 (0.8%)	3 (1.0%)	44 (0.9%)	21 (1.0%)
> 2 × ULN		10 (0.5%)	9 (0.4%)	9 (0.4%)	2 (0.7%)	20 (0.4%)	10 (0.5%)
ALP							
	N	1996	2187	2175	282	4644	1981
> 1.5 ULN		44 (2.2%)	52 (2.4%)	44 (2.0%)	7 (2.5%)	103 (2.2%)	40 (2.0%)
	N	1905	2196	2173	259	4628	1976
ALT > 3 × ULN + TBL > 1.5 × ULN							
ALT > 3 × ULN + TBL > 1.5 × ULN		0	0	0	0	0	0
ALT > 3 × ULN + TBL > 2 × ULN		0	1 (< 0.1%)	0	0	1 (< 0.1%)	0
	N	1890	2182	2148	251	4581	1950
AST > 3 × ULN + TBL > 1.5 × ULN		0	0	0	0	0	0
ALT > 3 × ULN + TBL > 2 × ULN		0	1 (< 0.1%)	0	0	1 (< 0.1%)	0
	N	1902	2190	2169	258	4617	1971
Hy's Law ALT > 3 × ULN + ALP < 2 × ULN + TBL ≥ 2 × ULN		0	0	0	0	0	0

Continues

Table 17-6						

Table 17-6 Dashboard Summary of Liver Function Tests and Liver-Related Adverse Events—Controlled Phase 2/3 Studies, Continued

		Placebo	ID = 5 mg	ID = 10 mg	ID = 15 mg	Total ID	Active Control
	N	1888	2181	2147	250	4578	1948
Hy's Law AST > 3 × ULN + ALP < 2 × ULN + TBL ≥ 2 × ULN		0	0	0	0	0	0
Liver-related Adverse Events							
	N	2200	2450	2400	325	5175	2225
ALT or AST > 3 × ULN + Nausea, Vomiting, Anorexia, Abdominal pain, or Fatigue[a]		0	1 (< 0.1%)	0	0	1 (< 0.1%)	0
Possible drug related hepatic-disorders— comprehensive search (SMQ)		11 (0.5%)	29 (1.2%)	24 (1.0%)	4 (1.2%)	57 (1.1%)	53 (2.4%)

SMQ = Standardised MedDRA Query; ID = investigational drug.

[a] To be included, the AE had to occur within +/− 14 days of ALT/AST values > 3 × ULN.

N = number of subjects; N = normal; H = above normal.

- The rate of subjects with a *normal* baseline TBL and *any* treatment value > 2 × ULN
- The rate of subjects with *normal* baseline ALP values and *any* treatment value > 1.5 × ULN
- The rate of subjects with a *normal* baseline ALT value and TBL and *any* treatment values of:
  - ALT > 3 × ULN + TBL > 1.5 × ULN
  - ALT > 3 × ULN + TBL > 2 × ULN
- The rate of subjects with a *normal* baseline AST and TBL values and *any* treatment values of:
  - AST > 3 × ULN + TBL > 1.5 × ULN
  - AST > 3 × ULN + TBL > 2 × ULN
- The rate of subjects with *normal* ALT, ALP values, and TBLS at baseline who meet the following criteria for Hy's Law during *any* treatment visit:
  - ALT > 3 × ULN + ALP < 2 × ULN + TBL ≥ 2 × ULN
- The rate of subjects with *normal* AST, ALP values, and TBLS at baseline who meet the following criteria for Hy's Law during *any* treatment visit:
  - AST > 3 × ULN + ALP < 2 × ULN + TBL ≥ 2 × ULN

- The rate of any subject with *normal* ALT or AST values at baseline and > 3 × ULN of ALT or AST at *any* treatment visit and any of the following AEs (MedDRA PTs): *Nausea, Vomiting, Anorexia, Abdominal pain, or Fatigue,* reported within +/− 14 days of the abnormal AT values.

  If the patient reported the same PT more than once, or reported more than one PT, e.g., *Nausea* and *Vomiting,* the subject is counted only once.

➡ **NOTE:** +/− 14 days is used to identify cases with a temporal association to the abnormal AT values, and also to ensure cases are included even if laboratory changes and AEs are not evaluated/reported at the same time. The selection of +/−14 days is arbitrary. One factor to consider is the time between study visits. The time frame and rationale for its use should be included in the methods section of the report.

- The rate of any subject who reported one or more AEs in the SMQ *Possible drug related hepatic-disorders—comprehensive search*. If the subject reported the same AE more than once or reported other AEs included in the same SMQ, the subject is counted only once.

➡ **NOTE:** The analyses for DILI shown here are based on subjects with *normal baseline values*. If this option is followed, a listing of *all* subjects with abnormal baseline ALT, AST, TBL, and/or ALP who otherwise met the criteria shown previously should be reviewed to ensure none of these subjects had a clinically significant change from baseline.

➡ **NOTE:** The DILI guidance document that these recommended analyses are based on is very helpful. Nevertheless, some gray areas remain. For instance, the document recommends analyzing "elevation of AT in temporal association with nausea, vomiting, anorexia, abdominal pain, or fatigue."[8,p 15] Does this mean any elevation of ALT or AST, or a clinically significant elevation, and if the latter, at what level— >3 ×, >5 × ULN, etc.? The time frame for temporal association as previously discussed is not specified either. Clinical judgment must be used. For these reasons, it is always a good idea to submit your analysis plan to the health authorities for their review and comment.

Table 17-6 is an example of a table display that summarizes these various analyses.

➡ **NOTE:** See Appendix II, "The Integrated Analysis of Safety for Mepro," where this table is duplicated and the table results summarized. Additional detective work is done to further investigate the results shaded in gray. The findings of this investigation are also discussed and provide a synthesis of the key points discussed in this chapter.

9. For any potential case of Hy's Law, a detailed narrative should be done and the following information included[8]:
   - Subject's age, sex, weight, and height
   - Discussion of signs and symptoms related to hepatotoxicity: type and timing to exposure
   - Relationship of exposure duration and dose to the development of the liver injury
   - Pertinent medical history
   - Concomitant drugs with dates and doses
   - Pertinent physical exam findings
   - Test results (e.g., laboratory data, biopsy data and reports, with dates and normal ranges)
   - Time course of serum enzyme and bilirubin elevations (consider tabular and/or graphical display of serial laboratory data)
   - A summary of all available clinical information including, if known:
     - Prior or current history of ethanol use
     - Presence of risk factors for NASH (Nonalcoholic steatohepatitis, e.g., obesity, diabetes, marked hypertriglyceridemia)
     - Evidence for pre- or coexisting viral hepatitis, or other forms of liver disease, prestudy AT values, if available
     - Symptoms and clinical course including follow-up to resolution
     - Special studies (i.e., ultrasound, radiologic examinations, liver biopsy results)
     - Presence or absence of possible confounders, including concomitant illness, and use of concomitant drugs that are known hepatotoxins, such as acetaminophen
   - Discussion of hepatotoxicity as supported by available clinical data and overall assessment of the treating physician, consultants, and applicants as to the likelihood of DILI
   - Treatment provided
   - Dechallenge and rechallenge results, if done
   - Outcomes and follow-up information
   - Copies of hospital discharge summaries, pathology, and autopsy reports

■ How to Summarize Clinical Laboratory Data—Postmarketing

1. Develop a detailed questionnaire for all cases of potential DILI, pancreatitis, acute renal failure, rhabdomyolysis, agranulocytosis, and aplastic anemia (see Chapter 11). The drug safety associates or call center personnel responsible for collecting postmarketing reports should be trained on these questionnaires so that maximum case information is collected when talking with the reporter.

2. Investigate any new safety signals, or any increases in the frequency or severity of lab-related adverse events compared to previous reporting periods, using the methods discussed in Chapters 5–9.

References

1. Chuang-Stein C. Summarizing laboratory data with different reference ranges in multicenter clinical trials. *Drug Inf J.* 1992;26:77–84.

2. Chuang-Stein C. Some issues concerning the normalization of laboratory values based on reference ranges. *Drug Inf J.* 2001;35:153–156.

3. International Conference on Harmonisation of Technical Requirements for Registration of Pharmaceuticals for Human Use. Structure and Content of Clinical Study Reports E3 ICH Secretariat, Geneva, Switzerland. November 1995. http://www.ich.org/cache/compo/276-254-1.html. Accessed March 16, 2010.

4. International Conference on Harmonisation of Technical Requirements for Registration of Pharmaceuticals for Human Use. The Common Technical Document for the Registration of Pharmaceuticals For Human Use—Efficacy—M4E (R1) Clinical Overview and Clinical Summary of Module 2 Module 5: Clinical Study Reports ICH Secretariat, Geneva, Switzerland. September 2002. http://www.ich.org/cache/compo/276-254-1.html. Accessed March 16, 2010.

5. "Guideline for the Format and Content of the Clinical and Statistical Sections of an Application" July 1988. www.fda.gov/downloads/Drugs/GuidanceComplianceRegulatoryInformation/Guidances/UCM071665.pdf. Accessed March 16, 2010.

6. Center for Drug Evaluation and Research, Food and Drug Administration, Department of Health and Human Services. Guideline for Conducting a Clinical Safety Review of a New Product Application and Preparing a Report on the Review. February 2005. http://www.fda.gov/downloads/Drugs/GuidanceComplianceRegulatoryInformation/Guidances/ucm072974.pdf. Accessed March 16, 2010.

7. Guidance for Industry: Cancer Drug and Biological Products—Clinical Data in Marketing Applications. US Department of Health and Human Services, Food and Drug Administration, Center for Drug Evaluation and Research (CDER), Center for Biologics Evaluation and Research (CBER). 2001. http://www.fda.gov/downloads/Drugs/GuidanceComplianceRegulatoryInformation/Guidances/ucm071323.pdf. Accessed March 16, 2010.

8. Guidance for Industry—Drug-Induced Liver Injury: Premarketing Clinical Evaluation. US Department of Health and Human Services, Food and Drug Administration, Center for Drug Evaluation and Research (CDER), Center for Biologics Evaluation and Research (CBER). 2009. http://www.fda.gov/downloads/Drugs/GuidanceComplianceRegulatoryInformation/Guidances/UCM174090.pdf. Accessed March 16, 2010.

9. Zimmerman HJ. Drug-induced liver disease. In: *Hepatotoxicity, The Adverse Effects of Drugs and Other Chemicals on the Liver.* New York, NY: Appleton-Century-Crofts; 1978; 351–353.

10. Zimmerman HJ. Drug-induced liver disease, in: *Hepatotoxicity, The Adverse Effects of Drugs and Other Chemicals* on the Liver. 2nd ed., Philadelphia, PA: Lippincott Williams & Wilkins; 1999;428–433.

18

The Analysis of Vital Signs, Physical Findings, and Other Observations Related to Safety

Vital signs or signs of life are measurements of key bodily functions that determine if we are alive or dead, and if alive, whether we are functioning normally. These measurements include blood pressure (BP), heart rate (HR) or pulse rate (PR), temperature (T), and respiratory rate (RR). Other observations related to safety include physical findings including body weight (BW), body mass index (BMI), physical examinations, and 12-lead electrocardiograms (ECGs). ECGs are discussed in Chapter 10 and Chapter 19.

■ The Measurement of Vital Signs and Body Weight

Vital signs should be measured using correct techniques. This chapter will outline those techniques.

Blood Pressure and Heart Rate

The proper way to measure blood pressure and heart rate is to have the patient rest comfortably for at least 5 minutes. Blood pressure and heart rate are usually measured in the sitting or supine (lying down) position or both (because they may differ). The brachial artery is used for the measurement of blood pressure. The blood pressure cuff is placed above the elbow to measure the blood

> **CAUTION:** The blood pressure cuff used should be the correct size and fit the patient's arm properly. If the blood pressure cuff is too small, the blood pressure readings will be artificially increased; conversely a cuff that is too large will result in readings that are erroneously lower. However, the cuff size used is rarely noted in the case report form. It is wise to note in the protocol that the appropriate (child, adult, obese, etc.) size cuff be used for measurements of blood pressure.

pressure, and the pulse (a measure of heart rate) is measured on the ventral surface (inner aspect) of the wrist, thumb side.

Blood pressure should also be measured for orthostatic changes. Blood pressure values that drop ≥ 20 mm Hg systolic or ≥ 10 mm Hg diastolic measured 3 minutes after the subject stands up are referred to as orthostatic hypotension or postural hypotension.[1] Dizziness, pre-syncope (feeling faint), or syncope (a faint) upon standing may be common presenting complaints in subjects experiencing orthostatic blood pressure changes.

RED HERRING ALERT: It is not unusual to see a healthy and strong football player who wants to donate blood suddenly pass out when he sees the needle! This type of syncope is not uncommon and has several names, which include vasovagal syncope, neurally mediated syncope, and neurocardiogenic syncope. Vasovagal syncope is often triggered in a setting of fear or anxiety, i.e., the drawing of blood. When blood pressure falls, the body's compensatory response is for the heart rate to go up. Paradoxically, fear and anxiety can result in the stimulation of the vagus nerve, which slows the heart rate. The *clue* that distinguishes vaso-vagal syncope from other types of syncope is the heart rate. It slows in vasovagal syncope rather than increases. Vasovagal syncope is not uncommon in healthy, nor-mal volunteers participating in Phase I clinical stud-ies—studies where there are many needle sticks and blood samples taken. These characteristic findings help to distinguish vasovagal syncope from drug-induced syncope.

Respiratory Rate

Respiratory rate is measured by counting the breaths a person takes per minute while the patient is at rest, usu-ally in the sitting position.

TIP: Because a subject can voluntarily control his or her respirations, it is a good idea to count res-pirations when the subject is unaware of it. This is often best done at the same time the heart rate or temperature is measured.

Temperature

Temperature can be measured at different anatomical locations. Oral, rectal, and axillary temperatures can differ by 1 or more degree. For this reason, the study protocol should instruct the investigator to use the same site for temperature measurement throughout the study and to document the method used in the study protocol; e.g., if oral temperatures are taken at baseline, all subsequent temperatures should be obtained the same way. For oral temperatures, subjects should be instructed to avoid any hot or cold beverages before the measurement is taken.

Height and Body Weight

In the measurement of height and body weight, what-ever method is used at baseline, i.e., with or without shoes, should be used throughout the study. If possible, the same scale should also be used throughout. Body mass index (BMI) is derived from height and body weight measurements.

■ Normal and Abnormal Values for Vital Signs and Body Mass Index

Tables 18-1 through 18-5 provide normal and abnormal ranges for blood pressure, heart rate, temperature, respi-rations, and BMI, respectively. Body weight is dependent on age, gender, and height, resulting in different weight categories. For this reason, body mass index values are shown instead.

Table 18-1 Resting Adult Blood Pressure Values[2-4]		
Category	Systolic BP (mm Hg)	Diastolic BP (mm Hg)
Hypotension	< 90	< 60
Normal	90 to < 120	60 to < 80
Prehypertension	120–139	80–89
Hypertension	≥ 140	≥ 90
Malignant hypertension	> 220	> 120

Table 18-2 Resting Adult Heart Rate Values[5]

Category	Heart Rate (bpm)
Bradycardia (slow heart rate)	< 60
Normal	60–100
Tachycardia (fast heart rate)	> 100

bpm = beats per minute.

Table 18-3 Adult Body Temperature Values[6-8]

Category	Centigrade (°C)	Fahrenheit (°F)
Hypothermia	< 35	< 95
Normal[a]	37	98.6
Fever (adult)[b]	> 38	> 100.4
Hyperthermia	> 40	> 104

[a] = average; [b] = rectal.

Table 18-4 Adult Resting Respiratory Rate Values[9]

Category	Respiratory Rate (bpm)
Bradypnea (slow breathing)	< 12
Normal	12–20
Tachypnea (fast breathing)	> 20

bpm = breaths per minute.

Table 18-5 Adult Body Mass Index Values[10,11]

Category	BMI Range (kg/m²)[a]
Underweight	< 18.5
Normal	18.5–24.9
Overweight	25–29.9
Obese	> 30
Morbidly obese	≥ 40

[a] Reference ranges for certain races, e.g., Asians are typically lower than shown in this table.

■ Physical Findings

Physical examinations are typically done at baseline and at the end of treatment, and sometimes during the study. Analyzing these data is usually challenging for the following reasons:

■ There is missing information. Although the protocol states certain examinations should be done (e.g., pelvic and rectal examinations), these are often not performed.

■ Different individuals perform the baseline and end-of-treatment physical examinations. This leads to variability in physical findings based on observer differences. Furthermore, a finding may be listed at the end-of-treatment examination and not during the baseline exam, even though the finding was undoubtedly there, e.g., an old surgical scar at the final exam that was not mentioned at baseline. This type of finding is not clinically important or useful in the determination of a drug effect.

■ The data are often incorrectly analyzed.

CAUTION: Physical examination data are often analyzed in clinically meaningless ways. One example is evaluating changes from baseline by calculating the rate of subjects with a normal exam at baseline and an abnormal exam at the final visit, and the rate of those with an abnormal baseline exam and a normal exam at final visit. Table 18-6 shows how this information is usually displayed.

At first glance this type of information looks useful. The table shows that the rate of subjects with normal baseline exams and abnormal final visit exams is similar to the rate for subjects with abnormal baseline exams and normal final visit exams. In addition, no difference is seen between treatment groups. The problem with this type of table is that abnormal can mean many different things, from the inconsequential—athlete's foot (tinea pedis)—to the clinically important—hepatosplenomegaly (enlarged liver and spleen).

For all these reasons, the aggregate analysis of physical examination findings is limited and usually provides little insight into the risk profile of drugs. A narrative summary of any physical finding that was serious or led to premature termination provides more useful information.

Table 18-6 **Incorrect Way to Summarize Physical Findings Data**

	Placebo N = 100	Investigational Drug N = 100
Normal baseline exam and abnormal final visit exam	10 (10%)	8 (8%)
Abnormal baseline exam and normal final visit exam	11 (11%)	10 (10%)

How to Approach and Handle Vital Signs, Body Weight, Body Mass Index, and Physical Findings Data— Clinical Trials

This section explains how to approach and handle vital signs, body weight, body mass index, and physical finding data from clinical trials. Appendix II, "The Integrated Analysis of Safety for Mepro," provides an example of how this information can be summarized in an integrated analysis of safety (IAS).

1. Review the Investigator's Brochure to understand the drug's mechanism of action and to determine if changes in vital signs, BW, etc. are expected. For example, beta-adrenergic receptor antagonists (beta blockers) block the effects of epinephrine and norepinephrine and decrease blood pressure and heart rate. If an investigational drug has similar properties, a comprehensive analysis of blood pressure and heart rate should be done, and a summary of the results should be included in the text of the report.

2. If the investigational drug belongs to a drug class that adversely affects vital signs, body weight, etc., proactively address this in the text. For instance, if the investigational drug is an atypical antipsychotic drug, a class of drugs associated with weight gain, the analysis results of body weight and BMI should be thoroughly discussed in the text, rather than buried in the appendix of the report.

3. Do the same types of analyses and use the same conventions (unless otherwise specified) described in Chapter 17, "The Analysis of Laboratory Data," for the analysis of BP, HR, T, RR, BW, and BMI. These include:

   - Determining the central tendency—i.e., mean or median changes from baseline for each treatment group
   - Categorical shifts—i.e., the rate of shifts from a category (below normal, normal, above normal) at baseline to another category during the treatment period (e.g., shifts from normal to below normal values, below normal to above normal values, etc.)
   - The rate of clinically significant or markedly abnormal changes. Table 18-7 summarizes clinically significant criteria to consider.

➡ **NOTE:** There is little published information regarding the criteria to use for determining clinically significant/markedly abnormal changes.[12] Some of the criteria used are based on clinical judgment, which is subjective. Because there is no one standard, there may be disagreement among various reviewers as to what constitutes a clinically significant change. Until standard criteria are established, the best that can be done is to clearly show what criteria were used to determine outliers. If a reviewer disagrees with the criteria used, the data can be reanalyzed based on the reviewer's preferred criteria.

   - Rates of adverse events (AEs) related to vital signs, body weight, and physical findings.

Table 18-7 Suggested Criteria for Clinically Significant Changes in Vital Signs

Parameter	Clinically Significant Value[a]	Change From Baseline[a]
Heart rate[12]	≥ 120 bpm	Increase of ≥ 15 bpm
	≤ 50 bpm	Decrease of ≥ 15 bpm
Systolic blood pressure[12]	≥ 180 mm Hg	Increase of ≥ 20 mm Hg
	≤ 90 mm Hg	Decrease of ≥ 20 mm Hg
Diastolic blood pressure[12]	≥ 105 mm Hg	Increase of ≥ 15 mm Hg
	≤ 50 mm Hg	Decrease of ≥ 15 mm Hg
Respiratory rate*	≥ 30 bpm	Increase of ≥ 10 bpm
	≤ 8 bpm	Decrease of ≥ 4 bpm
Body temperature[12]	≥ 38.3°C (101°F)	Increase of ≥ 1°C (2°F)
	≤ 96.8°F (36°C)	Decrease of ≥ 1°C (2°F)
Body weight[12]	None specified	Increase ≥ 7%
	None specified	Decrease ≥ 7%
BMI*	None specified	Increase to a higher BMI category[b]
	None specified	Decrease to a lower BMI category[b]

[a] To be counted in the rate, the subjects have to have a clinically significant treatment value (if specified) *and* the magnitude of change from baseline shown for each parameter.
[b] BMI categories include < 18.5, 18.5 to 25, > 25.
bpm = beats per minute (heart rate) and breaths per minute (respiratory rate); mm Hg = millimeters of mercury; * = clinically significant criteria based on clinical judgment.

Table 18-8 Summary of Some Suggested Combined Terms

Combined Term	Included MedDRA Preferred Terms
Hypertension	Accelerated hypertension; Blood pressure ambulatory increased; Blood pressure diastolic increased; Blood pressure increased; Blood pressure systolic increased; Diastolic hypertension; Essential hypertension; Hypertensive crisis; Hypertensive emergency; Labile hypertension; Malignant hypertension; Prehypertension; Systolic hypertension
Hypotension	Blood pressure ambulatory decreased; Blood pressure decreased; Blood pressure diastolic decreased; Blood pressure systolic decreased; Diastolic hypotension; Hypotension; Orthostatic hypotension
Bradycardia	Bradycardia; Heart rate decreased; Sinus bradycardia
Tachycardia	Heart rate increased; Sinus tachycardia; Tachycardia
Pyrexia	Pyrexia; Body temperature increased
Bradypnea	Bradypnea; Respiratory rate decreased
Tachypnea	Tachypnea; Respiratory rate increased
Weight increased	Abnormal weight gain; Weight increased
Weight decreased	Abnormal loss of weight; Weight decreased

TIP: Due to the convention used in the MedDRA dictionary to have separate Preferred Terms (PTs) for signs and symptoms and others for diagnoses, e.g., *Blood pressure decreased* versus *Hypotension*, it is recommended that some terms be combined in order to minimize any potential for underestimating rates. Table 18-8 provides some suggestions. Whether you use these combined terms or others doesn't matter as long as whatever terms you select are clearly documented. Whenever using a combined term, it should be flagged in the table as shown in Table 18-9. It is also recommended that combined terms be used for in-text summary tables only. AE summary tables located in appendices, referred to as *source* or *reference* tables, should show only the rates for individual (uncombined) PTs. This way the reviewer can refer to the source tables and understand how the rates for the combined terms were derived.

4. Use dashboard displays of the data in the text whenever possible. Table 18-9 provides an example of a dashboard summary of blood pressure changes. The combined terms shown in this table include the PT groupings suggested in Table 18-8.

➡ **NOTE:** Note that the Ns (number of subjects—the denominators) in this table for the calculation of AE rates differ from the Ns used in the mean change, categorical and clinically significant shift analyses. This difference is due to the fact that all subjects who received 1 or more doses of study medical are included in the AE analysis while subjects without a baseline and/or treatment blood pressure measurement are excluded from the blood pressure analyses. This table shows a small but consistent trend toward increased blood pressure in the active control group compared to placebo and the investigational drug group. This is also seen for hypertension-related AEs.

5. Review a listing of subjects included in the rate calculation for any combined term. The terms included in a combined term are not all equal (i.e., the AEs do not always have the same clinical relevance), and it is useful to know what specific events were reported. This is seen for the combined term *"Hypertension"* (shown in Table 18-8), which includes terms that

range from *"Blood pressure increased,"* a nonspecific term that can mean something relatively benign, to *"Malignant hypertension,"* a serious and potentially life-threatening condition.

6. Provide a brief in-text narrative (including subject number and study number) for any serious AE, or any AE that led to discontinuation considered treatment related (as judged by either the investigator or sponsor).

7. Review a listing or patient profile for all subjects who had 1 or more clinically significant changes. At a minimum, the listing should include values for the vital sign of interest for all visits, including baseline and posttreatment; all reported AEs by visit; and concomitant medications by visit. These types of listings can provide valuable information as shown in Tables 18-10 and 18-11 for 2 subjects with the same clinically significant blood pressure changes.

For Subject 1 (Table 18-10), clinically significant decreases in systolic and diastolic blood pressure and an increased heart rate are observed at only 1 visit (study day 56). Dizziness is also reported. The subject was started on the diuretic furosemide at the previous visit (study day 28) because of ankle swelling (coded to *Oedema peripheral*). Because of the decrease in blood pressure, increased heart rate, dizziness, and resolution of the ankle swelling, the furosemide was discontinued. On a subsequent visit, the blood pressure and heart rate were within the normal range and the subject was asymptomatic. The pattern of these changes associated with the use of furosemide suggests the changes in vital signs were due to either the furosemide alone or a potential drug interaction between furosemide and the investigational drug.

This is in contrast to Subject 2 (Table 18-11), who shows progressive decreases in blood pressure and increases in heart rate over time. The subject eventually develops a clinically significant drop in blood pressure associated with syncope (fainting), and the drug is discontinued. There are no other factors such as the use of concomitant medications that explain these findings. One week after the subject is discontinued from the investigational drug, the patient is asymptomatic and blood pressure and heart rate have normalized. These findings are consistent with a positive dechallenge; i.e., signs and symptoms resolve after the drug is discontinued, suggesting a potential drug-related blood pressure effect.

Table 18-9 Dashboard Summary of Blood Pressure Changes—Controlled Phase 2/3 Studies

	Placebo	ID = 5 mg	ID = 10 mg	ID = 15 mg	Total ID	Active Control
N	2122	2392	2305	305	5002	2124
SBP—supine (mm Hg)						
Baseline mean	122.3	122.7	122.3	122.2	122.5	122.4
Mean change[a]	−0.1	−0.1	−0.0	0.5	−0.0	2.4
H/N to L	70 (3.3%)	77 (3.2%)	71 (3.1%)	9 (3.0%)	157 (3.1%)	23 (1.1%)
L/N to H	323 (15.2%)	354 (14.8%)	341 (14.8%)	47 (15.4%)	742 (14.8%)	474 (22.3%)
Clinically significant:						
Decreases	1 (<0.1%)	0	1 (<0.1%)	0	1 (<0.1%)	0
Increases	6 (0.3%)	5 (0.2%)	9 (0.4%)	1 (0.3%)	15 (0.3%)	25 (1.2%)
DBP—supine (mm Hg)						
Baseline mean	77.7	78.2	77.6	77.4	77.9	78.0
Mean change[a]	0.5	0.6	0.4	0.2	0.5	1.0
H/N to L	11 (0.5%)	10 (0.4%)	15 (0.7%)	1 (0.3%)	26 (0.5%)	22 (1.0%)
L/N to H	108 (5.1%)	120 (5.0%)	111 (4.8%)	15 (4.9%)	246 (4.9%)	181 (8.5%)
Clinically significant:						
Decreases	2 (0.1%)	1 (<0.1%)	0	0	3 (0.1%)	0
Increases	2 (0.1%)	3 (0.1%)	2 (0.1%)	0	5 (0.1%)	17 (0.8%)
Orthostatic blood pressure changes	11 (0.5%)	13 (0.5%)	12 (0.5%)	1 (0.3%)	26 (0.5%)	9 (0.4%)
Blood pressure–related adverse events						
N	2200	2450	2400	325	5175	2225
Hypertension*	64 (2.9%)	76 (3.1%)	74 (3.1%)	10 (3.1%)	160 (3.1%)	129 (5.8%)
Hypotension*	11 (0.5%)	15 (0.6%)	14 (0.6%)	1 (0.3)%	30 (0.6%)	4 (0.2%)
Syncope	2 (0.1%)	1 (<0.1%)	2 (0.1%)	0	3 (0.1%)	2 (0.1%)

[a] Worst (i.e., the most extreme) treatment value.

ID = investigational drug; N = number of subjects; SBP = systolic blood pressure; mm Hg = millimeters of mercury; H = above normal range; L = below normal range; N = within normal range; * = combined terms (see Table 18-8 for the Preferred Terms included in the combined terms for Hypertension and Hypotension).

DBP = diastolic blood pressure;* = combined terms.

Table 18-10 Listing for Subject 1

Study Day	Sitting SBP (mm Hg)	Sitting DBP (mm Hg)	Sitting HR (bpm)	Adverse Events	Concomitant Medications
0 (baseline)	120	80	72	None	None
28	118	78	75	Oedema peripheral	None
56	85 (L, CS)	49 (L, CS)	105 (H)	Dizziness	Furosemide
84 (final)	125	82	78	None	None
91 (7 days posttreatment)	122	79	74	None	None

SBP = systolic blood pressure; DBP = diastolic blood pressure; mm Hg = millimeters of mercury; HR = heart rate; bpm = beats per minute; L = value below normal range; H = value above normal range; CS = clinically significant change.

Table 18-11 Listing for Subject 2

Study Day	Sitting SBP (mm Hg)	Sitting DBP (mm Hg)	Sitting HR (bpm)	Adverse Events	Concomitant Medications
0 (baseline)	120	80	72	None	None
28	110	72	85	Dizziness	None
42 (PT, final)	85 (L, CS)	49 (L, CS)	105 (H)	Syncope	None
51 (7 days posttreatment)	122	79	74	None	None

PT = premature termination; SBP = systolic blood pressure; DBP = diastolic blood pressure; mm Hg = millimeters of mercury; HR = heart rate; bpm = beats per minute; L = value below normal range; H = value above normal range; CS = clinically significant change.

Include in the text any relevant findings from the review of listings, e.g., Table 18-11 results. If no relevant findings are seen, indicate this in the text.

TIP: All cases of syncope should be thoroughly reviewed. Syncope has many causes and can range from the benign, such as fainting from seeing a needle, to events leading to death, e.g., torsades de pointes (a life-threatening arrhythmia). For this reason it is important to know the cause of any syncopal episodes and whether these events are considered drug related or not.

■ How to Approach and Handle Vital Signs, Body Weight, Body Mass Index, and Physical Findings Data—Postmarketing

This section explains how to approach and handle postmarketing vital signs, body weight, body mass index, and physical finding data.

1. Develop a detailed questionnaire or script for syncope and the following events that are serious and often life threatening: malignant hypertension; hyperthermia; hypothermia; and the respiratory events summarized in Chapter 11. The drug safety professionals or call center personnel responsible for collecting postmarketing spontaneous reports should be trained on these questionnaires so that maximum case information can be collected when talking with the reporter.

2. Do a search for the AEs listed in step 1 and include all sources of information, e.g., spontaneous reports, literature, reports received from regulatory agencies, postmarketing studies, registries, etc.

➡ **NOTE:** The US Periodic Adverse Drug Experience Report (PADER)[13,14] and the Periodic Safety Update Report for Marketed Drugs (PSUR)[15,16] used in the EU and elsewhere are different in format and content. For instance, for foreign reports, only those that are serious and unexpected are submitted in the PADER, while medically unconfirmed reports from consumers are usually excluded in the case evaluations and tabulations included in the PSUR. Regardless of these differences, it is recommended that all sources of information be used initially for purposes of signal detection and determining whether the frequency, intensity, or seriousness of AEs has changed from the previous reporting period. After this initial evaluation, narrower search criteria, e.g., excluding medically unconfirmed cases, can be used.

3. Utilizing the methods described in Chapters 5–8, determine whether any new safety signals have been identified, or whether the frequency, intensity, or seriousness of AEs related to vital signs, BW, BMI, or physical findings has changed from the previous reporting period.

4. If there is a change in the benefit–risk profile, consider following the options discussed in Chapter 8 that are best suited to your findings.

5. Summarize the results of your review in the periodic report according to the regulations, directives, and guidance documents relevant to your country.

References

1. The Consensus Committee of the American Autonomic Society and the American Academy of Neurology. Consensus statement on the definition of orthostatic hypotension, pure autonomic failure, and multiple system atrophy. *Neurology*. 1996;46:1470.

2. National Heart Lung and Blood Institute. Diseases and conditions index—Hypotension. Bethesda, MD: National Heart Lung and Blood Institute, September 2008. http://www.nhlbi.nih.gov/health/dci/Diseases/hyp/hyp_whatis.html. Accessed April 4, 2010.

3. National Heart Lung and Blood Institute. Diseases and conditions index—High blood pressure. Bethesda, MD: National Heart Lung and Blood Institute, November 2008. http://www.nhlbi.nih.gov/health/dci/Diseases/Hbp/HBP_WhatIs.html. Accessed April 4, 2010.

4. Bisognano JD. Hypertension, malignant. Omaha, NE: Medscape, April 13, 2010. http://emedicine.medscape.com/article/241640-overview. Accessed April 28, 2010.

5. Medline Plus. Pulse. Bethesda, MD: US National Library of Medicine, February 22, 2009. http://www.nlm.nih.gov/medlineplus/ency/article/003399.htm. Accessed April 4, 2010.

6. Medline Plus. Body temperature normals. Bethesda, MD: US National Library of Medicine, February 1, 2009. http://www.nlm.nih.gov/medlineplus/ency/article/001982.htm. Accessed April 4, 2010.

7. Edelstein JA, Li J, Silverberg MA, Decker W. Hypothermia. Omaha, NE: Medscape, October 29, 2009. http://emedicine.medscape.com/article/770542-overview. Accessed April 4, 2010.

8. Chan TC, Evans SE, Clark RF. Drug-induced hyperthermia. *Crit Care Clin.* 1997;13(4):785-808.

9. Goldberg, C. A practical guide to clinical medicine: Vital signs. San Diego: University of California, San Diego, June 11, 2009. http://meded.ucsd.edu/clinicalmed/vital.htm#Respiratory. Accessed April 4, 2010.

10. National Heart Lung and Blood Institute. Calculate your body mass index. Bethesda, MD: National Heart Lung and Blood Institute. http://www.nhlbisupport.com/bmi/. Accessed April 4, 2010.

11. World Health Organization (WHO). BMI classification. Geneva, Switzerland: WHO, April 28, 2010. http://apps.who.int/bmi/index.jsp?introPage=intro_3.html. Accessed April 28, 2010.

12. US Food and Drug Administration (FDA). Supplementary suggestions for preparing an integrated summary of safety information in an original NDA submission and for organizing information in periodic safety updates (Leber guidelines). Rockville, MD: FDA; 1987.

13. US Food and Drug Administration (FDA). Code of Federal Regulations title 21, Part 314—Applications for FDA approval to market a new drug, subpart B—Applications, sec. 314.80—Postmarketing reporting of adverse drug experiences. Silver Spring, MD: FDA, April 1, 2009. http://www.accessdata.fda.gov/scripts/cdrh/cfdocs/cfcfr/CFRSearch.cfm?fr=314.80. Accessed April 6, 2010.

14. US Food and Drug Administration (FDA). Draft guidance for industry: postmarketing safety reporting for human drug and biological products including vaccines. Washington, DC: FDA, March 2001. http://www.fda.gov/BiologicsBloodVaccines/Guidance

ComplianceRegulatoryInformation/Guidances/Vaccines/ucm074850.htm. Accessed April 6, 2010.

15. International Conference on Harmonisation of Technical Requirements for Registration of Pharmaceuticals for Human Use. *Clinical Safety Data Management: Periodic Safety Update Reports for Marketed Drugs E2C (R1)*. Geneva, Switzerland: ICH Secretariat; November 2005. http://www.ich.org/cache/compo/276-254-1.html. Accessed April 6, 2010.

16. Volume 9A of The Rules Governing Medicinal Products in the European Union—Guidelines on Pharmacovigilance for Medicinal Products for Human Use. September 2008. http://ec.europa.eu/enterprise/sectors/pharmaceuticals/documents/eudralex/vol-9/index_en.htm. Accessed April 6, 2010.

The Analysis of Electrocardiogram Data

In Chapter 10, we discussed 12-lead electrocardiograms (ECGs), including what is measured and what those measurements mean. The objective of this chapter is to provide approaches for the analysis of ECG data. Although the primary focus is on the integrated analysis of safety (IAS), the information presented in this chapter should also be relevant for clinical study reports (CSRs).

■ How to Approach and Handle ECG Data—Clinical Trials

This section explains how to approach and handle ECG data from clinical trials. Appendix II, "The Integrated Analysis of Safety for Mepro," provides an example of how ECG data can be summarized in an IAS.

1. Read Chapter 10, "12-Lead Electrocardiograms— What Is Measured; What It Means."

2. Review the Investigator's Brochure:

- For information from nonclinical cardiac and ECG studies, with a particular focus on whether the studies showed a potential for prolongation of the QT/QTc (QT corrected) interval.[1]

- For an understanding of the drug's pharmacological profile. If an investigational drug shows a drug-related effect on ECG parameters and this effect is dose-related, any interference with the metabolism and elimination of the investigational drug by another drug (a drug–drug interaction) may cause problems. See "The Terfenadine Story" in Chapter 20.

3. If a thorough QT/QTc study[2] was done, review the relevant study results for inclusion in the text of the IAS.

4. Determine if the investigational drug belongs to a drug class that adversely affects ECG parameters, and proactively address this in the text. For instance, if the investigational drug belongs to a class of drugs associated with prolongation of the pulse rate (PR) interval, discuss the analysis results for this parameter thoroughly in the text, rather than bury it in the appendix of the report.

5. Do the same types of analyses and use the same conventions (unless otherwise specified) described in Chapter 17 for the analysis of laboratory tests for the following ECG parameters: heart rate (HR), PR interval, and QRS complex. These analyses include:

■ Determining the central tendency; i.e., mean or median changes from baseline for each treatment group.

■ Categorical shifts; i.e., the rate of shifts from a category (below normal, normal, above normal) at baseline to another category during the treatment period (e.g., shifts from normal to below normal values, below normal to above normal values, etc.)

■ The rate of clinically significant or markedly abnormal ECG changes. Table 19-1 summarizes suggested clinically significant ECG criteria.

➡ **NOTE:** There is little published information regarding the criteria to use for determining clinically significant/markedly abnormal changes.[3] Most of the criteria used are based on clinical judgment, which is subjective. Because there is no one standard, there may be disagreement among various reviewers as to what constitutes a clinically significant change. Until standard criteria are established, the best that can be done is to clearly document the criteria used to determine outliers. If a reviewer disagrees, the data can be reanalyzed based on the reviewer's preferred criteria.

■ Rates of ECG-related adverse events (AEs).

TIP: Combining MedDRA Preferred Terms (PTs) that are medically alike, or are due to a similar underlying mechanism, is recommended. This minimizes under-estimating AE rates. Table 19-2 provides some suggestions for combined terms. Whether you use these combined terms or others doesn't matter, as long as whatever terms you select are clearly documented. Whenever using a combined term, this should be flagged in the table as a combined term as shown in Table 19-3. It is also recommended that combined terms be used for in-text summary tables only. AE summary tables located in appendices, referred to as *source* or *reference* tables, should show only the rates for individual (uncombined) PTs. In this way the reviewer can refer to the source tables and understand how the rates for the combined terms were derived.

Table 19-1 **Suggested Criteria for Clinically Significant ECG Changes (Excluding QTc)**

ECG Parameter	Clinically Significant Change
Heart rate[3]	120 bpm during treatment *and* an increase of ≥ 15 bpm from baseline
	50 bpm during treatment *and* a decrease of ≥ 15 bpm from baseline
PR interval*	< 120 ms (< 0.12 s) during treatment *and* a normal baseline value
	> 210 ms (> 0.21 s) during treatment *and* a normal baseline value
QRS complex*	> 110 ms (> 0.11 s) during treatment *and* a normal baseline value

ms = milliseconds; s = seconds; bpm = beats per minute.; * = clinically significant criteria based on clinical judgment.

Table 19-2 **Summary of Some Suggested Combined Terms**

Combined Term (CT)	Included MedDRA Preferred Terms
Bradycardia	Bradycardia; Heart rate decreased; Sinus bradycardia
Tachycardia	Heart rate increased; Sinus tachycardia; Tachycardia
Atrioventricular block	Atrioventricular block; Atrioventricular block first degree; Electrocardiogram PR interval prolonged; Atrioventricular block second degree; Atrioventricular block complete; AV dissociation
Bundle branch block	Bundle branch block; Bifascicular block; Bundle branch block bilateral; Bundle branch block left; Bundle branch block right; QRS complex prolonged; Trifascicular block

6. Review a listing of subjects included in the rate calculation for any combined term. Not all terms are equal. For instance, both "*Atrioventricular block first-degree*" and "*Atrioventricular block complete*" are included in the combined term "*Atrioventricular block*." The first event is often an incidental, non-serious finding requiring no treatment, while "*Atrioventricular block complete*" is a serious event requiring insertion of a pacemaker.

7. Provide a dashboard summary of the results of the ECG analyses as shown in Table 19-3 for the PR interval. This provides an overview of the data and aids in the identification of data trends.

➡ **NOTE:** Look at the Ns (number of subjects—denominators) for each analysis; they differ because the number of subjects included in each analysis is different. To be included in the mean and categorical ECG analyses, a subject has to have a minimum of a baseline ECG and at least one ECG during the treatment period, whereas any subject who received at least one dose of study medication is included in the

AE analysis. The Ns for the mean and categorical ECG analyses are less than the Ns for the AE analysis, indicating that some subjects did not have baseline and/or treatment ECGs. Furthermore, for the calculation of the rates of subjects with clinically significant changes, only subjects with normal baseline values are included in this table, and those with abnormal baseline values are excluded. Therefore, the Ns for the clinically significant analysis are less than the Ns for the mean change and categorical shift analyses.

RED HERRING ALERT: Be suspicious of heart rate data from ECGs and vital sign measurements that go in opposite directions. Heart rate changes should trend in the same direction in both analyses; e.g., if vital sign data show heart rate is trending up, so should heart rate data measured by an ECG, and vice versa.

Table 19-3	**Dashboard Summary of the PR Interval**					
		Placebo	ID = 5 mg	ID = 10 mg	ID = 15 mg	Total ID	Active Control
PR interval (ms)							
	N	2005	2254	2195	270	4719	2024
Baseline mean		161.4	159.8	160.4	159.0	160.1	160.8
Mean change[a]		0.9	0.8	0.9	0.9	0.9	0.8
	N	2005	2254	2195	270	4719	2024
L/N to H		24 (1.2%)	23 (1.0%)	24 (1.1%)	2 (0.7%)	49 (1.0%)	20 (1.0%)
	N	1956	2201	2134	265	4600	1998
Clinically significant increases[b]		4 (0.2%)	4 (0.2%)	9 (0.4%)	0	13 (0.3%)	6 (0.3%)
PR-related Adverse Events							
	N	2200	2450	2400	325	5175	2225
Atrioventricular block*		7 (0.3%)	10 (0.4%)	5 (0.2%)	7 (2.2%)	22 (0.4%)	9 (0.4%)

[a] Based on worst treatment value.

[b] Subjects with normal baseline values.

* Combined term and includes the Preferred Terms: *Atrioventricular block; Atrioventricular block complete; Atrioventricular block first degree; Atrioventricular block second degree; AV dissociation;* and *Electrocardiogram PR prolongation.*

N = number of subjects; ID = investigational drug; ms = milliseconds; L = below normal range; N = within normal range; H = above normal range.

8. To determine QT/QTc prolongation, the following conventions and analyses based on the guidance, *The Clinical Evaluation of QT/QTc Interval Prolongation and Proarrhythmic Potential for Non-Antiarrhythmic Drugs E14*, are recommended:[2]

➡ **NOTE:** More that one correction formula, e.g., Bazett, Fridericia, or others, should be used for each of these analyses.

- Mean change from baseline calculated for the largest time-matched mean treatment difference between the investigational drug and placebo. Another way to evaluate central tendency is to analyze the change from baseline that occurred around the Cmax (maximum concentration) of the investigational drug.

- Categorical analyses based on the following:
  - The rate of subjects with normal baseline values and any treatment value of > 450 milliseconds, > 480 milliseconds, and > 500 milliseconds.
  - The rate of subjects with above-normal baseline values and any treatment value > 450 milliseconds, > 480 milliseconds, and > 500 milliseconds.
  - The rate of subjects with normal baseline values and an increase of any treatment value of > 30 milliseconds and > 60 milliseconds from baseline.
  - The rate of subjects with above-normal baseline values and any treatment value of > 30 milliseconds and > 60 milliseconds from baseline.

➡ **NOTE:** In each of these analyses, if a subject had more than one treatment value in a specific category, e.g., > 450 milliseconds, the subject should be counted only once for that category. If a subject had treatment values in more than one category, the subject should be counted in the worst (i.e., the most extreme) category.

- Rates of QT/QTc-related AEs should be calculated for all subjects who reported one or more PTs included in the standardised MedDRA query (SMQ) *Torsade de pointe/QT prolongation*. If a subject reported the same PT more than once, the subject should only be counted once. If a subject reported more than 1 PT within the SMQ, the subject should only be counted once.

- Any subject with QTc values > 500 milliseconds should be identified by patient number, study number, and treatment group in the text of the report and a description of the finding should be provided.

A dashboard display of the QTc analysis results is recommended as shown in Table 19-4.

Table 19-4 shows a summary of the results using Bazett's correction formula for subjects with normal baseline QTc values. A separate analysis of subjects with abnormal baseline QTc values and categorical shifts during treatment also needs to be done. These analyses also have to be run using more than 1 correction formula, because results can differ using different correction formulas.

The gray areas highlight the results that require further investigation, i.e., the subject with a QTc value > 500 ms and all the subjects included in the SMQ *Torsade de pointes/QT prolongation*. The terms included in the SMQ can range from a nonspecific term such as syncope, which can be due to noncardiac causes, to torsades de pointes (TdP) and ventricular fibrillation (VF), which are life-threatening arrhythmias. For this reason, a listing or patient profile including, at the very least, the verbatim term of the event, whether the event was serious and/or led to discontinuation should be prepared and reviewed. The investigator's causality assessment should also be provided. An example of how this is done is shown in Appendix II, "The Integrated Analysis of Safety for Mepro."

9. Include in the text brief narratives for any serious AE, or any AE that led to premature discontinuation considered to be treatment related (as judged by either the investigator or sponsor).

10. Prepare and review listings/patient profiles for subjects with the following ECG/QTc findings:
- Clinically significant changes
- QTc values > 500 ms
- Any other finding that suggests a potential safety signal

At a minimum, the listing should include the values for the relevant ECG/QTc finding for all visits including

Table 19-4	**Summary of QTc (Bazett) Results—Controlled Phase 2/3 Studies**					
	Placebo	ID = 5 mg	ID = 10 mg	ID = 15 mg	Total ID	Active Control
N	2005	2254	2195	270	4719	2024
Mean Changes						
QTc ms (B)						
N	2005	2254	2195	270	4719	2024
Baseline mean	403.2	403.1	401.1	402.9	402.1	403.8
Mean change[a]	0.9	0.8	0.9	0.4	0.9	0.8
Categorical Shifts[b]						
N	1910	2105	1991	249	4345	1901
QTc (B) > 450[a]	29 (1.5%)	21 (1.0%)	24 (1.2%)	4 (1.6%)	49 (1.1%)	25 (1.3%)
QTc (B) > 480[a]	10 (0.5%)	8 (0.4%)	8 (0.4%)	1 (0.4%)	17 (0.4%)	6 (0.3%)
QTc (B) > 500[a]	1 (< 0.1%)	0	0	0	0	0
QTc(B) > 30[a]	27 (1.4%)	32 (1.5%)	24 (1.2%)	4 (1.6%)	60 (1.4%)	27 (1.4%)
QTc(B) > 60[a]	4 (0.2%)	6 (0.3%)	4 (0.2 %)	2 (0.8%)	12 (0.3%)	6 (0.3%)
Torsade de Pointes/QT Prolongation - Related AEs						
N	2200	2450	2400	325	5175	2225
Torsade de pointes/QT prolongation (SMQ)	2 (0.1%)	2 (0.1%)	1 (< 0.1%)	0	3 (0.1%)	2 (0.1%)

[a] Based on worst (i.e., most extreme) treatment value.
[b] Based on subjects with normal baseline values.
N = number of subjects; (B) = Bazett's correction. ID = investigational drug.

baseline and posttreatment; AEs reported during the study by visit; and concomitant medications reported by visit. Information organized in this fashion helps the reviewer identify data patterns that can suggest a drug effect. This is illustrated in Table 19-5 and Table 19-6 for 2 subjects—both with the same clinically significant change in PR interval.

In Table 19-5, a clinically significant PR interval is seen only on 1 day—study day 56. Because this is the only abnormal PR value noted, it is hard to form any firm conclusions from this case. Although the increased PR interval could conceivably be drug related, it appears to be transient (even with continued treatment), and there is no other information, e.g., adverse events or concomitant medications, that provides any more insight for the clinically significant change.

Table 19-6 shows a different pattern for Subject 2. Although there is only 1 abnormal value, the pattern of change in this case suggests a progressive incremental increase over time, with no alternative explanation for the change. Also, the PR interval returns to normal after treatment is stopped, indicating a positive dechallenge. This pattern of change is suggestive of a potential drug effect.

Include in the text any relevant findings from the review of listings, e.g., Table 19-6 results. If no relevant findings are seen, indicate this in the text.

11. For an IAS, the following information should be included in the ECG section of the report:
    - A summary of relevant ECG/QTc findings from nonclinical studies
    - A summary of the results from the "thorough QT/QTc study" (if one was done)
    - The results from the analysis of ECG data from Phase 2/3 studies
    - Any relevant Phase 1 findings
    - Any relevant postmarketing findings (if postmarketing data are available)

Table 19-5 Listing of PR Values for Subject 1

Study Day	PR Interval	Adverse Events	Concomitant Medications
0 (baseline)	180 ms	None	None
28	120 ms	None	None
56	240 ms (H, CS)	None	None
84 (last day of treatment)	160 ms	None	None
91 (7 days posttreatment)	180 ms	None	None

H = value above normal range; CS = clinically significant change; ms = milliseconds.

Table 19-6 Listing of PR Values for Subject 2

Study Day	PR Interval	Adverse Events	Concomitant Medications
0 (baseline)	120 ms	None	None
28	160 ms	None	None
56	200 ms	None	None
84 (last day of treatment)	240 ms (H, CS)	None	None
91 (7 days posttreatment)	180 ms	None	None

H = value above normal range; CS = clinically significant change; ms = milliseconds.

How to Approach and Handle ECG Data—Postmarketing

In this section, ways to approach and handle postmarketing data that may be ECG related are discussed.

1. Develop scripts or questionnaires for all cases of syncope, seizures, life-threatening ventricular arrhythmias (ventricular tachycardia including TdP, VF, ventricular flutter), cardiac arrest, and sudden death. The drug safety associates or call center personnel responsible for collecting postmarketing spontaneous reports should be trained on these questionnaires so that maximum case information can be collected.

2. Search all sources of postmarketing data, e.g., spontaneous reports, publications, reports received from regulatory agencies, postmarketing studies, registries, etc.

➡ **NOTE:** The US Periodic Adverse Drug Experience Report (PADER)[4,5] and the Periodic Safety Update Report for Marketed Drugs

(PSUR)[6,7] used in the European Union (EU) and elsewhere are different in format and content. For instance, for foreign reports, only those that are serious and unexpected are submitted in the PADER, while medically unconfirmed reports from consumers are usually excluded in the case evaluations and tabulations included in the PSUR. Regardless of these differences, it is recommended that all sources of information be used initially for purposes of signal detection and determining whether the frequency, intensity, or seriousness of AEs has changed from the previous reporting period. After this initial evaluation, narrower search criteria, e.g., excluding medically unconfirmed cases, can be used.

3. Search terms should include PTs found in the SMQ *Torsade de pointes/QT prolongation*. For other ECG-related events develop *ad hoc queries* (AHQs) as described in Chapter 4. Examples of terms to consider are those included in Table 19-2 for "*Atrioventricular block*" and "*Bundle branch block*".

4. Utilizing the methods described in Chapters 5–8, determine whether any new safety signals have been identified, or whether the frequency, intensity, or seriousness of ECG-related AEs has changed from the previous reporting period.

5. If there is a change in the benefit–risk profile, consider following the options discussed in Chapter 8 that are best suited to your findings.

6. Summarize the results of your review in the periodic report according to the regulations, directives, and guidance documents relevant to your country.

References

1. International Conference on Harmonisation of Technical Requirements for Registration of Pharmaceuticals for Human Use. *The Nonclinical Evaluation of the Potential for Delayed Ventricular Repolarization (QT Interval Prolongation) by Human Pharmaceuticals S7B*. Geneva, Switzerland: ICH Secretariat, May 2005. http://www.ich.org/cache/compo/276-254-1.html. Accessed April 6, 2010.

2. International Conference on Harmonisation of Technical Requirements for Registration of Pharmaceuticals for Human Use. *The Clinical Evaluation of QT/QTc Interval Prolongation and Proarrhythmic Potential for Non-Antiarrhythmic Drugs E14*. Geneva, Switzerland: ICH Secretariat, May 2005. http://www.ich.org/cache/compo/276-254-1.html. Accessed April 6, 2010.

3. Supplementary suggestions for preparing an integrated summary of safety information in an original NDA submission and for organizing information in periodic safety updates (Leber guidelines). Rockville, MD: US Food and Drug Administration; 1987.

4. US Food and Drug Administration (FDA). Code of Federal Regulations title 21, Part 314—Applications for FDA approval to market a new drug, subpart B–Applications, sec. 314.80—Postmarketing reporting of adverse drug experiences. Silver Spring, MD: FDA, April 1, 2009. http://www.accessdata.fda.gov/scripts/cdrh/cfdocs/cfcfr/CFRSearch.cfm?fr=314.80. Accessed April 6, 2010.

5. US Food and Drug Administration (FDA). Draft guidance for industry: postmarketing safety reporting for human drug and biological products including vaccines. Rockville, MD: FDA, March 2001. http://www.fda.gov/BiologicsBloodVaccines/GuidanceComplianceRegulatoryInformation/Guidances/Vaccines/ucm074850.htm. Accessed April 6, 2010.

6. International Conference on Harmonisation of Technical Requirements for Registration of Pharmaceuticals for Human Use. *Clinical Safety Data Management: Periodic Safety Update Reports for Marketed Drugs E2C(R1)*. Geneva, Switzerland: ICH Secretariat, November 2005. http://www.ich.org/cache/compo/276-254-1.html. Accessed April 6, 2010.

7. Volume 9A of The Rules Governing Medicinal Products in the European Union—Guidelines on Pharmacovigilance for Medicinal Products for Human Use. September 2008. http://ec.europa.eu/enterprise/sectors/pharmaceuticals/documents/eudralex/vol-9/index_en.htm. Accessed April 6, 2010.

Safety in Special Groups and Situations—Intrinsic Factors, Extrinsic Factors, and Drug Interactions

There are many factors that can affect a drug's risk profile. These can be divided into 2 broad categories—intrinsic factors and extrinsic factors.

Intrinsic factors are those factors internal or inherent to an individual, many of which are often genetically determined. Examples include:

- Age
- Gender
- Race
- Weight
- Diseases such as renal and hepatic impairment

Even individuals who share similar demographic characteristics may show considerable variability in their response to a drug in terms of efficacy and safety. This variability in response may be due to genetic polymorphism or human biodiversity due to genetic variation. An example of genetic polymorphism is the difference in blood types—A, B, AB, O—in the population. Genetic polymorphism plays a significant role in the individual variations seen in the metabolism of drugs. A slow metabolizer (someone whose liver has a certain set of enzymes

that metabolize drugs more slowly than others) may be at greater risk of developing an adverse event (AE) because of higher-than-predicted drug levels, while a rapid metabolizer may experience less benefit from treatment because the drug is metabolized quickly and becomes inactive or disappears too soon to help.

Extrinsic factors are those that are external to an individual but nevertheless may still influence the drug's benefit–risk profile. These factors include:

- Concomitant use of other drugs, e.g., drugs that inhibit, activate, or induce enzymes involved in the metabolic pathway of the investigational drug.
- The presence or absence of food when a drug is taken.
- Habits such as smoking and alcohol consumption.
- Cultural/medical practice differences, e.g., circumcision and reduced risk of AIDS virus transmission,[1–3] which could theoretically influence the efficacy outcome of an AIDS vaccine study.
- Geographic regions; e.g., the rate of drug-related photosensitivity may be increased in areas of high sun exposure (so-called sun allergy) in countries close to the equator versus countries far north of the equator.

Pharmacokinetics and Pharmacodynamics

Pharmacokinetics (PK) is the study of the absorption, distribution, metabolism, and excretion of a drug. Pharmacodynamics (PD) refers to the study of the biochemical, biomechanical, or physiological effects (function) of the drug. An example of a PD study is the evaluation of a drug's affect on the QT/QTc interval (an ECG parameter). Prolongation of the QT/QTc interval increases the risk for torsades de pointes (TdP; a life-threatening rhythm disturbance) and sudden death. A variety of different interaction studies (e.g., drug–drug, drug–demographic) are usually done as part of the clinical development program.[4–8] These studies determine if the investigational drug's PK and PD properties are affected by the intrinsic/extrinsic factors listed previously. Sometimes the investigational drug can affect the PK and PD properties of other drugs—this, too, is important to identify.

The Terfenadine Story

There are many examples where the use of a drug in combination with the intrinsic and extrinsic factors summarized previously can result in increased risk to patients. A classic case is terfenadine. Terfenadine is an antihistamine that is no longer on the market. It is actually a prodrug, meaning that it first has to be metabolized to its active form, fexofenadine, before it is active. The prodrug has no antihistaminic effect until it is metabolized to an active form. At therapeutic concentrations, terfenadine can increase the QTc interval. When terfenadine is taken with other drugs such as erythromycin or ketoconazole that compete for the same enzyme in the CYP3A4 metabolic pathway (the pathway that is involved in the metabolism of the drug), less terfenadine is metabolized to fexofenadine, resulting in higher terfenadine levels. Higher terfenadine drug levels are associated with greater increases in the QTc interval and a greater risk of developing TdP and sudden death. These findings resulted in the market withdrawal of terfenadine.[9] Consequently, the QT/QTc findings due to terfenadine and other drugs led to the requirement of more rigorous evaluation of nonclinical and clinical drug–drug interaction and QT/QTc prolongation studies as part of a drug's clinical development program.[10,11]

Population Pharmacokinetics

In addition to interaction studies, it is also important to know whether the intrinsic and extrinsic characteristics of the clinical trials' study population are similar to the targeted real-world population that will be taking the marketed drug. If so, the results from clinical trials can be extrapolated to the real world with greater confidence. If not, the benefit–risk profile from clinical trials may not be generalizable to populations with different intrinsic/extrinsic profiles. Substantial differences between the clinical trials' and real world populations can exist; e.g., 2% Blacks in the clinical study population compared to an estimated 24% of Blacks in the population targeted to receive the drug once marketed. This disparity can lead to nonapproval of the drug or a requirement to do a postmarketing study in individuals representative of the targeted population.

It is good practice to obtain blood samples at steady state (when drug levels are neither going up nor down) from patients in large, Phase 3 studies. Usually it is not practical to obtain a complete PK profile from each patient and a sparse sampling technique is used, where a limited number of blood samples are taken from each patient. PK information obtained from these blood samples is referred to as population pharmacokinetics. This information can provide additional insight into potential demographic-related PK differences found in the study population.

How to Approach and Handle Drug Interaction Data—Clinical Trials

This section explains how to approach and handle drug interaction data from clinical trials. Appendix II, "The Integrated Analysis of Safety for Mepro," provides an example of how this information can be summarized in an integrated analysis of safety (IAS).

1. Review the Investigator's Brochure for the results of nonclinical evaluations. These studies provide important insights into potential interactions before exposure in humans. In vitro tests screen for drugs that are metabolized by the cytochrome P450 system or other metabolic pathways and determine the potential for enzyme induction and inhibition leading to lower or greater drug levels, respectively.

   The results of nonclinical evaluations also guide what interaction studies in humans will be required. If in vitro testing suggests that drug elimination is not dependent on hepatic metabolism, many of the drug–drug interaction studies that evaluate inhibition, activation, and induction of the various enzymes in the hepatic metabolic pathway may not be required.

2. Review the guidance documents and other reference materials to determine the types of interaction studies required for the investigational product or disease under development (see references).[4-8] The types of interaction studies routinely done include the following pharmacokinetic (PK) studies:

- Drug-demographic studies
  - Nonelderly versus the elderly
  - Males versus females
  - Different racial or ethnic groups
- Drug–drug interaction studies to evaluate inhibition, activation, or induction of enzymes involved in metabolism of the investigational drugs and other drugs that may be used concomitantly. The types of drugs used are based on the metabolic pathway of the investigational drug. Some examples of drugs that are tested in these studies are ketoconazole (an inhibitor) and rifampin (an inducer).
- Drug–disease interaction studies
  - Normal versus hepatically impaired
  - Normal versus renally impaired
- The effect of taking the drug with food versus the fasting state
- The effect of other substances, such as grapefruit and smoking, on the investigational drug's PK properties

3. Obtain blood samples at steady state from patients in large, Phase 3 studies so PK information of the study population can be determined.

4. Do a subgroup analysis based on the rates of adverse events and the rates of other safety findings (e.g., labs, vital signs, ECGs), if warranted. Subgroup analyses are typically reserved for large studies or the IAS where data are pooled across studies. Subgroup analyses cannot be done in small studies because there are too few subjects to divide into different subgroups.

   Based on the available data, do subgroup analyses on a variety of intrinsic and extrinsic factors such as age, race, gender, and geographic regions. One approach to determine if 1 subgroup differs from another is to calculate the attributable risk ratio (ARR) for subgroup differences as follows:

   $$\begin{aligned} ARR = &(AE \text{ rate of investigational drug}_x \\ &- AE \text{ rate of placebo}_x) \\ &/(AE \text{ rate of investigational drug}_y \\ &- AE \text{ rate of placebo}_y), \end{aligned}$$

where x and y are different subgroups, e.g., males and females for gender differences.[12]

This calculation is reserved for common adverse drug reactions (AEs considered drug related) and the rates of other common potentially drug-related safety findings, such as labs. This analysis cannot be done for rare events because there would be too few events to analyze.

Example

The rate for nausea (an event considered to be related to the investigation drug) is 12% in Caucasians and 6% in Blacks in the investigational drug group and 4% in Caucasians and 3% in Blacks in the placebo group.

$$\begin{aligned} ARR &= (12\% - 4\%)_{\text{Caucasians}} /(6\% - 3\%)_{\text{Blacks}} \\ &= 8/3 = 2.7, \end{aligned}$$

indicating that Caucasians have more than 2 times the rate of nausea compared to Blacks.

CAUTION: An important assumption in any subgroup analysis is that all other factors between the subgroups are equal (i.e., subgroups on average are the same age, same weight, etc.); this is often not true. Also, comparing subgroups where there is an imbalance between subgroups, e.g., a small number of patients in 1 subgroup compared to a large number of patients in the other subgroup, may be difficult. For instance, the results from a comparison of the rate of an adverse event in 970 Caucasians versus 30 Blacks can be confusing and potentially misleading because of the small number of Blacks in the subgroup. For reasons such as these, it is important to consult with your statistician to decide the best analysis to do based on the data available.

---

5. Be alert for similar factors across cases when reviewing less common adverse reactions. For example, your AE review shows 3 cases of thrombocytopenia and further review of listings or patient profiles shows 2 of these 3 patients were taking the same concomitant medication. This observation can be a *clue* there may be an interaction between the investigational drug and the concomitant medication; it may be due to the concomitant medication alone, or it may just be a coincidental finding

and mean nothing at all. In this example there is simply insufficient information to make any conclusions from the data, but it should serve as an alert and prompt you to list this finding as one you will track over time.

6. For the IAS, present the information in a comprehensive, logical, and integrated way. All relevant information should be summarized in the text of the report in the following order:

   ■ Nonclinical studies
   ■ Clinical interaction studies
   ■ Population pharmacokinetic data
   ■ Subgroup analyses for common adverse drug reactions and other safety findings (if applicable) from Phase 2/3 studies
   ■ Identification of similar factors in a case series
   ■ Postmarketing interaction information (if available)

The greater the consistency in findings across different evaluations, the greater the likelihood the finding is drug related.

■ How to Approach and Handle Drug Interaction Data—Postmarketing

This section explains how to approach and handle posttmarketing drug interaction data. Appendix IV, "6-Month Periodic Safety Update Report—Mepro," provides examples of how these data can be summarized in the Periodic Safety Update Report for Marketed Drugs (PSUR).

1. Do specific searches to identify cases of potential drug interactions and adverse events in special groups. Table 20-1 provides suggestions for search criteria and data sorting to help with the identification of relevant cases. This is a starting point—the searches summarized in the table may have to be widened or narrowed, or additional searches may need to be done.

TIP: In order to search the postmarketing safety database for potential drug interactions, it is important that all suspect and concomitant drugs be coded (i.e., assigned a standardized term) so that cases can be identified, retrieved, and sorted in a consistent fashion. Similarly, to be able to identify subjects with organ impairment, it is important to code medical histories. If this is not planned for and coding of these data elements are not done, the types of searches summarized in Table 20-1 cannot be done automatically. Time, resources, costs, and error rates increase with manual review of the data. If the volume of cases is large, a manual review is nearly impossible to do.

2. For searches, use all sources of information, e.g., spontaneous reports, publications, reports received from regulatory agencies, postmarketing studies, registries, etc.

➡ **NOTE:** The US Periodic Adverse Drug Experience Report (PADER)[13,14] and the PSUR[15,16] used in the European Union (EU) and elsewhere are different in format and content. For instance, for foreign reports, only those that are serious and unexpected are submitted in the PADER, while medically unconfirmed reports from consumers are usually excluded in the case evaluations and tabulations included in the PSUR. Regardless of these differences, it is recommended that all sources of information be used initially for purposes of signal detection and determining whether the frequency, intensity, or seriousness of adverse events has changed from the previous reporting period. After this initial evaluation, narrower search criteria, e.g., excluding medically unconfirmed cases, can be used.

3. Group cases by variable of interest, e.g., concomitant medication, age, gender, geographic location, etc. to identify any new potential drug interactions.

4. Utilizing the methods described in Chapters 5–8, determine whether any new safety signals have been identified, or whether the frequency, intensity, or seriousness of AEs in special groups (e.g., children, elderly, organ impaired) has changed from the previous reporting period.

5. If there is a change in the benefit–risk profile, consider following the options discussed in Chapter 8 that are best suited to your findings.

Table 20-1 Suggested Search/Sorting Criteria for Identification of Drug Interactions and Adverse Events in Special Groups

Potential interaction	Search/sorting criteria
Interactions (type of interaction not specified)	MedDRA High-Level Term (HLT)—*Interactions*
Drug–drug interactions	Search for cases by the same suspect (i.e., other than the marketed drug) or concomitant drugs
Interactions in the renally impaired	Search for cases by medical history included in the MedDRA HLTs: *Nephropathies* or *Renal disorders (excl. nephropathies)*
Interactions in the hepatically impaired	Search for cases by medical history included in the MedDRA High-Level Group Term (HLGT) *Hepatic and hepatobiliary disorders*
Age	Sort cases by the following age categories: < 2, 2-11, 12-16, and ≥ 65 to determine if pattern, frequency, intensity, or seriousness of AEs is different than those of patients between the ages of >16 years and 64 years
Race	Sort cases by the following racial categories: Caucasians, Blacks, Asians, and other races, e.g., Native American, to see if pattern, frequency, intensity, or seriousness of AEs is different across races
Gender	Sort cases by gender to see if pattern, frequency, intensity, or seriousness of AEs is different between genders
Geographic region	Sort cases by geographic regions to see if pattern, frequency, intensity, or seriousness of AEs is different among geographic regions

6. Summarize the results of your review in the periodic report according to the regulations, directives, and guidance documents relevant to your country.

References

1. Auvert B, Taljaard D, Lagarde E, Sobngwi-Tambekou J, Sitta R, Puren A. Randomized, controlled intervention trial of male circumcision for reduction of HIV infection risk: the ANRS 1265 trial. *PLoS Med.* 2005;2(11):e298. Erratum in: *PLoS Med.* 2006;3(5):e298.

2. Bailey RC, Moses S, Parker CB, et al. Male circumcision for HIV prevention in young men in Kisumu, Kenya: a randomised controlled trial. *Lancet.* 2007;369(9562):643–656.

3. Gray RH, Kigozi G, Serwadda D, et al. Male circumcision for HIV prevention in men in Rakai, Uganda: a randomised trial. *Lancet.* 2007;369 (9562):657–666.

4. Department of Health and Human Services, U.S. Food and Drug Administration, Center for Drug Evaluation and Research, Center for Biologics Evaluation and Research. Drug metabolism/drug interaction studies in the drug development process: Studies in vitro. April 1997. http://www.fda.gov/downloads/Drugs/fda.gov/Guidances/ucm072104.pdf. Accessed March 29, 2010.

5. Department of Health and Human Services, US Food and Drug Administration, Center for Drug Evaluation and Research, Center for Biologics Evaluation and Research. In vivo drug metabolism/drug interaction studies—Study design, data analysis, and recommendations for dosing and labeling. November 1999. http://www.fda.gov/downloads/Drugs/fda.gov/Guidances/UCM072119.pdf. Accessed March 29, 2010.

6. International Conference on Harmonisation of Technical Requirements for Registration of Pharmaceuticals for Human Use. *Studies in Support of Special Populations: Geriatrics E7.* Geneva, Switzerland: ICH Secretariat, June 1993. http://www.ich.org/cache/compo/276-254-1.html. Accessed March 29, 2010.

7. International Conference on Harmonisation of Technical Requirements for Registration of Pharmaceuticals for Human Use. *Studies in Support*

of Special Populations: Geriatrics E7 Questions and Answers. Geneva, Switzerland: ICH Secretariat, September 2009. http://www.ich.org/cache/compo/276-254-1.html. Accessed March 29, 2010.

8. International Conference on Harmonisation of Technical Requirements for Registration of Pharmaceuticals for Human Use. *General Considerations for Clinical Trials E8.* Geneva, Switzerland: ICH Secretariat, July 1997. http://www.ich.org/cache/compo/276-254-1.html. Accessed March 29, 2010.

9. Hoechst Marion Roussel, Inc., and Baker Norton Pharmaceuticals, Inc. Terfenadine; Proposal To Withdraw Approval of Two New Drug Applications and One Abbreviated New Drug Application; Opportunity for a Hearing. *Federal Register.* 1997; 62(9): 1889–1892.

10. International Conference on Harmonisation of Technical Requirements for Registration of Pharmaceuticals for Human Use. *The Nonclinical Evaluation of the Potential for Delayed Ventricular Repolarization (QT Interval Prolongation) by Human Pharmaceuticals S7B.* Geneva, Switzerland: ICH Secretariat, May 2005. http://www.ich.org/cache/compo/276-254-1.html. Accessed April 6, 2010.

11. International Conference on Harmonisation of Technical Requirements for Registration of Pharmaceuticals for Human Use. *The Clinical Evaluation of QT/QTc Interval Prolongation and Proarrhythmic Potential for Non-Antiarrhythmic Drugs E14.* Geneva, Switzerland: ICH Secretariat, May 2005. http://www.ich.org/cache/compo/276-254-1.html. Accessed April 6, 2010.

12. Center for Drug Evaluation and Research, US Food and Drug Administration, US Department of Health and Human Services. Guideline for conducting a clinical safety review of a new product application and preparing a report on the review. 2005. http://www.fda.gov/downloads/Drugs/GuidanceComplianceRegulatoryInformation/Guidances/ucm072974.pdf. Accessed March 29, 2010.

13. US Food and Drug Administration (FDA). Code of Federal Regulations Title 21, Part 314—Applications for FDA Approval to Market a New Drug, Subpart B—Applications, Sec. 314.80—Postmarketing reporting of adverse drug experiences. Silver Spring, MD: FDA, April 1, 2009. http://www.accessdata.fda.gov/scripts/cdrh/cfdocs/cfcfr/CFRSearch.cfm?fr=314.80. Accessed April 6, 2010.

14. US Food and Drug Administration (FDA). Draft guidance for industry: Postmarketing safety reporting for human drugs and biological products including vaccines. Rockville, MD: FDA, March 2001. http://www.fda.gov/BiologicsBloodVaccines/GuidanceComplianceRegulatoryInformation/Guidances/Vaccines/ucm074850.htm. Accessed April 6, 2010.

15. International Conference on Harmonisation of Technical Requirements for Registration of Pharmaceuticals for Human Use. *Clinical Safety Data Management: Periodic Safety Update Reports for Marketed Drugs E2C(R1).* Geneva, Switzerland: ICH Secretariat, November 2005. http://www.ich.org/cache/compo/276-254-1.html. Accessed April 6, 2010.

16. Volume 9A of The Rules Governing Medicinal Products in the European Union—Guidelines on Pharmacovigilance for Medicinal Products for Human Use. September 2008. http://ec.europa.eu/enterprise/sectors/pharmaceuticals/documents/eudralex/vol-9/index_en.htm. Accessed April 6, 2010.

Use in Pregnancy and Lactation

It is important to understand the effects of taking a drug during conception, pregnancy, or lactation and the risks involved. The factors that should be considered for conception and pregnancy include[1,2]:

Maternal/Paternal Risk

- Fertility (female and male)
- Effect on the actual pregnancy (females)
- Effect on labor and delivery (parturition) (females)

Fetal Risk

- Structural abnormalities (congenital malformations and birth defects)
- Fetal and infant mortality
- Impaired physiologic function (e.g., locomotor activity, learning, and memory)
- Alterations to growth (e.g., body weight and length)

For lactation, the risks that should be considered include the following:

Maternal Risk

- Effect on the quality and quantity of breast milk

Infant Risk

- The amount and consequences of drug that gets passed to the nursing infant.

The majority of information of a drug's risk to pregnancy and lactation prior to market authorization is based on animal reproductive and developmental studies.[3] Even with extensive animal testing, it is still considered unethical in almost all cases to expose pregnant or lactating women to investigational drugs. This is because a drug's risk during pregnancy and lactation cannot be adequately predicted from animal studies alone. Situations where it can be acceptable to treat pregnant woman include times when the pregnant mother is desperately sick (e.g., cancer) or if there is an illness or disease in the fetus that calls for experimental procedures (e.g., drugs or surgery). There is also an ethical issue of consent because the fetus cannot give informed consent. Although there is a great desire to know whether a drug can be used if needed in pregnant women, no one has come up with a way of testing such drugs without posing significant potential risk to mother and fetus. For this reason, birth control use or documented history of loss of childbearing potential (e.g., hysterectomy, menopause) and periodic pregnancy testing during a clinical trial are required.

Information on lactation is also usually limited to animal studies, though it is possible to test the drug on lactating women.[4] In reality, clinical trials specifically looking at a drug's effect on milk production, the drug levels in milk relative to plasma levels, and the amount passed to nursing infants are uncommon and typically not prospectively studied in humans either before or after a drug is marketed.

Even though pregnancy prevention during clinical trials is required, a few women invariably do get pregnant. This information is important but of limited use because:

- There are too few cases to adequately determine risk.
- For ethical reasons, once pregnancy is discovered, the patient is discontinued from the study—usually during the earlier stages of pregnancy. This results in little or no information about the drug's effect on the later stages of pregnancy, labor, delivery, or lactation.

Once the drug is marketed, more information becomes available through the following:

- Spontaneous reporting of pregnancy/lactation cases.
- Epidemiology studies.
- Pregnancy registries.
- Prospective studies in lactating females and nursing infants. (These types of studies, as mentioned previously, can also be done during the premarketing period if indicated).[4]

Each of these postmarketing sources of information has strengths and weaknesses. Information gained from these evaluations can potentially lead to changes in the drug's benefit–risk profile. A new and clinically important risk will require labeling changes and likely result in revisions to a drug's risk management plan.

■ Collection of Pregnancy Information

A pregnancy and lactation case report form (CRF) should be part of the CRFs developed for clinical trials and should include the following:

- Patient ID, study number, and center
- Age and race
- Dose and duration of study drug

- Concomitant medications
- Coexistent illnesses
- Last menstrual period
- Estimated fetal exposure to drug
- Pregnancy outcome
- Any postnatal follow-up to determine if there are any infant growth and developmental issues
- Information on previous pregnancies and their outcomes
- Information on any birth defects in the family and any history of any genetic associations for cases of congenital anomalies (birth defects)
- For lactation cases include any information regarding:
  - The quality and quantity of breast milk
  - Any breastfeeding difficulties
  - Any adverse events reported in breastfeeding infants

➥ **NOTE:** Pregnancy and lactation information should be collected even if the pregnancy outcome is normal. Pregnancy information should also be obtained on any pregnant partner of a male participating in a clinical trial. This is important because a drug can cause genetic changes/damage to the sperm of the male patient. This could result in an adverse pregnancy outcome. This information, in practice, is often difficult to obtain.

A similar form should be developed and used by drug safety associates or call center personnel responsible for collecting information on postmarketing cases of pregnancy and lactation.

TIP: Pregnancies in either the pre- or postmarketing setting are *not* considered serious events unless the pregnancy results in a serious outcome for either the mother and/or the infant e.g., a death, hospitalization, a congenital anomaly, etc.

■ Estimating Reproductive and Developmental Risks

Because of limited human experience prior to drug approval, reproductive and developmental risks largely rely on nonclinical data and extrapolation of these data to humans. One approach is to compare *relative drug exposure ratios.* Relative drug exposure ratios (animals:humans) compare the dose causing a reproductive toxic effect in animals to the therapeutic dose in humans, normalized to the doses causing a response common to both animals and humans. This information may be hard to find and compare, especially if the drug is dosed by body weight in animals and fixed doses in human adults. Examples of different methodologies used in the calculation of relative drug exposure ratios include maximum concentration, minimum concentration, body surface area, adjusted dose, etc. Once calculated, relative drug exposure ratios are in general classified as follows[1]:

- ≤ 10—increased concern
- > 10 and < 25—no change in concern
- ≥ 25—decreased concern

TIP: Some *clues* that increase the weight of evidence that animal findings may be relevant to humans include[1]:

- Similar findings are found in more than 1 animal species.
- The same types of adverse effects are seen in more than 1 reproductive and/or developmental study.
- Adverse effects are seen during multiple stages of the reproductive or developmental process rather than at a single, discrete period of time.
- Findings that occur in the fetus in the absence of maternal toxicity. Maternal toxicity itself can be the cause of abnormal findings in the fetus. Absence of maternal toxicity suggests a direct fetal effect.
- A dose–response relationship exists.
- Rare events are observed. Reproductive and development studies are typically not large enough to detect rare adverse events. If rare events occur, suspicions should be raised.
- There is little separation between the therapeutic dose and the dose associated with reproductive or developmental toxicities.
- The reproductive or developmental toxicological mechanisms are similar to or are an exaggeration of the pharmacologic effect of the drug. For example, an increase in the delivery time of a newborn due to a drug that has a pharmacological effect of decreasing uterine contraction.
- The pharmacokinetic (absorption, distribution, metabolism, elimination) profiles of the

affected animal species are similar to humans.

- The relative drug exposure ratio of animals:humans is ≤ 10.
- A class-associated effect exists, i.e., similar findings have been reported with drugs belonging to the same drug class.

How to Approach and Handle Pregnancy and Lactation Data— Clinical Trials

This section explains how to approach and handle pregnancy and lactation data from clinical trials. Appendix II, "The Integrated Analysis of Safety of Mepro," provides an example of how pregnancy/lactation data can be summarized in an integrated analysis of safety (IAS). Appendix III, "Company Core Safety Information for Mepro," is an example of how pregnancy and lactation data are summarized in the company's core safety information (CCSI).

1. Review the Investigator's Brochure (IB) for nonclinical information with a focus on the following:
   - Evidence of genotoxicity. Is the drug mutagenic (causes mutations or changes in the normal nucleic acid sequence of genes)? Is it clastogenic (resulting in chromosomal damage or breakage)?
   - Any adverse effects on female or male fertility in animals?
   - Any evidence the drug is a teratogen (an agent that causes abnormal development of the embryo or fetus), e.g., skeletal malformations, septal defects of the heart, or other congenital anomalies or birth defects?
   - Any increase in miscarriages or a decrease in embryo/fetal and neonatal survival rates?
   - Any physiologic impairment of the fetus?
   - Whether the drug crosses the placenta.
   - Whether the drug is found in breast milk. If so, what is the concentration in breast milk relative to plasma—increased, decreased, or the same?
2. Determine the *relative drug exposure ratios.* This can be complicated and a clinical pharmacologist should be consulted.
3. Specify in the clinical study protocol that the investigator must notify the sponsor immediately of any pregnancies and must complete a pregnancy CRF.

The sponsor should check to make sure complete and accurate pregnancy data from any patient or partner of a patient who becomes pregnant in a clinical trial are obtained. If the pregnancy information received is incomplete, follow-up information should be aggressively sought.

4. Prepare a full narrative summarizing the relevant information obtained from the pregnancy/lactation CRF, including those from patients who received placebo or an active control. Placebo and active control information is useful for comparison purposes. Prepare narratives for all pregnancy cases, even those with normal outcomes.

5. Include the following information in the pregnancy and lactation section of an IAS:

   ■ Relevant, nonclinical information including any adverse effects on reproduction and parturition. Also include the relative drug exposure ratios between animals and humans.

   ■ A table listing all pregnancies in all treatment groups (see Appendix II, "The Integrated Analysis of Safety of Mepro," for an example).

   ■ A brief in-text narrative of each pregnancy or, if the submission is electronic, a hyperlink to the narrative.

   ■ A statement of any known risks to pregnancy or lactation in other members of a drug class to which the investigational drug belongs. For example, NSAIDs are associated with the premature closure of the ductus arteriosus (a duct that connects the pulmonary artery with the aortic arch). Normal closure occurs soon after the baby is born. If specific information about the drug in question does not exist, class labeling is used. For NSAIDs, recommended class labeling states: "Because of the known effects of nonsteroidal anti-inflammatory drugs on the fetal cardiovascular system (closure of ductus arteriosus), use during pregnancy (particularly late pregnancy) should be avoided."[5, p. 6].

   ■ Include a summary of any postmarketing pregnancy/lactation information (if available).

How to Approach and Handle Pregnancy and Lactation Data— Postmarketing

This section explains how to approach and handle pregnancy and lactation data in the postmarketing setting. Appendix IV, "6-Month Periodic Safety Update Report—

Mepro," provides sample text of how these data can be summarized for the Periodic Safety Update Report (PSUR).

1. Complete a pregnancy report form, including the data elements described previously, for all spontaneously reported cases of pregnancy and lactation.

TIP: Pregnancy/lactation information received by the drug company is often incomplete. This happens even more in the postmarketing setting. To maximize collection of this information, develop a script or questionnaire and train call center personnel and drug safety professionals on its use. These questionnaires are designed to maximize the information obtained from the reporter by prioritizing and directing questions to ensure key case information is received.

---

2. Search for all cases found in the MedDRA system organ class (SOC) "*Pregnancy, puerperium, and perinatal conditions*," and include all sources of information (e.g., spontaneous reports, publications, reports received from regulatory agencies, postmarketing studies, registries, etc.).

NOTE: The US Periodic Adverse Drug Experience Report (PADER)[6,7] and the PSUR[8,9] used in the European Union (EU) and elsewhere are different in format and content. For instance, for foreign reports, only those that are serious and unexpected are submitted in the PADER, while medically unconfirmed reports from consumers are usually excluded in the case evaluations and tabulations included in the PSUR. Regardless of these differences, it is recommended that all sources of information be used.

3. Utilizing the methods described in Chapters 5–8, determine whether any new safety signals have been identified.

4. If there is a change in the benefit–risk profile, consider following the options discussed in Chapter 8 that are best suited to your findings.

5. Summarize the results of your review in the periodic report according to the regulations, directives, and guidance documents relevant to your country.

To get a somewhat different point of view of how pregnancy and lactation information can be used, look at the Web site from the Children's Hospital of Toronto (University of Toronto), which has a special unit and section on pregnancy and has many comments on drugs and pregnancy. Note that this is not a US site, and the labeling and uses provided do *not* fall under US labeling, medical practice, etc. The URL is www.motherisk.org; the specific section on drugs is at www.motherisk.org/women/drugs.jsp.[10,11]

References

1. US Food and Drug Administration (FDA). Reviewer guidance: Integration of study results to assess concerns about human reproductive and developmental toxicities. Rockville, MD: FDA, October 2001. http://www.fda.gov/downloads/GuidanceComplianceRegulatoryInformation/Guidances/UCM079240.pdf. Accessed March 30, 2010.

2. European Medicines Agency, Committee for Medicinal Products for Human Use. Guideline on risk assessment of medicinal products on human reproduction and lactation: From data to labelling. 2008. http://www.emea.europa.eu/pdfs/human/swp/20392705enfin.pdf. Accessed March 30, 2010.

3. International Conference on Harmonisation of Technical Requirements for Registration of Pharmaceuticals for Human Use. *ICH Harmonised Tripartite Guideline "Detection of Toxicity to Reproduction for Medicinal Products & Toxicity to Male Fertility S5(R2)."* Geneva, Switzerland: ICH Secretariat, November 2005. http://www.ich.org/cache/compo/276-254-1.html, March 30, 2010.

4. US Food and Drug Administration. Guidance for industry: Clinical lactation studies—Study design, data analysis, and recommendations for labeling. Rockville, MD: FDA, February 2005. http://www.fda.gov/RegulatoryInformation/Guidances/ucm127484.htm. Accessed March 30, 2010.

5. US Food and Drug Administration (FDA). Proposed NSAID package insert labeling template1. Rockville, MD: FDA, 2005. http://www.fda.gov/downloads/Drugs/DrugSafety/downloads/ucm106230.pdf. Accessed March 30, 2010.

6. US Food and Drug Administration (FDA). Code of Federal Regulations Title 21, Part 314—Application for FDA approval to market a new drug, subpart B—Applications, Sec. 314.80—Postmarketing reporting of adverse drug experiences. Silver Spring, MD: FDA, April 1, 2009. http://www.accessdata.fda.gov/scripts/cdrh/cfdocs/cfcfr/CFRSearch.cfm?fr=314.80. Accessed April 6, 2010.

7. US Food and Drug Administration (FDA). Draft guidance for industry: Postmarketing safety reporting for human drug and biological products including vaccines. Rockville, MD: FDA, March 2001. http://www.fda.gov/BiologicsBloodVaccines/GuidanceComplianceRegulatoryInformation/Guidances/Vaccines/ucm074850.htm. Accessed April 6, 2010.

8. International Conference on Harmonisation of Technical Requirements for Registration of Pharmaceuticals for Human Use. *Clinical Safety Data Management: Periodic Safety Update Reports for Marketed Drugs E2C(R1).* Geneva, Switzerland: ICH Secretariat, November 2005. http://www.ich.org/cache/compo/276-254-1.html. Accessed April 6, 2010.

9. Volume 9A of The Rules Governing Medicinal Products in the European Union—Guidelines on Pharmacovigilance for Medicinal Products for Human Use. September 2008. http://ec.europa.eu/enterprise/sectors/pharmaceuticals/documents/eudralex/vol-9/index_en.htm. Accessed April 6, 2010.

10. The Hospital for Sick Children. http://www.motherisk.org. Accessed April 6, 2010.

11. The Hospital for Sick Children. Drugs in Pregnancy. http://www.motherisk.org/women/drugs.jsp. Accessed April 6, 2010.

Overdose

An *overdose* is the consumption (voluntarily or not) of more than the prescribed or approved dose of a drug. Note that the prescribed dose by the physician may exceed the approved dose in some cases. This sometimes adds ambiguity to the definition. The importance of having overdose information is twofold: (1) to understand the known and theoretical risks of drug overdose and (2) how best to treat the overdose.

In terms of risk, an overdose can provide *clues* to dose-related toxicity. That is, at the normal dose, an adverse event may not appear or may appear in a mild or subclinical form. At a dose that exceeds the recommended dose range, the toxic effects of a drug can emerge. This is obviously not a good way to go about understanding a drug's risk profile, but, because overdoses do occur, it is critical to review this information to gain insight into the type of toxicities that occur and the doses associated with these risks. This information is then included as part of the prescribing information of the drug to provide guidance regarding the expected outcomes of overdose and their treatments.

Until the drug is marketed and its use and misuse in the real world are better understood, the known and potential risks of overdose come from animal toxicology and clinical studies. During clinical development, only a few cases of overdose are typically reported. With few reported cases, an understanding of the potential toxicities and the best treatment to use in overdose situations is extremely limited. Without clinical overdose information available, review of animal data, the drug's pharmacologic profile, and the drug's dose-related effects can provide some insight into potential consequences of overdoses and how best to treat those who have overdosed.

Nonclinical Versus Clinical Data

Nonclinical safety studies are a requirement of drug development and can provide important *clues* for the types of toxicologic findings that might develop in humans.[1]

> **CAUTION:** Always use extreme caution in interpreting animal data. How the drug is handled in animals can be species specific and not correlated to humans. For instance, rats may form a toxic metabolite to a drug that is not formed in humans or vice versa. For these reasons, clinical data supersede animal data in assessing risk.

The relevance of animal data and potential risk to humans is strengthened if the following are found[2]:

- Similar findings are found in more than 1 animal species.
- The same types of adverse effects are seen in more than 1 nonclinical safety study.
- Rare events are observed. Nonclinical safety studies are typically not large enough to detect rare adverse events. If rare events occur, suspicions should be raised.
- There is little separation between the clinical therapeutic dose and the *no observed adverse effect levels (NOAELs)*, i.e., the dose or concentration where no adverse effects are seen in animals.
- The toxicologic mechanisms are similar to or are an exaggeration of the pharmacologic effect of the drug.
- The pharmacokinetic (absorption, distribution, metabolism, elimination) profiles of the affected animal species are similar to humans.
- A class-associated effect exists, i.e., similar findings have been reported with drugs belonging to the same drug class.

The Pharmacologic Properties of the Drug

The pharmacologic properties of the drug in humans provide insight into potential consequences of overdose. For examples, drugs with a long half-life, large molecules, drug distributed in fat, and those that are highly protein bound will take longer to be metabolized or eliminated from the body, resulting in a greater risk of toxicity. Drugs that cross the blood–brain barrier, form toxic metabolites, and accumulate in the kidney are more likely to increase the risk for central nervous system, hepatic, and renal toxicities, respectively.

If the pharmacologic effect of the drug is dose related, an exaggerated drug effect can be anticipated in overdose situations. For example, if an antihypertensive drug is overdosed, there is a greater risk for hypotension (low blood pressure) and syncope (fainting). If adverse drug reactions are dose related, more frequent and severe events can also be expected.

Other Things to Consider

Drug overdose can be accidental or intentional. If it is intentional, this can be a *clue* the drug may be associated with an increased risk of depression/suicidality or have abuse potential. For accidental overdoses, it is important to explore the reasons why they happened. For example, it could be that the name, appearance, or packaging of the drug was similar to another drug the patient was taking.

Overdose Treatment

Some drugs have antidotes (specific agents that reverse or neutralize the effects of the overdose). Examples include the use of n-acetylcysteine (e.g., Mucomyst) for overdose of acetaminophen and naloxone (e.g., Narcan), which is used to reverse the effects of narcotic overdose.[3,4] Most drugs, however, do not have specific antidotes, and treatment is based on the following:

- Prevention of absorption and enhanced elimination of the drug from the body as rapidly as possible. Examples include gastric lavage (pumping out the stomach), administration of activated charcoal to prevent gastric absorption, and hemodialysis/hemoperfusion to remove excess drug and toxic substances from the blood. Whether or not these strategies are successful depends on the pharmacologic profile of the drug.
- Support of life functions with focus on the ABCs—airway, breathing, and circulation—until the drug and its effects are gone.
- Anticipation and treatment of the known effects of the drugs. These effects are likely to be more frequent and severe with overdoses. For example, anticipate the need to treat hypoglycemia (low blood sugar) after an overdose of insulin or other hypoglycemic agents.

Because there are usually only a few overdoses reported during clinical development, specific advice on effective treatment is often lacking. Understanding the drug's pharmacologic profile provides guidance for potential treatment strategies. For example, large molecules, drugs distributed in fat, and drugs highly protein bound are less likely to be cleared from the body by hemodialysis/hemoperfusion because little of the drug will be found free in the blood and therefore cannot be easily filtered or removed from the blood. In such cases, treatment recommendations should include a statement that hemodialysis and hemoperfusion are unlikely to be effective treatments and the reasons stated; e.g., > 99% protein bound. Another example of a treatment recommendation based on pharmacologic properties is drugs that are weak acids (these drugs have higher hydrogen concentrations compared to nonacidic drugs). An example of a drug that is a weak acid is acetylsalicylic acid (aspirin). Alkalinization of the urine with bicarbonate, a substance that lowers the urine's hydrogen concentration or acidity, helps eliminate acetylsalicylic acid and other weak acids and should be considered in overdoses of drugs that are weak acids.[5]

How to Approach and Handle Overdose Information— Clinical Trials

This section explains how to approach and handle overdose information from clinical trials. Appendix II, "The Integrated Analysis of Safety for Mepro," provides sample text for overdose data for an integrated analysis of safety (IAS). Appendix III, "Company Core Safety Information for Mepro," provides sample text of overdose information for inclusion in a company's core safety information (CCSI).

1. Review the Investigator's Brochure:
   - For results of nonclinical safety studies with respect to extent of exposure, NOAELs, and toxicities that occurred.
   - To understand the pharmacology of the drug and gain an understanding of the potential expected risks of overdose and empiric treatment options if the investigational drug is first in class.

2. Review the results from clinical studies where the highest doses of study medication were given or higher than normal blood/plasma drug levels occurred. These include:
   - Individuals who received the highest doses in clinical trials. This information is typically found in Phase 1 dose-ranging studies where the highest maximum tolerated dose is determined.
   - Interaction studies where high blood levels can occur due to:
     - Drug–drug interactions
     - Drug–disease interactions
     - Drug–demographic interactions

   Although these results should be reviewed because they may provide some *clues* about potential toxicity, these types of studies remain of limited value. This is a result of the short duration of exposure, i.e., some of these studies are single-dose studies, and even the highest doses given are likely to fall below the total amount of drug taken in an overdose.

3. Collect the following information for all cases of overdose:
   - Patient ID, study number/center
   - Age, gender, race
   - Relevant medical history, e.g., history of depression
   - Any precipitating factors, such as loss of job, recent divorce, the drug looked like another drug the patient was taking, etc.
   - Concomitant medications
   - The date and time of the overdose
   - The total amount of study medication taken
   - Whether the overdose was accidental or intentional
   - The safety findings associated with the overdose, e.g., adverse events (including the intensity), changes in physical examination, laboratory test results, vital signs, and ECG values
   - Whether the overdose resulted in any serious outcomes; i.e., the patient died, was hospitalized, etc.
   - The disposition of the patient (e.g., continued in the study, discontinued, whether the drug was stopped temporarily or the dose reduced,

and whether the next scheduled dose was given)

- The treatment the patient received for the overdose
- Outcome of the overdose (e.g., recovered, recovered with sequelae, ongoing, or died)

TIP: Even if the subject is asymptomatic from the overdose, complete information of the overdose should still be collected. If many and/or large overdoses occur without toxicity, this argues strongly for the safety of the drug and a wide therapeutic margin, indicating that increases in the dose do not necessarily increase toxicity significantly.

---

4. Aggressively pursue follow-up information in real time until complete information is received.
5. Write a complete narrative of the relevant information collected for all overdose cases. Include in the narrative any known or suspected reasons for the overdose.

➡ **NOTE:** An overdose may not result in a serious outcome or require expediting reporting. Nevertheless, a narrative of each case of overdose should be included in the clinical study report and the IAS.

6. Summarize in the overdose section of the IAS the following information:
   - Relevant nonclinical safety findings including the NOAELs observed in these studies. Relevant nonclinical findings were discussed previously and should be summarized in this section.
   - The highest dose level (drug concentration) reported in clinical trials and any relevant safety findings seen at that dose/concentration.
   - Provide a summary table of all overdose cases (unless there are only a few cases, e.g., < 3) and include the following information:
     - Patient ID, study/center number
     - Age, gender, and race
     - Total dose of study medication taken

- Date and time of day of overdose
- Whether or not the overdose was serious
- What action was taken; e.g., the subject was withdrawn from the study, study medication was temporarily held, etc.
- Outcome of the overdose
- A brief description of the signs and symptoms associated with the overdose
- Include a brief in-text narrative of each overdose and treatment received.
- If the drug is marketed, summarize any overdose experience including treatment.
- Provide recommendations for the treatment of overdoses.
  - If the investigational drug is a new chemical entity, treatment recommendations should be based on the pharmacologic properties of the drug as discussed in the previous section.
  - If the investigational drug is part of a drug class where there are already drugs on the market, use similar recommendations found in the prescribing information for these drugs unless the investigational drug has different pharmacologic properties.

7. If the number of intentional overdoses seems to be more than expected, do a search using the MedDRA standardised MedDRA queries (SMQs) "*Depression and suicide/self-injury*" and "*Drug abuse*" and compare rates across treatment groups. A higher rate of depression/suicide or drug abuse in the investigational drug group compared to placebo may be a *clue* of an increased risk of depression, or an indication the drug may have abuse potential.

■ How to Approach and Handle Overdose Information— Postmarketing

This section explains how to approach and handle overdose information in the postmarketing setting. Appendix IV, "6-Month Periodic Safety Update Report— Mepro," provides sample text of how overdose information can be summarized in the Periodic Safety Update Report (PSUR).

1. Collect the information described in the previous section for all overdoses.

TIP: Develop a script or questionnaire for cases of overdose and train call center personnel and drug safety professionals on its use. These questionnaires are designed to maximize the information obtained from the reporter by prioritizing and directing questions to ensure key case information is received.

2. Search for, and review, all cases that are found in the MedDRA High-Level Group Term (HLGT) *Medication errors*. This search category not only includes overdoses but also includes terms associated with medication errors—a potential source for accidental overdose. Also search the database for cases of drug abuse and intentional drug misuse, because drug overdose can be a consequence of these types of events. Include all sources for overdose cases, e.g., spontaneous reports, publications, reports received from regulatory agencies, postmarketing studies, registries, etc.

➡ **NOTE:** The US Periodic Adverse Drug Experience Report (PADER)[6,7] and the PSUR[8,9] used in the European Union (EU) and elsewhere are different in format and content. For instance, for foreign reports, only those that are serious and unexpected are submitted in the PADER, while medically unconfirmed reports from consumers are usually excluded in the case evaluations and tabulations included in the PSUR. Regardless of these differences, it is recommended that all sources of information be used initially for purposes of signal detection and determining whether the frequency, intensity, or seriousness of adverse events has changed from the previous reporting period. After this initial evaluation, narrower search criteria, e.g., excluding medically unconfirmed cases, can be used.

TIP: Poison control centers can be a good source for overdose information.

3. Look for a dose response. That is, look at the amount of drug taken and whether the toxic events seemed to differ by dose. Was a tachycardia faster with an overdose of a full bottle of tablets compared to a 1-tablet overdose? This type of information may provide some insight into how wide the safety margin is between the recommended dose and a toxic dose.

4. Determine whether the information in the current and approved prescribing information is still valid based on the new overdose cases received by the company; if not, the label should be revised.

5. If there is a change in the benefit–risk profile, consider following the options discussed in Chapter 8 that are best suited to your findings.

6. Summarize the results of your review in the periodic report according to the regulations, directives, and guidance documents relevant to your country.

References

1. International Conference on Harmonisation of Technical Requirements for Registration of Pharmaceuticals for Human Use. *Guidance on Nonclinical Safety Studies for the Conduct of Human Clinical Trials and Marketing Authorization for Pharmaceuticals M3(R2)*. Geneva, Switzerland: ICH Secretariat, June 2009. http://www.ich.org/cache/compo/276-254-1.html. Accessed March 31, 2010.

2. US Food and Drug Administration (FDA). Draft guidance: Reviewer guidance integration of study results to assess concerns about human reproductive and developmental toxicities. Rockville, MD: FDA, October 2001. http://www.fda.gov/downloads/GuidanceComplianceRegulatoryInformation/Guidances/UCM079240.pdf. Accessed March 31, 2010

3. Prescott LF, Park J, Ballantyne A, Adriaenssens P, Proudfoot AT. Treatment of paracetamol (acetaminophen) poisoning with N-acetylcysteine. *Lancet*. 1977;2(8035):432–434.

4. Handal KA, Schauben JL, Salamone FR. Naloxone. *Ann Emerg Med*. 1983;12(7):438–445.

5. Kreplick LW. Toxicity, salicylate. eMedicine: December, 2009. http://emedicine.medscape.com/article/818242-overview. Accessed March 31, 2010.

6. US Food and Drug Administration (FDA). Code of Federal Regulations title 21, Part 314—Applications for FDA approval to market a new drug, subpart

B—Applications, sec. 314.80—Postmarketing reporting of adverse drug experiences. Silver Spring, MD: FDA, April 1, 2009. http://www.accessdata.fda.gov/scripts/cdrh/cfdocs/cfcfr/CFRSearch.cfm?fr=314.80. Accessed April 6, 2010.

7. US Food and Drug Administration (FDA). Draft guidance for industry: Postmarketing safety reporting for human drugs and biological products including vaccines. Rockville, MD: FDA, March 2001. http://www.fda.gov/BiologicsBloodVaccines/GuidanceComplianceRegulatoryInformation/Guidances/Vaccines/ucm074850.htm. Accessed April 6, 2010.

8. International Conference on Harmonisation of Technical Requirements for Registration of Pharmaceuticals for Human Use. *Clinical Safety Data Management: Periodic Safety Update Reports for Marketed Drugs E2C(R1)*. Geneva, Switzerland: ICH Secretariat, November 2005. http://www.ich.org/cache/compo/276-254-1.html. Accessed April 6, 2010.

9. Volume 9A of The Rules Governing Medicinal Products in the European Union—Guidelines on Pharmacovigilance for Medicinal Products for Human Use. September 2008. http://ec.europa.eu/enterprise/sectors/pharmaceuticals/documents/eudralex/vol-9/index_en.htm. Accessed March 31, 2010.

Drug Abuse

Abuse potential "refers to a drug that is used in nonmedical situations, repeatedly or even sporadically, for the positive psychoactive effects it produces."[1, p. 4] Although substance abuse is associated with inappropriate use of psychoactive drugs (drugs that are mind or mood altering), performance-enhancing drugs such as anabolic steroids (e.g., testosterone) and erythropoietin (which increases red blood cell counts), although lacking psychoactive effects, are also drugs that are used inappropriately and for nonmedical reasons.

Addiction is defined as "a primary, chronic, neurobiologic disease, with genetic, psychosocial, and environmental factors influencing its development and manifestations. It is characterized by behaviors that include one or more of the following: impaired control over drug use, compulsive use, continued use despite harm, and craving."[2] *Physical dependence* is the body's adaptation to the effects of certain drugs given chronically and the development of unwanted signs and symptoms after the substance is suddenly stopped or the dose reduced.

Psychoactive drugs, because they can provide a sense of well-being, euphoria, or mood alteration, often make the user dependent on the substance in order to maintain these feelings, resulting in *psychological dependence*.

Substances typically associated with abuse/addiction are alcohol, amphetamines, barbiturates, benzodiazepines, cocaine, methaqualone, and opium alkaloids.[3]

Based on the pharmacology of the drug and nonclinical studies, drugs with abuse potential are usually identified prior to drug approval. Further clinical testing to determine the proper labeling of the drug and whether it needs to be scheduled as a controlled substance are also required. But the true abuse potential of a drug can still be masked before it is marketed. An example of this occurred with the drug OxyContin (oxycodone hydrochloride controlled release) which, as an opioid, was abused, and serious and fatal adverse events associated with its use were reported. The FDA and other federal agencies became involved, leading to labeling changes for the product.[4] The current prescribing information for OxyContin contains a statement regarding abuse and addiction potential. Similar text is also included in the prescribing information of other drugs with the potential for abuse.[4]

Once approved, the way a drug with abuse potential is being used in the real world must be carefully monitored (as FDA and other health agencies note) to ensure it is not being misused.

How to Approach and Handle Drug Abuse Data—Clinical Trials

This section explains how to approach and handle drug abuse data from clinical trials. Appendix II, "The Integrated Analysis of Safety for Mepro," provides an example of how to summarize drug abuse data for an integrated analysis of safety.

1. Review the guidance document "*Assessment of Abuse Potential of Drugs.*"[1] This will provide you with a checklist of what data to collect and summarize.

2. Review the Investigator's Brochure to learn about the abuse potential of the drug based on the pharmacology of the investigational drug (e.g., whether or not it has central nervous system activity) and the results of nonclinical studies, including in vitro receptor binding studies and animal behavior studies.

3. Determine if the investigational drug belongs to a drug class with known abuse potential.

4. Review the results of any clinical drug abuse studies.

5. Review all cases of intentional overdose to determine if there is any evidence the overdoses were due to potential drug abuse.

6. Look for any cases of possible withdrawal after the abrupt discontinuation of the investigational drug. Withdrawal symptoms can be a *clue* of physical dependence.

7. Prepare a narrative of any case suggestive of drug abuse.

8. Select AEs that can be signs and symptoms of potential abuse, such as events affecting mental activity (e.g., confusional state) and mood alteration (e.g., euphoric mood). In addition, include any preferred term (PT) from the Standardised MedDRA Query (SMQ) *Drug abuse.*

> ➡ **NOTE:** The selection of these AEs is arbitrary, based on clinical judgment, and can vary from company to company. This should not be a

concern. As long as it is clear what terms are selected, reviewers can determine for themselves what terms to include, exclude, or add for their own analysis. An example of a list of AEs to evaluate can be found in Appendix II, "The Integrated Analysis of Safety for Mepro."

Determine the rates of these events and compare across treatment groups for treatment differences. In the calculation of rates, if the patient reports the same PT more than once, the patient should be counted only once.

9. Include in the drug abuse section of the integrated analysis of safety (IAS) the following:[1]

   ■ A summary of the pharmacological profile of the drug as it relates to the potential for drug abuse (e.g., the drug crosses the blood brain barrier)

   ■ A summary of the key results from nonclinical investigations relevant to abuse potential (e.g., receptor binding, animal behavioral studies, etc.)

   ■ A summary of the key results from any clinical drug abuse study

   ■ The results of the AE analysis of pooled Phase 2/3 data evaluating the rates of abuse potential AEs across treatment groups

   ■ A narrative of any drug abuse reports, abrupt withdrawals, and intentional overdoses suggestive of drug abuse

   ■ Any postmarketing drug abuse data (if available)

   ■ A summary statement and an assessment of risk of drug abuse based on these data

How to Approach and Handle Drug Abuse Potential Data—Postmarketing

This section explains how to approach and handle postmarketing drug abuse data. Appendix IV, "6-Month Periodic Safety Update Report—Mepro," provides an example of how drug abuse and misuse cases can be summarized in the Periodic Safety Update Report for Marketed Drugs (PSUR).

1. Develop scripts or questionnaires for cases of drug abuse and train call center personnel and drug safety professionals on their use. These questionnaires are designed to maximize the information obtained from the reporter by prioritizing and directing questions to ensure key case information is received.

2. Do a search using the adverse event terms included in the SMQ *Drug abuse* involving the drug in question. Also search for all cases of intentional overdose and withdrawal. Include all sources for drug abuse information, e.g., spontaneous reports, publications, reports received from regulatory agencies, postmarketing studies, registries, etc.

→ **NOTE:** The US Periodic Adverse Drug Experience Report (PADER)[5,6] and the PSUR[7,8] used in the European Union (EU) and elsewhere are different in format and content. For instance, for foreign reports, only those that are serious and unexpected are submitted in the PADER, while medically unconfirmed reports from consumers are usually excluded in the case evaluations and tabulations included in the PSUR. Regardless of these differences, it is recommended that all sources of information be used initially for purposes of signal detection and determining whether the frequency, intensity, or seriousness of adverse events has changed from the previous reporting period. After this initial evaluation, narrower search criteria, e.g., excluding medically unconfirmed cases, can be used.

TIP: In addition to the usual sources of postmarketing data, another potential source for drug abuse cases is the Internet. Increased chatter regarding the recreational use of a drug or its street value (the amount of money that the drug would fetch if sold illegally) can be a *clue* of potential drug abuse. Any evidence of doctor shopping for prescriptions and prescription tampering are additional *clues* of potential abuse. It is also possible that the marketing and sales departments will be aware of unusual uses or areas where sales are out of proportion to the expected need. While this may be totally innocent,

it may also be a *clue* to misuse or abuse. It may be difficult, however, to get this information.

---

3. Utilizing the methods described in Chapters 5–8, determine whether any new safety signals have been identified, or whether the frequency, intensity, or seriousness of drug abuse cases has changed from the previous reporting period.

4. If there is a change in the benefit–risk profile, consider following the options discussed in Chapter 8 that are best suited to your findings.

5. Summarize the results of your review in the periodic report according to the regulations, directives, and guidance documents relevant to your country.

References

1. US Food and Drug Administration (FDA). Guidance for industry: Assessment of the abuse potential of drugs. Washington, DC: FDA, January 2010. http://www.fda.gov/downloads/Drugs/Guidance ComplianceRegulatoryInformation/Guidances/UCM198650.pdf. Accessed April 8, 2010.

2. American Academy of Pain Medicine, American Pain Society, American Society of Addiction Medicine. Definitions related to the use of opioids for the treatment of pain. American Academy of Pain Medicine, American Pain Society, American Society of Addiction Medicine, 2001. http://www.painmed .org/pdf/definition.pdf. Accessed April 8, 2010.

3. National Institute on Drug Abuse (NIDA). Commonly abused drugs. Rockville, MD: NIDA, March 9, 2010. http://www.nida.nih.gov/DrugPages/DrugsofAbuse.html. Accessed April 8, 2010.

4. OxyContin [package insert]. Stamford, CT: Purdue Pharma; 2009. http://www.purduepharma.com/PI/Prescription/Oxycontin.pdf. Accessed April 8, 2010.

5. US Food and Drug Administration (FDA). Code of Federal Regulations title 21, Part 314—Applications for FDA approval to market a new drug, subpart B—Applications, sec. 314.80—Postmarketing reporting of adverse drug experiences. Silver Spring, MD: FDA, April 1, 2009. http://www.accessdata.fda.gov/scripts/cdrh/cfdocs/cfcfr/CFRSearch.cfm?fr=314.80. Accessed April 6, 2010.

6. US Food and Drug Administration (FDA). Draft guidance for industry: Postmarketing safety reporting for human drugs and biological products including vaccines. Rockville, MD: FDA, March 2001. http://www.fda.gov/Biologics BloodVaccines/GuidanceComplianceRegulatory Information/Guidances/Vaccines/ucm074850.htm. Accessed April 6, 2010.

7. International Conference on Harmonisation of Technical Requirements for Registration of Pharmaceuticals for Human Use. *Clinical Safety Data Management: Periodic Safety Update Reports for Marketed Drugs E2C(R1).* Geneva, Switzerland: ICH Secretariat, November 2005. http://www .ich.org/cache/compo/276-254-1.html. Accessed April 6, 2010.

8. Volume 9A of The Rules Governing Medicinal Products in the European Union—Guidelines on Pharmacovigilance for Medicinal Products for Human Use. September, 2008. http://ec.europa.eu/ enterprise/sectors/pharmaceuticals/documents/ eudralex/vol-9/index_en.htm. Accessed April 6, 2010.

Withdrawal and Rebound

Withdrawal refers to the signs and symptoms that develop when drug administration is suddenly stopped, doses are missed, or the dose is reduced. This is typically seen with drugs that are given chronically and cause a physical dependence to the drug. With physical dependence, the body adapts to the drug's effect over time and becomes tolerant to (gets used to) the treatment. When treatment is suddenly stopped, the body may not have sufficient time to adapt, and signs and symptoms may surface. Examples of such drugs include recreational drugs (e.g., heroin, cocaine, and amphetamines), alcohol, antidepressants, and tranquilizers (benzodiazepines). With many drugs, sudden withdrawal may result in little more than patient discomfort, but with certain drugs, such as alcohol, sudden cessation of treatment (also referred to as *going cold turkey*) can result in life-threatening conditions and even death.

In chronic alcoholics, the sudden stopping of alcohol can result in the development of *delirium tremens*. Delirium tremens is often associated with visual hallucinations (e.g., seeing snakes crawling on the walls), tremors (shaking), fever, high blood pressure, tachycardia (fast heart rate), tachypnea (rapid breathing), and sometimes seizures. Delirium tremens is a medical emergency and can lead to death if not appropriately treated.[1]

Another withdrawal syndrome worth mentioning is the *selective serotonin reuptake inhibitors (SSRI) discontinuation syndrome*. This syndrome, although not life threatening, is important because of the extensive use of SSRIs for the treatment of depression, and other conditions. Signs and symptoms vary and can include flu-like symptoms, insomnia, nausea, imbalance, paresthesias (tingling sensations), electric shock–like sensations, anxiety, and agitation. Risks for developing this syndrome vary among the different SSRIs. A higher risk is seen in shorter-acting SSRIs such as paroxetine with a half-life of 21 hours compared to longer acting agents such as fluoxetine (half-life of 84 to 144 hours).[2]

Rebound is the return of the condition being treated in an exaggerated or severe form, after treatment is stopped. Examples include severe angina after beta blocker therapy is stopped, and rebound headaches with nonsteroidal anti-inflammatory drug (NSAID) withdrawal. To avoid withdrawal and rebound effects in such drugs, decreasing the dose of a drug over time (tapering) rather than stopping it abruptly is recommended.

Withdrawal and rebound effects can be important risks. Identification of these effects prior to marketing is important so that prescribing information can alert health professionals and patients of these risks and advise how to avoid these effects. An example of prescribing information regarding withdrawal and rebound effects can be found in the US prescribing information for Xanax (alprazolam), a drug used in the treatment of anxiety and panic disorders.[3]

■ How to Approach and Handle Withdrawal and Rebound Information—Clinical Trials

This section explains how to approach and handle withdrawal and rebound information from clinical trials. Appendix II, "The Integrated Analysis of Safety for Mepro," provides an example of how withdrawal and rebound information can be summarized in an integrated analysis of safety (IAS).

1. Compare the safety findings in patients who stopped the drug abruptly compared to those patients who had their dose tapered before stopping.

TIP: To be able to do this evaluation, a study has to be prospectively designed to evaluate tapering versus not tapering the dose. Many studies are not designed in this way.

2. Estimate the *residual effect* of the drug. The residual effect of the drug, as discussed in Chapter 15, is the period after the last dose of drug when drug levels are still detectable. The length of the effect is dependent on a number of factors including the drug's half-life and how quickly the drug is cleared from the body.

Consult a clinical pharmacologist for guidance regarding how long the residual effect period is estimated to be.

TIP: In Chapter 15, "Adverse Events Part 1: Common Adverse Events," a treatment-emergent adverse event was defined as an AE that occurred during the treatment period or the period of residual effect of

the drug, or an AE present at baseline that worsened in intensity during the treatment period or period of residual effect. For drugs that are cleared quickly, the time of residual effect should be negligible and close to the time of the last dose. The period of residual effect becomes more of a factor in the evaluation of treatment-emergent AEs for drugs that are cleared slowly and have persistent and relevant drug levels. In determining the potential for withdrawal/rebound, the opposite is true. A drug with a long residual effect has a lower potential for withdrawal or rebound effects, whereas a drug with a short residual effect has a greater potential for these events.

3. Define the posttreatment period based on the estimated period of residual effect, e.g., the day following the last dose of drug (for drugs with short/minimal/no residual effect), 7 days after the last day of treatment (for drugs with an estimated residual effect of 7 days), etc. The evaluation of posttreatment AEs over a short period of time (e.g., ≤ 7 days) can miss withdrawal/rebound events if the drug's period of residual effect is long and exceeds the observation period. The evaluation of posttreatment AEs over a longer period e.g., ≥ 14 days for drugs with a short residual effect period can lead to confounding results (confusion) since the risk of capturing nontreatment-related AEs (e.g., intercurrent illnesses) increases with time. The optimal time period to analyze posttreatment AEs should be made in collaboration with a clinical pharmacologist.

4. Summarize all new onset AEs or those that worsened in intensity during the posttreatment period (i.e., based on the definition of the posttreatment period determined in step 3) and compare rates across treatment groups.

CAUTION: This type of analysis is limited if the drug has a long residual effect and the study protocol did not specify a long enough posttreatment follow-up period. Another limitation to this type of evaluation is if AEs were not consistently and reliably captured posttreatment.

5. Pay particular attention to serious and severe AEs that were first reported during the posttreatment period or AEs that were present during the treatment period and became severe/serious posttreatment.

6. Provide a narrative for any AE suspected of being due to a withdrawal or a rebound effect. For drugs with a high potential for withdrawal/rebound, if many events are reported, an aggregate analysis comparing the rates of these events across treatment groups should be considered rather than a narrative description of each event.

How to Approach and Handle Withdrawal and Rebound Effects—Postmarketing

This section explains how to summarize postmarketing withdrawal and rebound information.

1. Develop scripts or questionnaires for cases of withdrawal and rebound, and train call center personnel and drug safety professionals on its use. These questionnaires are designed to maximize the information obtained from the reporter by prioritizing and directing questions to ensure key case information is received.

2. Search the postmarketing safety database for all adverse event terms found in the standardized MedDRA query (SMQ) *Drug withdrawal*. Review all the cases identified in the search. The search should include all sources of information, e.g., spontaneous reports, publications, reports received from regulatory agencies, postmarketing studies, registries, etc.

➡ **NOTE:** The US Periodic Adverse Drug Experience Report (PADER)[4,5] and the Periodic Safety Update Report for Marketed Drugs (PSUR)[6,7] used in the European Union (EU) and elsewhere are different in format and content. For instance, for foreign reports, only those that are serious and unexpected are submitted in the PADER, while medically unconfirmed reports from consumers are usually excluded in the case evaluations and tabulations included in the PSUR. Regardless of these differences, it is recommended that all sources of information be used initially for purposes of signal detection and determining whether the frequency, intensity, or seriousness of adverse events has changed from the previous reporting period. After this

initial evaluation, narrower search criteria, e.g., excluding medically unconfirmed cases, can be used.

3. Utilizing the methods described in Chapters 5–8, determine whether any new safety signals have been identified, or whether the frequency, intensity, or seriousness of cases of withdrawal or rebound has changed from the previous reporting period.

4. If there is a change in the benefit–risk profile, consider following the options discussed in Chapter 8, that are best suited to your findings.

5. Summarize the results of your review in the periodic report according to the regulations, directives, and guidance documents relevant to your country.

References

1. Burns M, Price J, Lekawa ME. Delirium tremens. eMedicine, 2008. http://emedicine.medscape.com/article/166032-overview. Accessed April 1, 2010.

2. Warner CH, Bobo W, Warner C, Reid S, Rachal J. Antidepressant discontinuation syndrome. *Am Fam Physician*. 2006;74:449–457. http://www.aafp.org/afp/20060801/449.html. Accessed April 1, 2010.

3. Xanax [package insert]. New York, NY: Pfizer, 2006. www.pfizer.com/files/products/uspi_xanax.pdf. Accessed April 1, 2010.

4. US Food and Drug Administration (FDA). Code of Federal Regulations title 21, Part 314—Applications for FDA approval to market a new drug, subpart B—Applications, sec. 314.80—Postmarketing reporting of adverse drug experiences. Silver Spring, MD: FDA, April 1, 2009. http://www.accessdata.fda.gov/scripts/cdrh/cfdocs/cfcfr/CFRSearch.cfm?fr=314.80. Accessed April 6, 2010.

5. US Food and Drug Administration (FDA). Draft guidance for industry: Postmarketing safety reporting for human drugs and biological products including vaccines. Rockville, MD: FDA, March 2001. http://www.fda.gov/BiologicsBloodVaccines/GuidanceComplianceRegulatoryInformation/Guidances/Vaccines/ucm074850.htm. Accessed April 6, 2010.

6. International Conference on Harmonisation of Technical Requirements for Registration of Pharmaceuticals for Human Use. *Clinical Safety*

Data Management: Periodic Safety Update Reports for Marketed Drugs E2C(R1). Geneva, Switzerland: ICH Secretariat, November 2005. http://www .ich.org/cache/compo/276-254-1.html. Accessed April 6, 2010.

7. Volume 9A of The Rules Governing Medicinal Products in the European Union—Guidelines on Pharmacovigilance for Medicinal Products for Human Use. September 2008. http://ec.europa.eu/ enterprise/sectors/pharmaceuticals/documents/ eudralex/vol-9/index_en.htm. Accessed April 6, 2010.

25

Effects on Ability to Drive or Operate Machinery or Impairment of Mental Ability

A ny known drug-related adverse effects on mental impairment and the ability to drive a vehicle and operate machinery safely must be included in the drug's prescribing information.

Drugs with central nervous system (CNS) activity such as sedatives, hypnotics (sleep-producing drugs), antidepressants, antipsychotics, alcohol, and recreational drugs can have adverse effects on mental alertness and coordination. Other drugs may in fact heighten awareness (e.g., caffeine or theophylline) and have effects that alter mental function in a way that might be viewed as beneficial, these should also be kept in mind. It is also possible that drugs will have a mixed picture in heightening awareness but altering judgment (e.g., LSD). Some drugs might produce effects after a night's sleep (if taken before bed) making driving in the morning problematic.

Some drugs may not alter the central nervous system, yet have other effects that will make operating machinery or driving unsafe. For example, some drugs such as pilocarpine, which causes pupil constriction, and atropine, which dilates the pupil, can cause blurry vision.[1,2]

An example of prescribing information for a drug that can cause mental impairment and result in the inability to drive or operate machinery safely can be found in the US prescribing information for Ambien CR (zolpidem tartrate extended release) tablets, a hypnotic with CNS depressant effects.[3]

◼ How to Approach and Handle the Effects on the Ability to Drive or Operate Machinery or Impairment of Mental Ability Information—Clinical Trials

This section describes how to approach and handle a drug's effects on mental ability and the ability to drive or operate machinery. Appendix II, "The Integrated Analysis of Safety for Mepro," provides an example of how to summarize this information in an integrated analysis of safety (IAS).

1. Review the Investigator's Brochure to understand the drug's mechanism of action (e.g., whether it causes sedation or affects coordination or vision).

2. Include in the IAS the following:

   ■ A summary of nonclinical data indicating any adverse central nervous system, coordination, or eye effects. Central nervous system effects in animals are seen indirectly in such things as performance tests (e.g., rats or mice running through a maze) or in learning to do a task (e.g., pushing a button to get food).

   ■ Select AEs that may be signs and symptoms of mental impairment, coordination problems, or visual disturbance. For completeness, also look for the rate of accident-related events because mental impairment and disturbances in coordination and vision increase the risk for accidental injuries. MedDRA terms to consider include the following:

   ▫ **For mental impairment**—High-Level Terms (HLTs) *Confusion and disorientation, Disturbance in consciousness NEC*, and *Mental impairment* (*excl dementia* and *memory loss*)

   ▫ **For coordination-related events**—HLTs *Cerebellar coordination and balance disorders*, and *Vertigo NEC*

   ▫ **For visual impairment**—The High-Level Group Term (HLGT) *Vision disorders*

   ▫ **For accident-related events**—Preferred Terms (PTs) *Accident, Accident at work, Accident at home, Road-traffic accident,* and *Fall*

TIP: This list of recommended, specified HLGTs, HLTs, and PTs is subjective, based on clinical judgment, and likely to vary from company to company. For this reason, the terms selected should be clearly documented. Reviewers can then determine if they want to use the selected search terms as is, or add or delete terms.

---

3. Determine the rates of these events from pooled Phase 2/3 studies and compare across treatment groups for treatment differences. In the calculation of rates, if the patient reports more than 1 PT included in the HLGT or HLT, the patient should be counted only once. If the patient reports the same PT more than once, he or she should be counted only once for that PT. An example of a table summarizing the rates of these events is shown in Appendix II, "The Integrated Analysis of Safety for Mepro."

4. If any rate differences are observed, prepare and review a patient listing to determine if any common findings across patients are identified.

5. Include a brief narrative in the text for any AE judged by either the investigator or the sponsor to be treatment related that was serious or resulted in premature discontinuation.

■ How to Approach and Handle the Effects on the Ability to Drive or Operate Machinery or Impairment of Mental Ability—Postmarketing

This section explains how to approach and handle postmarketing information on a drug's effect on mental ability and the ability to drive or operate machinery.

1. If the company's core safety information (CCSI) already includes impairment of mental ability and caution when driving or operating machinery as a drug risk, review all sources of postmarketing data (e.g., spontaneous reports, publications, reports from regulatory agencies, postmarketing studies, registries, etc.) to determine if the frequency, pattern, intensity, or seriousness of events has changed from the previous reporting period. For drugs that have shown no previous adverse effect on mental impairment, driving, or operating machinery, search all sources of postmarketing data using the search criteria recommended in the previous section to identify any new signals.

➡ **NOTE:** The US Periodic Adverse Drug Experience Report (PADER)[4,5] and the Periodic Safety Update Report for Marketed Drugs (PSUR)[6,7] used in the European Union (EU) and elsewhere are different in format and content. For instance, for foreign reports, only those that are serious and unexpected are submitted in the PADER, while medically unconfirmed reports from consumers are usually excluded in the case evaluations and tabulations included in the PSUR. Regardless of these differences, it is recommended that all sources of information be used initially for purposes of signal detection and determining whether the frequency, intensity, or seriousness of adverse events has changed from the previous reporting period. After this initial evaluation, narrower search criteria, e.g., excluding medically unconfirmed cases, can be used.

2. Utilizing the methods described in Chapters 5–8, determine whether any safety signals have been identified suggesting a new risk for driving or operating heavy equipment. For drugs known to have this risk, determine whether the frequency, intensity, or seriousness of the risk has changed from the previous reporting period.

3. If there is a change in the benefit–risk profile, consider following the options discussed in Chapter 8 that are best suited to your findings.

4. Summarize the results of your review in the periodic report according to the regulations, directives, and guidance documents relevant to your country.

References

1. Medline Plus. Pilocarpine ophthalmic. Bethesda, MD: The American Society of Health, February 1, 2009. http://www.nlm.nih.gov/medlineplus/drug info/meds/a682874.html. Accessed April 1, 2010.

2. Medline Plus. Atropine ophthalmic. Bethesda, MD: The American Society of Health, February 1, 2009. http://www.nlm.nih.gov/medlineplus/druginfo/meds/a682487.html. Accessed April 1, 2010.

3. AmbienCR [prescribing information]. Bridgewater, NJ: Sanofi aventis, 2010. http://products.sanofi-aventis.us/ambien_cr/ambienCR.html. Accessed April 1, 2010.

4. US Food and Drug Administration (FDA). Code of Federal Regulations title 21, Part 314—Applications for FDA approval to market a new drug, subpart B—Applications, sec. 314.80—Postmarketing reporting of adverse drug experiences. Silver Spring, MD: FDA, April 1, 2009. http://www.accessdata.fda.gov/scripts/cdrh/cfdocs/cfcfr/CFRSearch.cfm?fr=314.80. Accessed April 6, 2010.

5. US Food and Drug Administration (FDA). Draft guidance for industry: Postmarketing safety reporting for human drugs and biological products including vaccines. Rockville, MA: FDA, March 2001. http://www.fda.gov/BiologicsBloodVaccines/GuidanceComplianceRegulatoryInformation/Guidances/Vaccines/ucm074850.htm. Accessed April 6, 2010.

6. International Conference on Harmonisation of Technical Requirements for Registration of Pharmaceuticals for Human Use. *Clinical Safety Data Management: Periodic Safety Update Reports for Marketed Drugs E2C (R1)*. Geneva, Switzerland: ICH Secretariat, November 2005. http://www.ich.org/cache/compo/276-254-1.html. Accessed April 6, 2010.

7. Volume 9A of The Rules Governing Medicinal Products in the European Union—Guidelines on Pharmacovigilance for Medicinal Products for Human Use. September 2008. http://ec.europa.eu/enterprise/sectors/pharmaceuticals/documents/eudralex/vol-9/index_en.htm. Accessed April 6, 2010.

Introducing Mepro—
A Fictitious Drug

We have created a fictitious drug with fictitious data in order to illustrate and apply some of the key concepts that are covered in this book. The fictitious drug is meproamine dihydroacetate (Mepro), a nonsteroidal anti-inflammatory drug (NSAID) for the treatment of rheumatoid arthritis. The commercial (brand, invented) name for Mepro is MEPRO. This introduction provides a brief overview of the drug's key nonclinical and clinical findings at various stages of its life cycle from nonclinical evaluation, to clinical development, to marketed product.

This introduction is followed by:

■ Appendix II, "The Integrated Analysis of Safety for Mepro"

■ Appendix III, "Company Core Safety Information for MEPRO (Meproamine Dihydroacetate)"; this is the CCSI that was produced at time of drug approval

■ Appendix IV, "6-Month Periodic Safety Update Report—Mepro"

■ Appendix V, "Clinically Significant Criteria for Laboratory, Vital Signs, Body Weight, Body Mass Index, and Electrocardiogram Parameters"

Remember this is all fictitious information!

■ Background

Meproamine dihydroacetate (Mepro) is a new generation NSAID that preferentially inhibits the cyclooxygenase 2-beta ($COX-2_\beta$) receptor. In nonclinical studies, inhibition of the $COX-2_\beta$ receptor showed significant decreases in inflammatory biomarkers and decreases in the signs and symptoms of inflammation in rats, mice, dogs, rabbits, mini pigs, and monkeys. Significantly less ($p \leq 0.05$) inhibition of renal and gastrointestinal prostaglandins was seen in these same species with Mepro treatment compared to those treated with active comparators that were nonselective or selective COX-2 NSAIDs. Correspondingly, significantly ($p \leq 0.05$) lower rates of gastrointestinal perforations, ulcers, and bleeds (PUBs), renal toxicity, and fluid retention were also seen with treatment with Mepro compared to nonselective and selective COX-2 NSAIDs. Based on Mepro's pharmacologic profile, Mepro was evaluated for the treatment of rheumatoid arthritis.

■ Nonclinical Safety Findings

Nonclinical data revealed no special hazards for humans based on studies of safety, pharmacology, repeated dose toxicity, genotoxicity, and carcinogenic potential. In determining reproductive risks to humans, relative exposure ratios were used in an attempt to correlate the findings in animals to those in humans by comparing dose causing a reproductive toxic effect in animals to the therapeutic dose in humans, normalized to the doses causing a response common to both animals and humans. Once calculated, relative drug exposure ratios were classified as follows[1]:

- ≤ 10—increased concern
- > 10 and < 25—no change in concern
- ≥ 25—decreased concern

Mutagenesis, Impairment of Fertility

Mepro was not mutagenic in an Ames test. It was not clastogenic in a chromosome aberration assay in Chinese hamster ovaries or in an in vivo test in mice bone marrow.

Mepro did not impair male and female fertility in rats at oral doses of up to 50 mg/kg/day (relative exposure ratio of 35).

Teratogenic Effects

Mepro caused an increased incidence of ventricular septal defect of the heart—a rare event—at oral doses of > 85 mg/kg/day (relative exposure ratio 60), and embryo lethality at oral doses of 45 mg/kg/day (relative exposure ratio of approximately 30) when rabbits were treated through organogenesis. A dose-dependent increase in skeletal abnormalities including fused ribs and misshapen vertebrae was observed at Mepro oral doses of ≥ 60 mg/kg/day (relative exposure ratio > 40) in rats treated through organogenesis.

Nonteratogenic Effects

Mepro caused pre- and postimplantation losses and reduced live births and neonatal survival at oral doses of > 55 mg/kg/day (relative exposure ratio of approximately > 40) when rats were treated through the late gestation and lactation period. These changes were expected with inhibition of prostaglandin synthesis and were not considered the result of permanent alterations of female reproductive function. NSAIDs as a class are known to induce closure of the ductus arteriosus, but this has not been studied in Mepro clinical trials.

Mepro was also observed to cross the placenta barrier in rats.

Labor and Delivery

Mepro produced no evidence of delayed labor or parturition in rats treated with oral doses of up to 42 mg/kg/day (relative exposure ratio of 30).

Lactation

Mepro is excreted in the milk of lactating rats at concentrations 1.5 times greater than those found in plasma.

■ Pharmacology Profile in Humans

Key findings from pharmacokinetic, pharmacodynamic, and other pharmacology studies showed that:

- Mepro is almost completely (> 99%) absorbed after oral administration and is approximately 99.4% protein bound.
- No differences in apparent volumes of distribution after intravenous and oral administration are observed.
- Mepro crosses the blood–brain barrier.
- Peak concentration is generally attained within 1.4–1.5 hours.
- Half-life is approximately 24 hours.
- Pharmacokinetic properties show linearity across the dose range of 1.25 mg to 15 mg/day.
- Mepro is almost completely metabolized in the liver to 3 inactive metabolites (the major metabolite is 6'-carboxy-meproamine) via the P450 2C9 pathway.

- Studies with radio-labeled drug have demonstrated that up to 95% of the orally administered dose is recovered in urine. Very little (< 1%) is excreted unchanged in urine. Urinary excretion is in the form of inactive metabolites.

Key Points of Benefit Profile (Based on Phase 3 Efficacy Studies)

Mepro was statistically and clinically significantly superior to placebo in the treatment of rheumatoid arthritis at the recommended doses of 5 mg and 10 mg given once daily for 6 months (Study MP3002). It should be noted that both the Mepro and placebo groups received etanercept 50 mg (given once weekly) concomitantly.

Mepro was shown to be equivalent to COX (a marketed NSAID drug) in the treatment of rheumatoid arthritis in 2 studies, a 6-month (MP3001) study and 12-month (MP3003) study. The Mepro doses evaluated were 5 mg and 10 mg given once daily. The COX dose used in these 2 studies was the lowest recommended dose of 25 mg. Although these studies were not designed to show superiority of Mepro, in both studies, Mepro showed trends toward greater efficacy in the evaluation of the primary and secondary end points of the studies. One can argue that this may be due to the fact that the lowest recommended dose of COX was used (25 mg); however, the lower dose of COX was chosen so as not to unfairly bias the safety results because the adverse reactions associated with COX treatment are dose dependent.

Key Points of Risk Profile (Based on the Integrated Analysis of Safety)

Twenty-eight studies were included in the integrated analysis of safety (IAS). Any subject who received one or more doses of study medication was included in the analysis of safety. A total of 5783 subjects were exposed to Mepro, and 5410 of these subjects participated in Phase 2/3 studies. Person–years exposure in Phase 2/3 studies was 2933.2. In Phase 2/3 studies 2871 and 113 subjects received Mepro for ≥ 24 weeks and ≥ 52 weeks respectively. Key findings showed that:

- Common adverse reactions were GI-related, dose-related, and expected. However, rates of events in the Mepro group were consistently lower than those in the COX group.

- Rates of PUBs were dose-related in the Mepro group, but the rates at Mepro recommended doses were less than those for COX. The pattern of onset was also different between the two treatment groups. In the Mepro group, most of the PUBs occurred within 4–24 weeks and no PUBs occurred after 36 weeks, whereas the events in the COX group had a later onset and increased over time. More long-term data are needed to determine if PUBs show a second peak in onset after longer Mepro exposure.

- In the Mepro group, the risk for strokes and other cardiovascular events was similar to placebo; whereas the risk in COX was slightly higher.

- The rates for anemia and hemorrhage were greater in the Mepro and COX groups compared to placebo, but the rates for these events were greater in the COX group compared to Mepro. Most of the anemia and hemorrhage cases were due to GI bleeds.

- Risks for other NSAID class effects such as hypertension, congestive heart failure, and fluid retention were similar to placebo or less than for COX.

➡ **NOTE:** Like the efficacy results, studies were not designed to prove a better safety profile with Mepro compared to COX, but consistent trends comparing the 2 treatments suggest this.

- There was 1 case of well-documented mania.
- There was 1 case of Stevens-Johnson syndrome confounded by the concomitant use of penicillin in an Asian female who tested positive for the B*1502 allele of HLA-B, a gene associated with an increased risk for Stevens-Johnson syndrome in subjects exposed to phenytoin and carbamazepine.
- There were 5 photosensitivity reactions in Caucasians with exposure of 3 months or more—all were nonserious and resolved, although 1 subject discontinued treatment.
- Higher plasma levels were found in females than in males, in subjects with mild to moderate hepatic impairment, and in subjects who received Mepro and concomitant administration of fluconazole.
- Females taking Mepro had a maximum concentration approximately 50% greater than that of males. The rates of PUBs are dose related. Females should therefore be at greater risk for PUBs than males. However, the rate and attributable risk ratio for PUBs

were essentially no different between males and females; this finding was therefore unexpected. There are insufficient data at this time to determine if this finding is real or due to the relatively small number of PUBs. Also in a subgroup analysis, the rate and attributable risk ratio for PUBs showed no relevant differences between the elderly and nonelderly. It should be noted, however, that historically, the elderly are at greater risk of developing PUBs with NSAID use. More data are required to determine if the risk for PUBs in the elderly is any different than for the nonelderly.

- Lithium levels were increased with concomitant administration of Mepro.

Based on the efficacy results and the risk profile seen in the IAS, on July 31, 2008, the FDA approved Mepro 5 mg and 10 mg given once daily for the treatment of rheumatoid arthritis.

Key Points of the Risk Management Plan

In addition to routine postmarketing pharmacovigilance, questionnaires were developed, and call center personnel and drug safety associates were trained to maximize the collection of information reported during calls to the manufacturer for the following events:

- Any cases of mania or changes in mood
- Photosensitivity reactions
- Any serious skin condition suggestive of erythema multiforme, Stevens-Johnson syndrome, or toxic epidermal necrolysis
- Any cases of aplastic anemia, agranulocytosis, hepatotoxicity, renal toxicity, torsades de pointes/QT prolongation

Because the results of the IAS suggested a better safety profile for Mepro compared to COX, it was decided to conduct a prospective, randomized, long-term, active-controlled study to evaluate cardiovascular risk and the risk of PUBs as the primary end points. Secondary end points include evaluation of risk of hypertension, renal disease, and congestive heart failure. Features of the study include:

- 15,000 patients—10,000 subjects to receive Mepro (5,000 to receive 5 mg and 5,000 to receive 10 mg) and 5,000 subjects to receive COX 25 mg
- Study duration 3 years
- 400 sites in the United States, Canada, and the European Union
- Powered to show a reduction of > 30% in the risk of strokes, cardiovascular events, and PUBs compared to COX
- The number of Caucasians will be limited to ≤ 50% of patients randomized in order to determine the safety profile in other races.

Company Core Safety Information

Based on the results from the IAS, NSAID class labeling, and nonclinical information, the company core safety information (CCSI) was prepared and was used as the reference information for the 6-month PSUR.

Key Safety Findings From the 6-Month Periodic Safety Update Report

After approval it took 3 months to launch the drug; therefore, the first PSUR covering the first 3-month period after marketing authorization contained no adverse events. The 6-month PSUR showed the following:

- The majority of cases reported were GI related, including PUBs, consistent with the findings summarized in the CCSI.
- Two more cases of photosensitivity reactions were reported in Caucasians after 78–84 days of exposure. Both were nonserious and resolved within 2 weeks while the subjects continued Mepro treatment.
- No cases of serious skin reactions were reported.
- There was 1 serious case of exacerbation of mania in a subject with bipolar disease. The case was confounded because the subject stopped taking her lithium 2 weeks before onset.

■ One subject with suicide intent overdosed and took 10, 10 mg tablets = 100 mg of Mepro. The subject experienced nausea, vomiting, and abdominal pain. He underwent gastric lavage and received activated charcoal. He was admitted to the hospital for observation and suicide precautions. The subject recovered from the overdose with no sequelae; he is still being evaluated/treated in the psychiatric ward.

■ One subject nursed her baby and complained the infant would not breastfeed. No other adverse events were reported.

Based on the information received during the reporting period of the 6-month PSUR, no new drug-related risks were identified, and the benefit–risk profile remained essentially unchanged. No changes were made to the CCSI.

Reference

1. Center for Drug Evaluation and Research, Food and Drug Administration, Department of Health and Human Services. Draft guidance: Reviewer guidance integration of study results to assess concerns about human reproductive and developmental toxicities. October 2001. http://www.fda.gov/downloads/GuidanceComplianceRegulatoryInformation/Guidances/UCM079240.pdf. Accessed April 21, 2010.

The Integrated Analysis of Safety for Mepro

➡ **NOTE:** In this appendix, the text portion of an integrated analysis of safety (IAS) based entirely on fictitious data is presented. It is designed to show how the key concepts discussed in this book can be applied. Although simplified and abbreviated in some parts of the text, this sample should help guide you in the preparation of the safety summaries required for drug approval. Reference should be made to *The Common Technical Document for the Registration of Pharmaceuticals For Human Use—Efficacy—M4E (R1) Clinical Overview and Clinical Summary of Module 2 Module 5: Clinical Study Reports*, and *Guideline for the Format and Content of the Clinical and Statistical Sections of an Application*, for specific requirements for both content and format for the Summary of Clinical Safety (SCS) and the Integrated Summary of Safety (ISS), respectively.[1,2]

Throughout the text, references are made to appendices (this simulates how it is done in study reports and in the ISS/SCS) where key data are extracted from the appendices and shown in the text. In these reports the appendix table number should be referenced in the text (and hyperlinked for electronic submissions) so the appendix table can be easily located and the entire table reviewed. It should be noted that the format of this sample IAS and the numbering of sections and appendices used in this example are different than those used in the aforementioned guidance documents. In preparing an SCS/ISS for regulatory submissions, the format and numbering specified in the guidelines should be followed. Please also note that although references to appendices are made throughout the text, none of these are provided in this sample report—only sample text is provided.

Contents

Lastly, there are 3 important caveats to remember:

- **Caveat No. 1**—Regulations, directives, and guidance documents are different across countries and you need to follow the ones that are relevant to your country.
- **Caveat No. 2**—Regulations keep changing and new guidances are issued over time. What is relevant today can be outdated tomorrow.
- **Caveat No. 2**—One size doesn't fit all. There are many approaches in the way data can be analyzed, summarized, displayed, and interpreted. Some of the approaches included in this book may not be the best fit for your drug. Or different types of analyses not mentioned in this book will be required. Some may also disagree with the approaches that are recommended. For these reasons, the analysis plan for the IAS should be discussed with the regulatory agency's reviewing division well before you plan to submit your registration dossier.

■ The Integrated Analysis of Safety for Mepro

Meproamine dihydroacetate (Mepro) is a new-generation nonsteroidal anti-inflammatory drug (NSAID) that preferentially inhibits the cyclooxygenase 2-beta (COX-2_β) receptor. In nonclinical studies, inhibition of the COX-2_β receptor showed significant decreases in inflammatory biomarkers and decreases in the signs and symptoms of inflammation in rats, mice, dogs, rabbits, mini pigs, and monkeys. Significantly less ($p \leq 0.05$) inhibition of renal and gastrointestinal prostaglandins was seen in these same species with Mepro treatment compared to those treated with active comparators that were nonselective or selective COX-2 NSAIDs. Correspondingly, significantly ($p \leq 0.05$) lower rates of gastrointestinal perforations, ulcers, and bleeds (PUBs) as well as those of renal toxicity and fluid retention were also seen with treatment with Mepro compared to nonselective and selective COX-2 NSAIDs. Based on its pharmacologic profile, Mepro was evaluated for the treatment of rheumatoid arthritis.

■ 1 Exposure to Drug

1.1 Studies Included in the IAS

This integrated analysis of safety (IAS) presents safety data from 28 completed studies (9 Phase 2/3 studies and 19 Phase 1 studies). Two studies were ongoing at the time of the data cutoff date of December 31, 2006. Because these studies are still blinded and no serious adverse events were reported, the only information included in the IAS is the estimated exposure from these studies and a brief narrative of the study designs.

1.1.1 Tabular Description of Clinical Studies That Provided Safety Data

Table AII1-1 is a summary of completed studies included in the IAS and includes: protocol number; location of study sites; age range of study subjects; the dose(s) of study medication and study controls; the number of subjects who participated in the study; the treatment duration; and in which dataset the study was included for analysis.

Table AII1-2 is a summary of the 2 studies that were ongoing at time of the data cutoff date of December 31, 2006.

> ➡ **NOTE:** Please note Tables AII1-1 and AII1-2 are *simplified* tables. Reference should be made to *The Common Technical Document for the Registration of Pharmaceuticals for Human Use—Efficacy—M4E (R1) Clinical Overview and Clinical Summary of Module 2 Module 5: Clinical Study Reports* and *Guideline for the Format and Content of the Clinical and Statistical Sections of the Application* for more information of what should be included in these tables.[1,2]

1.1.2 Narrative Description of Safety Studies

The following is a brief description of each of the completed studies and ongoing studies shown in Tables AII1-1 and AII1-2, respectively. Information for each of the completed studies can be found in Appendix CSR. The number of subjects in each study is shown in parentheses.

Completed Phase 1 Studies

- Study MP1001 was a maximum tolerated, single-dose, placebo-controlled, pharmacokinetic (PK) study evaluating Mepro 1.25 mg (6), Mepro 2.5 mg (6), Mepro 5 mg (6), and placebo (6).
- Study MP1002 was a maximum tolerated, single-dose, placebo-controlled, PK study evaluating Mepro 10 mg (12), Mepro 15 mg (12), Mepro 30 mg (12), and placebo (6).
- Study MP1003 was a maximum tolerated, multiple-dose (7-day), placebo-controlled, PK study evaluating Mepro 5 mg (12), Mepro 10 mg (12), and placebo (6).

Table AII1-1   Summary of Completed Clinical Studies

Protocol No.	Study Site Locations	Age Range	Dose/Controls	No. of Subjects	Treatment Duration	Data Set
			Phase 1 studies			
MP1001	United States	19–44	Mepro 1.25 mg, 2.5mg, 5.0 mg; placebo	Mepro—18; placebo—6	Single dose	Phase 1 studies
MP1002	United States	18–47	Mepro 10 mg, 15 mg, 30 mg; placebo	Mepro—36; placebo—6	Single dose	Phase 1 studies
MP1003	United States	20–60	Mepro 5 mg, 10 mg; placebo	Mepro—24; placebo—6	7 days	Phase 1 studies
MP1004	United States	18–57	Mepro 15 mg, 30 mg; placebo	Mepro—24; placebo—6	7 days	Phase 1 studies
MP1005	United Kingdom	21–51	Mepro 5 mg	Mepro—12	Single dose each period	Phase 1 studies
MP1006	United States	18–73	Mepro 5 mg	Mepro—24	Single dose	Phase 1 studies
MP1007	United States	12–16	Mepro 2.5 mg, 5.0 mg, 10 mg; placebo	Mepro—36; placebo—6	Single dose	Phase 1 studies
MP1008	Canada	19–62	Mepro 10 mg	Mepro—12	7 days	Phase 1 studies
MP1009	United States	22–55	Mepro 5 mg	Mepro—24	Single dose	Phase 1 studies
MP1010	United States	22–60	Mepro 30 mg; moxifloxacin 400 mg; placebo	Mepro—35; moxifloxacin—35; placebo—35	7 days	Phase 1 studies
MP1011	France	24–57	Mepro 5 mg	Mepro—12	Single dose	Phase 1 studies
MP1012	France	19–62	Mepro 5 mg	Mepro—12	Single dose	Phase 1 studies
MP1013	United States	23–55	Mepro 10 mg; digoxin 0.25 mg	Mepro/digoxin—12	Digoxin alone—7 days followed by digoxin and Mepro for 7 days	Phase 1 studies
MP1014	Canada	19–61	Mepro 10 mg; lithium 600 mg 3× daily	Mepro/lithium—12	Lithium alone—7 days followed by lithium + Mepro for 7 days	Phase 1 studies
MP1015	United States	18–59	Mepro 10 mg; fluconazole 150 mg	Mepro/fluconazole—12	Single dose of fluconazole alone; single dose of Mepro alone; single dose of Mepro + fluconazole	Phase 1 studies

MP1016	United States	25–49	Mepro 10 mg; methotrexate 7.5 mg	Mepro/methotrexate—12	Methotrexate single dose, followed by single dose of Mepro + methotrexate	Phase 1 studies
MP1017	United States	20–46	Mepro 10 mg; warfarin 5 mg	Mepro/warfarin—12	Warfarin given alone for 7 days followed by warfarin + Mepro for 7 days	Phase 1 studies
MP1018	United States	18–58	Mepro 5 mg	Mepro—8	7 days for each of 2 periods	Phase 1 studies
MP1019	United States	2–11	Mepro 1.25 mg, 2.5 mg; 5 mg placebo	Mepro—36; placebo—6	Single dose	Phase 1 studies
Phase 2 studies						
MP2001	United States	18–80	Mepro 2.5 mg, 5.0 mg + etanercept 50 mg (given once a week); placebo + etanercept 50 mg (given once a week)	Mepro—50; placebo—25	6 weeks	Controlled Phase 2/3 studies; all Phase 2/3 studies
MP2002	United States	18–78	Mepro 5 mg, 10 mg, 15 mg + etanercept 50 mg (given once a week); placebo + etanercept 50 mg (given once a week)	Mepro—75; placebo—25	6 weeks	Controlled Phase 2/3 studies; all Phase 2/3 studies
MP2003	United States, Canada, United Kingdom, France, Germany, Belgium	18–71	Mepro 5 mg, 10 mg, 15 mg; COX 25 mg	Mepro—450; COX—150	12 weeks	Controlled Phase 2/3 studies; all Phase 2/3 studies
MP2003X	United States, Canada, United Kingdom, France, Germany, Belgium	18–71	Mepro 5 mg, 10 mg, 15 mg	Mepro—125	Patients participated until they dropped out or study ended.	All Phase 2/3 studies

Continues

Table AII1-1 Summary of Completed Clinical Studies, Continued

Protocol No.	Study Site Locations	Age Range	Dose/Controls	No. of Subjects	Treatment Duration	Data Set
MP2004	United States, Canada, United Kingdom, France, Germany, Poland, Netherlands	18–75	Mepro 5 mg, 10 mg, 15 mg + etanercept 50 mg (given once a week); placebo + etanercept 50 mg (given once a week)	Mepro—450; placebo—150	12 weeks	Controlled Phase 2/3 studies; all Phase 2/3 studies
MP2004X	United States, Canada, United Kingdom, France, Germany, Poland, Netherlands	18–75	Mepro 5 mg, 10 mg, 15 mg + etanercept 50 mg (given once a week)	Mepro 110	Patients participated until they dropped out or study ended	All Phase 2/3 studies
Phase 3 studies						
MP3001	United States, Canada, United Kingdom, France, Italy, Germany, Spain, Portugal, Sweden, Denmark, Netherlands, Belgium, Norway, Greece, Poland Czech Republic	18–80	Mepro 5 mg, 10 mg; COX 25 mg	Mepro—2000; COX—2000	6 months	Controlled Phase 2/3 studies; all Phase 2/3 studies
MP3002	United States, Canada, United Kingdom, France, Italy, Germany, Spain, Portugal, Sweden, Denmark, Netherlands, Belgium, Norway, Greece, Poland Czech Republic	18–80	Mepro 5 mg, 10 mg, + etanercept 50 mg (given once a week); placebo + etanercept 50 mg (given once a week)	Mepro—2000; placebo—2000	6 months	Controlled Phase 2/3 studies; all Phase 2/3 studies
MP3003	United States, Canada, United Kingdom, France, Germany, Italy, Spain	18–81	Mepro 5 mg, 10 mg; COX 25 mg	Mepro—150; COX—75	12 months	Controlled Phase 2/3 studies; all Phase 2/3 studies

Source: Appendix CSRs.

Table AII1-2 **Summary of Ongoing Clinical Studies**

Protocol No.	Study Site Locations	Age Range	Dose/Controls	No. of Subjects	Treatment Duration
MP2006	United States	12–15	Mepro 2.5 mg, 5.0 mg, 5.0 mg + etanercept 0.8 mg/kg (given once weekly); placebo + etanercept 0.8 mg/kg (given once weekly)	Mepro—50; placebo—25	12 weeks
MP2007	United States	3–10	Mepro 1.25 mg, or 2.5 mg; COX 6.25 mg, or 12.5 mg	Mepro—50; COX—50	12 weeks

Source: Appendix Ongoing Studies1.0.

- Study MP1004 was a maximum tolerated, multiple-dose (7-day), placebo-controlled, PK study evaluating Mepro 15 mg (12), Mepro 30 mg (12), and placebo (6).

- Study MP1005 was a single-dose, crossover study in 12 subjects evaluating the effect on PK parameters of Mepro 5 mg given in a fasting condition and in a fed state.

- Study MP1006 was a single-dose study evaluating the effect on PK parameters of Mepro 5 mg (12) given to the elderly (age ≥ 65 years old) and Mepro 5 mg (12) given to the nonelderly (age < 65 years old).

- Study MP1007 was a maximum tolerated, single-dose, placebo-controlled, Mepro study evaluating Mepro 2.5 mg (12), Mepro 5 mg (12), Mepro 10 mg (12), and placebo (6) in 12–16 year-olds.

- Study MP1008 was a study evaluating PK levels in joint fluid after 7 days of daily dosing with Mepro 10 mg (12).

- Study MP1009 was a single-dose study evaluating the effect on PK parameters of Mepro 5 mg (12) given to female subjects compared to Mepro 5 mg (12) given to male subjects.

- Study MP1010 was a multiple-dose, placebo- and active-controlled study evaluating the QTc interval in subjects given Mepro 30 mg (35), placebo (35), or moxifloxacin 400 mg (35) for 7 days.

- Study MP1011 was a single-dose study evaluating the effect on PK parameters in subjects given Mepro 5 mg with mild to moderate hepatic impairment (6) and normal subjects (6).

- Study MP1012 was a single-dose study evaluating the effect on PK parameters in subjects given Mepro 5 mg with mild to moderate renal impairment (6) and normal subjects (6).

- Study MP1013 was a drug interaction study evaluating the PK parameters of digoxin 0.25 mg daily given alone for 7 days (12) and in combination with Mepro 10 mg for 7 days.

- Study MP1014 was a drug interaction study evaluating the PK parameters of lithium 600 mg given 3 times a day for 7 days (12) alone and in combination with Mepro 10 mg for 7 days.

- Study MP1015 was a 3-period, crossover, drug interaction study in 12 subjects evaluating the PK parameters of fluconazole and Mepro after a single dose of fluconazole 150 mg, a single dose of Mepro 10 mg, and a single dose of fluconazole 150 mg given in combination with a single dose of Mepro 10 mg.

- Study MP1016 was a drug interaction study evaluating the PK parameters of a single dose of methotrexate 7.5 mg given alone (12) and in combination with a single dose of Mepro 10 mg.

- Study MP1017 was a drug interaction study evaluating the PK parameters of warfarin 5 mg given alone for 7 days (12) and in combination with Mepro 10 mg for 7 days.

- Study MP1018 was a multiple-dose, crossover study in 8 subjects evaluating the bioavailability of Mepro 5 mg liquid formulation given for 7 days versus Mepro 5 mg tablet formulation given for 7 days.

- Study MP1019 was a single dose maximum tolerated placebo-controlled study evaluating the effect on PK parameters in children (2–11 year-olds) receiving the liquid formulation of Mepro 1.25 mg (12), Mepro 2.5 mg (12), Mepro 5 mg (12), and placebo (6) based on body surface area.

Completed Phase 2 Studies

- Study MP2001 was a 6-week, randomized, placebo-controlled study evaluating Mepro 2.5 mg (25), Mepro 5 mg (25), and placebo (25) in combination with etanercept 50 mg (given once a week) for treatment of rheumatoid arthritis.
- Study MP2002 was a 6-week, randomized, placebo-controlled study evaluating Mepro 5 mg (25), Mepro 10 mg (25), Mepro 15 mg (25 mg), and placebo (25) in combination with etanercept 50 mg (given once a week) for treatment of rheumatoid arthritis.
- Study MP2003 was a 12-week, randomized, active-controlled study evaluating Mepro 5 mg (150), Mepro 10 mg (150), Mepro 15 mg (150), and COX 25 mg (150) for treatment of rheumatoid arthritis.
- MP2003X was an open, long-term extension study to MP2003 evaluating Mepro 5 mg (75) and Mepro 10 mg (50). Patients randomized to COX in study 2003 could roll over and receive Mepro 5 mg in study 2003X.
- MP2004 was a 12-week, randomized, placebo-controlled study evaluating Mepro 5 mg (150), Mepro 10 mg (150), Mepro 15 mg (150), and placebo (150) in combination with etanercept 50 mg (given once weekly) for treatment of rheumatoid arthritis.
- MP2004X was an open long-term extension study to MP2004 evaluating Mepro 5 mg (40), Mepro 10 mg (60), and Mepro 15 mg (10). Patients randomized to placebo in study MP2004 could roll over and receive Mepro 5 mg in study MP2004X.

Completed Phase 3 Studies

- Study MP3001 was a 6-month, randomized, active-controlled study evaluating Mepro 5 mg (1000), Mepro 10 mg (1000), and COX 25 mg (2000) for treatment of rheumatoid arthritis.
- Study MP3002 was a 6-month, randomized, placebo-controlled study evaluating Mepro 5 mg (1000), Mepro 10 mg (1000), and placebo (2000)

in combination with etanercept 50 mg (given once a week), for treatment of rheumatoid arthritis.
- Study MP3003 was a 12-month, randomized, active-controlled study evaluating Mepro 5 mg (75), Mepro 10 mg (75), and COX 25 mg (75) for treatment of rheumatoid arthritis.

Ongoing Studies (as of the Data Cut-Off Date of December 31, 2006)

- Study MP2006 is a 12-week, randomized placebo-controlled study in adolescents (ages 12–16 years old) evaluating Mepro 2.5 mg (25), Mepro 5 mg (25), and placebo (25) in combination with etanercept 0.8 mg/kg/week for treatment of juvenile rheumatoid arthritis. Mepro doses are based on body surface area.
- Study MP2007 is a 12-week, randomized, active-controlled study in children (ages 2–11 years old) evaluating the liquid formulation of Mepro 1.25 mg or 2.5 mg (50) and the liquid formulation of COX 6.25 mg or 12.5 mg (50) for treatment of juvenile rheumatoid arthritis. Mepro and COX doses are based on body surface area.

1.2 Analysis Methods

The analysis methods and conventions used in the IAS are briefly summarized in this section. In Appendix IASSAP1.0 the detailed statistical analysis plan for the IAS can be found.

Any subject from the 28 completed studies who received 1 or more doses of study medication is included in the IAS. With the exception of the completed studies MP1018, MP1019, and the ongoing study MP2007, which used the liquid formulation of Mepro, all subjects received the oral tablet formulation of Mepro at doses that ranged from 1.25 mg to 30 mg given once daily. The active control used in Phase 2/3 studies was COX, a marketed NSAID approved for the treatment of rheumatoid arthritis. The dose of COX used in the active controlled studies was 25 mg once daily—one of the recommended doses according to the product's prescribing information. For placebo-controlled Phase 2/3 studies, etanercept 50 mg given once weekly was given concomitantly to patients randomized to the placebo and Mepro groups.

In all 28 studies, safety was assessed by collection of adverse events (AEs), clinical laboratory evaluations, vital signs, and body weight measurements. In addition, 12-lead electrocardiograms (ECGs) were obtained in all studies except for study MP1019.

The data were pooled into the following 3 data sets:

- Controlled Phase 2/3 studies
- All Phase 2/3 studies
- Phase 1 studies

In Table AII1-1 the studies included in each data set are shown.

> **NOTE:** Which studies to pool and which studies to discuss separately can be complex and are based on a number of different factors including dose, duration, study design, and indication. For instance, if the study populations are similar and the doses of study medication and study durations are similar across studies, the data can be pooled. If, however, the characteristics of the study populations are different, e.g., an antibiotic used for the treatment of skin infections in non-hospitalized patients versus the treatment of sepsis (a life-threatening infection) in hospitalized patients, pooling these studies can yield confusing results. Decisions of what studies to pool should be made in collaboration with a statistician and discussed with the regulatory agency that will be reviewing the IAS. In this sample IAS, there is only 1 indication and similar study designs, which made pooling decisions more straightforward as you will see.

1.2.1 Exposure

The Mepro dose groups in Phase 2/3 studies included: ≤ 5 mg, 10 mg, 15 mg, and all Mepro doses combined. Because only 25 patients received Mepro doses < 5 mg the inclusion of these patients in the 5 mg dose group was considered too small to lead to any false conclusions regarding the 5 mg dose.

For subjects who received placebo or COX in a short-term study and then received Mepro in a long-term extension study, Mepro exposure was calculated from the time the subject received the first dose of Mepro in the long-term extension study to the last dose of Mepro received. For subjects who received Mepro in a short-term study and continued to receive Mepro in a long-term extension study, exposure was calculated from the time the subject received the first dose of Mepro in the

short-term study to the last dose of Mepro received in the long-term extension study.

Person-years exposure (PYE) was calculated by totaling the number of days subjects received study drug and then dividing the number of days by 365 days/year.

Concomitant medications were coded using the World Health Organization Drug Dictionary Enhanced (WHO-DDE) version March 1, 2006. The Medical Dictionary for Regulatory Activities (MedDRA) version 12.0 was used to code medical history terms.

For disposition, if a subject was listed as discontinuing because of both an adverse event and lack of efficacy, the subject was included in the adverse event category and was counted only once. If the investigator listed on the adverse event case report form, "Disease progression," Worsening disease," "Rheumatoid arthritis," "Rheumatoid arthritis aggravated," or "Rheumatoid arthritis flare up," and the event led to premature discontinuation from treatment, the event was included in the adverse event category.

1.2.2 Adverse Events

Adverse event (AE) terms included in the AE summary tables were coded using the Medical Dictionary for Regulatory Activities (MedDRA) version 12.0.

Treatment-emergent AEs were defined as (1) AEs that occurred during the treatment period or within 7 days posttreatment (the estimated period of the drug's residual effect); or (2) AEs that were present at baseline but increased in severity during the treatment period or within 7 days of the last dose of study drug. Posttreatment AEs were defined as those that occurred > 7 days after the last dose.

> **NOTE:** For Mepro we indicate that the drug's residual effect is approximately 7 days. For many drugs the residual effect is negligible and the posttreatment period starts after the last dose of drug received. For drugs with slow elimination times, the residual effect can be significant and this needs to be taken into to account when defining the posttreatment period.

In the calculation of AE rates:

- If a subject reported the same MedDRA Preferred Term (PT) more than once, the subject was counted only once in the calculation of the PT rate.

- If a subject reported more than 1 PT within the same System Organ Class (SOC), High Level Group Term (HLGT), or High Level Term (HLT), the subject was counted only once in the calculation of the rate of the respective SOC, HLGT, or HLT.

- If a subject reported the same PT more than once or reported more than 1 PT in a Standardised MedDRA Query (SMQ), modified SMQ (mSMQ), or ad hoc query (AHQ), the subject was counted only once in the rate of the respective SMQ, mSMQ, or AHQ. An mSMQ refers to an SMQ where PTs have been added to or deleted from the original SMQ. An AHQ refers to a list of PTs selected by Brie Pharmaceuticals for a defined medical condition.

AEs were considered unrelated to treatment if the investigator assigned none or unlikely to the AE relationship assessment, and were considered related if the relationship to study drug was listed as possible, probable, or definite. If a subject reported the same event more than once and both related and not related were listed, the AE was considered related to treatment. If relationship to treatment was missing, the AE was considered related to treatment.

Intensity was categorized as mild, moderate, or severe. If the AE was reported more than once, and different intensities were listed, the strongest intensity was chosen. If the intensity of the AE was missing, severe was listed. If the AE onset date was missing, the date assigned for the AE was the first day of treatment. If the end date of the AE was missing, the AE was considered ongoing during the last day of treatment.

Common was defined as a rate of ≥ 5%. Adverse events were considered to be potential adverse reactions (i.e., drug related) to Mepro if the event met 1 or more of the following criteria: (1) the event rate in the total Mepro group was ≥ 5% and twice the rate in the placebo group; (2) a dose relationship was seen; and/or (3) the event was considered to be related to Mepro based on clinical judgment. Adverse events were considered to be potential adverse reactions (i.e., drug related) to COX if the event met 1 or both of the following criteria: (1) the event rate for the COX group was ≥ 5% and twice the rate in the placebo group; and/or (2) the event was considered to be related to COX based on clinical judgment.

Known risks of NSAIDs include gastrointestinal PUBs. The rate of PUBs was calculated based on any PT found in the MedDRA HLGTs *Gastrointestinal haemorrhages NEC* and *Gastrointestinal ulceration and perforation*. If a subject experienced the same PT more than once or reported more than 1 PT in either or both HLGTs, the subject was counted only once in the rate calculation for PUBs.

1.2.3 Clinical Laboratory Tests

Laboratory parameters were grouped into the following categories:

- **Hematology**: white blood cells (WBCs, including differential WBC count), red blood cells (RBCs), hemoglobin (Hb), hematocrit (Hct), mean corpuscular volume (MCV), mean corpuscular hemoglobin concentration (MCHC), and platelets

- **Clinical chemistry**

  - **Hepatic profile**: alanine aminotransferase (ALT), aspartate aminotransferase (AST), total bilirubin levels (TBLs), and alkaline phosphatase (ALP)
  - **Renal profile**: creatinine, blood urea nitrogen (BUN), total protein, and albumin
  - **Lipid profile**: cholesterol (C), High-density lipoprotein (HDL) cholesterol, low-density lipoprotein (LDL) cholesterol, and triglycerides (TGs)
  - **Metabolic and muscle profile**: glucose, creatine kinase (CK), sodium (Na), potassium (K), chloride (Cl), bicarbonate (HCO_3), calcium (Ca), inorganic phosphorus, and uric acid

- **Urinalysis**: specific gravity, glucose, ketones, protein, albumin, RBCs, WBCs, crystals, casts (RBC, WBC, hyaline, waxy, broad and granular)

The following 4 types of analyses were done for the analysis of laboratory parameters (excluding liver function tests and urinalysis):

- Mean change from baseline
- Categorical shifts
- Clinically significant changes
- Rates of laboratory-related adverse events

For the mean change, categorical shift, and clinically significant change analyses, subjects were included in the analysis if the subject had a baseline value and at least 1 treatment value. Baseline was defined as the last value obtained before treatment was started. Any subject who took 1 or more doses of study medication was included in the analysis of laboratory-related AEs.

1.2.3.1 Mean Change From Baseline

Laboratory values were normalized based on the methodology described in Appendix IASSAP1.0. Mean change from baseline was calculated for each visit, worst (i.e., most extreme) treatment value, and at end point i.e., last treatment value.

1.2.3.2 Categorical Shift Analysis

For the categorical analysis, rates were calculated for:

- Any subject with a value that shifted from above normal (H) or normal (N) at baseline to a below normal (L) value during any visit during the treatment period.

- Any subject with a value that shifted from L or N at baseline to an H value during the treatment period.

- If a subject had more than one L/N to H shift or more than one H/N to L shift, the subject was counted only once in the rates for the respective shift categories.

- If a subject had both a H/N to L and a L/N to H shift, the subject was counted in the rates for both types of shifts.

1.2.3.3 Clinically Significant Change

A clinically significant change was defined as a normal value at baseline and a clinically significant value any time during the treatment period. Clinically significant values for each laboratory value can be found in Appendix IASSAP1.0.

> ➡ **NOTE:** Suggested clinically significant laboratory values can be found in Appendix V of this book.

Calculation of rates of subjects with clinically significant changes was based on the following conventions:

- If a subject had more than 1 clinically significant change for a given laboratory parameter, the subject was counted only once, if the changes were in the same direction, e.g., both increased.

- If a subject had both a clinically significant increased change and a clinically significant decreased change, the subject was counted in the rates for both types of clinically significant changes.

A listing was prepared and medically reviewed for all subjects with clinically significant values (including the subjects with abnormal baseline values who were excluded from the clinically significant change analysis). The listings included:

- Subject ID, study number, treatment assignment, age, gender, and race

- All baseline, treatment, and posttreatment values by date and study day

- Any concurrent adverse event(s) at time of clinically significant change

- Any concomitant medication(s) at time of clinically significant change

> ➡ **NOTE:** Although the clinically significant change analysis includes only subjects with normal baseline values, these listings include all subjects with clinically significant treatment values—even those with abnormal baseline values. This is to ensure that subjects with preexisting abnormalities who have clinically significant changes during treatment are identified and discussed in the text of the report if warranted.

1.2.3.4 Laboratory-Related Adverse Events

The same methodology and conventions described in Section 1.2.2 for the calculation of AE rates were also used in the calculation of lab-related AEs.

1.2.3.5 Liver Function Tests

The conventions used and the analyses performed for liver function tests (LFTs) were based on the FDA guidance document *Drug-Induced Liver Injury: Premarketing Clinical Evaluation* and included:[3]

- The rate of subjects with a normal baseline ALT value and a treatment value $\geq 3 \times$ upper limit of normal (ULN), $\geq 5 \times$ ULN, $\geq 10 \times$ ULN, and $\geq 20 \times$ ULN*

- The rate of subjects with a normal baseline AST value and a treatment value $\geq 3 \times$ ULN, $\geq 5 \times$ ULN, $\geq 10 \times$ ULN, and $\geq 20 \times$ ULN*

- The rate of subjects with normal baseline ALT and AST values with treatment values $\geq 3 \times$ ULN, $\geq 5 \times$ ULN, $\geq 10 \times$ ULN, and $\geq 20 \times$ ULN* for both ALT and AST

- The rate of subjects with a normal baseline TBL and a treatment value above normal (H)

- The rate of subjects with a normal baseline TBL and a treatment value $> 2 \times$ ULN

- The rate of subjects with a normal baseline ALP values and a treatment value $> 1.5 \times$ ULN

- The rate of subjects with a normal baseline ALT value and TBL, and treatment values of:
  - ALT $> 3 \times$ ULN + TBL $> 1.5 \times$ ULN
  - ALT $> 3 \times$ ULN + TBL $> 2 \times$ ULN

---

* If a subject had more than 1 treatment value within the same category, e.g., $\geq 10 \times$ ULN, the subject was only counted once for that category. If a subject had treatment values in more than one category, the subject was counted in the worst (i.e., the most extreme) category.

- The rate of subjects with a normal baseline AST value and TBL, and treatment values of:
  - AST > 3 × ULN + TBL > 1.5 × ULN
  - AST > 3 × ULN + TBL > 2 × ULN
- The rate of subjects with normal ALT, ALP values, and TBLs at baseline who met the following criteria for Hy's Law during treatment:
  - ALT > 3 × ULN + ALP < 2 × ULN + TBL ≥ 2 × ULN
- The rate of subjects with normal AST, ALP values, and TBLs at baseline who met the following criteria for Hy's Law during treatment:
  - AST > 3 × ULN + ALP < 2 × ULN + TBL ≥ 2 × ULN
- The rate of any subject with normal ALT and/or AST values at baseline and > 3 × ULN at any treatment visit and any of the following PTs: *Nausea, Vomiting, Anorexia, Abdominal pain*, or *Fatigue*, reported within +/− 14 days of the abnormal ALT and/or AST values. If the patient reported the same PT more than once, or reported more than one PT, e.g., *Nausea* and *Vomiting*, the subject was counted only once.

> **NOTE:** +/− 14 days is used to identify cases with a temporal association to the abnormal ALT/AST values, and also to ensure cases are included even if laboratory changes and adverse events were not evaluated/reported at the same time. The selection of +/−14 days is arbitrary. One factor to consider is the time frame between study visits. Whatever time frame you choose, be sure to provide the rationale for it and include it in the methods section of the report.

- The rate of any subject who reported a PT included in the SMQ *Possible drug related hepatic-disorders—comprehensive search*. If the subject reported the same PT more than once or reported more than one PT included in the SMQ, the subject was counted only once.

Listings of subjects were prepared and medically reviewed for subjects with normal and abnormal baseline values and treatment values of:

ALT, AST values > 3 × ULN, TBL > 1.5 × ULN, and/or ALP values > 1.5 × ULN. Listings for subjects with abnormal baseline values were included to determine if any subjects with preexisting abnormalities developed clinically significant changes during the treatment period.

1.2.3.6 Urinalysis   For urinalysis the following analyses were done:

- Rates of clinically significant changes (according to the conventions described in Section 1.2.3.3). The criteria for clinically significant changes can be found in Appendix IASSAP1.0.

> **NOTE:** Suggested criteria for clinically significant changes in urinalysis parameters are provided in Appendix V of this book.

- Rates of urinary-related AEs (according to the conventions described in Section 1.2.2).

1.2.4 Vital Signs, Physical Findings, and Other Observations Related to Safety

Vital signs measurements included systolic blood pressure (SBP), diastolic blood pressure (DBP), heart rate (HR), and temperature (T). Measurements were obtained at rest and for SBP, DBP, and HR, in the supine and standing positions. Body weight (BW) and body mass index (BMI) are summarized with vital signs.

1.2.4.1 Vital Signs, Body Weight, and Body Mass Index

The methodologies and conventions described in Section 1.2.3 for laboratory parameters, unless otherwise specified, were also used in the analysis of vital signs, BW, and BMI.

1.2.4.1.1 Clinically Significant Changes   A clinically significant change was defined as a clinically significant treatment value and a change from baseline that reached the values shown in Table AII1-3.

> **NOTE:** Some of the criteria shown in this table and tables summarizing clinically significant changes in other sections of the report are based on published recommendations,[4] while others are based on clinical judgment; i.e., subjective rather than absolute objective criteria. Because there is no one standard, there may be disagreement among various reviewers as to what constitutes a clinically significant change. Until standard criteria are established, the best that can be done is to clearly show what criteria were used to determine outliers. If a reviewer disagrees, the data can be reanalyzed based on the reviewer's preferred criteria.

Table AII1-3 Criteria for Clinically Significant Changes in Vital Signs, Body Weight, and Body Mass Index*[4]

Parameter	Clinically Significant Treatment Value	Change From Baseline
Heart rate	≥ 120 bpm	Increase of ≥ 15 bpm
	≤ 50 bpm	Decrease of ≥ 15 bpm
Systolic blood pressure	≥ 180 mmHg	Increase of ≥ 20 mmHg
	≤ 90 mmHg	Decrease of ≥ 20 mmHg
Diastolic blood pressure	≥ 105 mmHg	Increase of ≥ 15 mmHg
	≤ 50 mmHg	Decrease of ≥ 15 mmHg
Body temperature	≥ 38.3°C (101°F)	Change of ≥ 1°C (2°F)
	≤ 36°C (96.8°F)	Change of ≥ 1°C (2°F)
Body weight	Not specified	Increase ≥ 7%
	Not specified	Decrease ≥ 7%
Body mass index	Not specified	Increase to a higher BMI category[a]

* Some criteria based on clinical judgment
[a] BMI categories include < 18.5, 18.5 to 25, and > 25.
Source: Appendix IASSAP1.0.

1.2.4.1.2 Orthostatic Blood Pressure Changes Orthostatic blood pressure change was defined as a drop in systolic blood pressure ≥ 20 mmHg or a drop in diastolic blood pressure ≥ 10 mmHg from supine values 3 minutes after standing.[5]

1.2.4.2 Electrocardiograms
The ECG parameters analyzed included: heart rate (HR), PR interval, QRS complex and QT interval corrected (QTc).

1.2.4.2.1 Electrocardiogram Data (Excluding QTc) The methodologies and conventions described in Section 1.2.3 for laboratory parameters, unless otherwise specified, were also used in the analysis of ECG parameters (excluding QTc).

The criteria for clinically significant changes for HR, PR interval, and QRS complex are summarized in Table AII1-4.

1.2.4.2.2 QTc The evaluation of the QTc interval was based on the ICH guidance for industry *Clinical Evaluation of QT/QTc Interval Prolongation and Proarrhythmic Potential for Non-Antiarrhythmic Drugs E14.*[6]

Baseline was defined as the mean of all baseline measurements obtained on the same day before treatment was started. To be included in the analysis a subject had to have at least 1 baseline and 1 treatment ECG. QTc was evaluated for mean change from baseline, categorical/clinically significant shifts, and QTc-related adverse events. QTc was calculated using 2 correction formulas—Bazett and Fridericia.

Table AII1-4 Clinically Significant Changes in Heart Rate, PR Interval, and QRS Complex*[5]

ECG Parameter	Clinically Significant Change
Heart rate	≥ 120 bpm during treatment *and* an increase of ≥ 15 bpm from baseline
	≤ 50 bpm during treatment *and* a decrease of ≥ 15 bpm from baseline
PR interval	≤ 120 ms during treatment *and* a normal baseline value
	≥ 210 ms during treatment *and* a normal baseline value
QRS complex	≥ 110 ms during treatment *and* a normal baseline value

* Some criteria based on clinical judgment.
Source: Appendix IASSAP1.0.

1.2.4.2.2.1 Mean Change From Baseline Mean change from baseline was calculated for each visit, worst (i.e., most extreme) treatment value, and at end point.

1.2.4.2.2.2 Categorical/Clinically Significant Shifts Rates of subjects with QTc categorical/clinically significant shifts were based on the following:

- Subjects with normal baseline values and a treatment value > 450 milliseconds, > 480 milliseconds, and > 500 milliseconds. If a subject had more than 1 treatment value within the same category, e.g., > 450 milliseconds, the subject was only counted once for that category. If a subject had treatment values in more than one category, the subject was counted in the worst (i.e., the most extreme) category.

- Subjects with above normal baseline values and a treatment value > 450 milliseconds, > 480 milliseconds, and > 500 milliseconds. If a subject had more than 1 treatment value within the same category, e.g., > 450 milliseconds, the subject was counted only once for that category. If a subject had treatment values in more than one category, the subject was counted in the worst (i.e., the most extreme) category.

- Subjects with normal baseline values and an increase of > 30 milliseconds and > 60 milliseconds from baseline during treatment. If a subject had more than 1 treatment value within the same category, e.g., > 30 milliseconds, the subject was counted only once for that category. If a subject had treatment values in both categories, the subject was counted in the worst (i.e., the most extreme) category.

- Subjects with above normal baseline values and an increase of > 30 milliseconds and > 60 milliseconds from baseline during treatment. If a subject had more than 1 treatment value within the same category, e.g., > 30 milliseconds, the subject was counted only once for that category. If a subject had treatment values in both categories, the subject was counted in the worst (i.e., the most extreme) category.

1.2.4.2.2.3 QTc-Related AEs

- Rates of QTc-related AEs were calculated for all subjects who reported 1 or more PT included in the SMQ *Torsades de pointes/QT prolongation*. If a subject reported the same PT more than once, or reported more than 1 PT included in the SMQ, the subject was counted only once.

1.2.5 Safety in Special Groups and Situations

The attributable risk ratio (ARR) for the subgroups of age, gender, race, and geographic regions were calculated for those events identified as common potential adverse reactions (see Section 1.2).

Attributable risk ratio (ARR) was calculated based on the following equation:[7]

$$\text{ARR} = (\text{AE rate of investigational drug}_x - \text{AE rate of placebo}_x)/(\text{AE rate of investigational drug}_y - \text{AE rate of placebo}_y)$$

Where x and y are different groups within the same subgroup, e.g., males and females for gender differences.

➡ **NOTE:** In this sample IAS the ARR was calculated only for common potential adverse reactions. For other drug-related findings, e.g., labs, vital signs, etc., calculation of the ARR is also recommended.

1.3 Overall Extent of Exposure

1.3.1 Enumeration of Subjects

Table AII1-5 summarizes the number of subjects who received at least 1 dose of study medication in completed studies included in the IAS.

For the Phase 2/3 placebo-controlled studies, both the placebo and Mepro groups received etanercept 50 mg/week as concomitant treatment. In 5 Phase 1 studies, a total of 60 Mepro subjects also received concomitant digoxin (12), lithium (12), fluconazole (12), methotrexate (12), and warfarin (12) in studies MP1013, MP1014, MP1015, MP1016, and MP1017, respectively.

Table AII1-6 summarizes the number of subjects from completed studies by data sets.

The controlled Phase 2/3 studies and all Phase 2/3 studies are similar except that the latter data set includes the long-term extension studies MP2003X and MP2004X.

The total numbers of subjects who received Mepro, placebo, COX, and other drugs in completed studies are 5783, 2271, 2225, and 95, respectively (Table AII1-5). It should be noted that these totals include subjects who participated in more than 1 study and include:

- 25 subjects who received COX in study MP2003 and received Mepro 5 mg in the long-term extension study MP2003X

- 100 Mepro subjects who received Mepro in study MP2003 and continued in the long-term extension study MP2003X at the same Mepro dose

- 10 subjects who received placebo in study MP2004 received Mepro 5 mg in the long-term extension study MP2004X

- 100 Mepro subjects who participated in study MP2004 and continued in the long-term extension study MP2004X at the same Mepro dose

The number of unique subjects who received Mepro by data set is shown in Table AII1-7. The total number of unique subjects who received Mepro is 5210 for Phase 2/3 studies (uncontrolled and controlled studies combined) and 373 for Phase 1 studies for a total of 5583 unique Mepro subjects.

1.3.3 Exposure—Ongoing Studies
At the time of the data lock date of December 31, 2006, 2 blinded studies were ongoing. The estimated exposure as of the data cutoff date is shown in Table AII1-8.

1.3.4 Exposure by Dose
Table AII1-9 summarizes the number of subjects by dose and data set for all completed studies.

The 5-mg and 10-mg doses were the most common doses given in all 3 data sets.

➡️ **NOTE:** In this example, all studies were fixed-dose studies, making summarization of dose groups easier. For dose-titration studies, dose groups can be based on mean doses, most frequent dose used, or cumulative doses. Whatever approach is used should be clearly stated.

1.3.2 Exposure by Dose and Duration
Table AII1-10 and Table AII1-11 summarize exposure by dose and treatment duration for the controlled Phase 2/3 studies and all Phase 2/3 studies, respectively.

Table AII1-5 **Enumeration of Subjects in Completed Studies—Data Cutoff Date of December 31, 2006**

Study Number	Placebo[a]	Mepro[b]	COX	Other[c]
Phase 2/3 Studies				
Placebo-Controlled Studies				
MP2001	25	50		
MP2002	25	75		
MP2004	150	450		
MP3002	2000	2000		
Active Controlled Studies				
MP2003		450	150	
MP3001		2000	2000	
MP3003		150	75	
Total controlled Phase 2/3 studies	2200	5175	2225	
Uncontrolled (open) Studies				
MP2003X		125[d]		
MP2004X		110[e]		
Total Phase 2/3	2200	5410[d,e]	2225	
Phase 1 Studies				
Single-Dose Studies				
MP1001	6	18		
MP1002	6	36		
MP1005		12[f]		
MP1006		24		
MP1007	6	36		
MP1009		24		
MP1011		12		
MP1012		12		
MP1015		12[f,g]		12[g]
MP1016		12[g]		12[g]
MP1019	6	36		

Continues

Table AII1-5 Enumeration of Subjects in Completed Studies—Data Cutoff Date of December 31, 2006, Continued

Multiple-Dose Studies

MP1003	6	24		
MP1004	6	24		
MP1008		12		
MP1010	35	35		35
MP1013		12[g]		12[g]
MP1014		12[g]		12[g]
MP1017		12[g]		12[g]
MP1018		8[f]		
Total Phase 1	71	373[f,g]		95
Grand Total	2271	5783[d,e,f,g]	2225	95[g]

[a] Includes patients taking placebo + etanercept.

[b] Includes patients taking Mepro + etanercept.

[c] Other includes moxifloxacin, digoxin, lithium, fluconazole, methotrexate, and warfarin.

[d] There were 25 and 100 patients who received COX and Mepro, respectively, in study MP2003, and who received Mepro in study MP2003X.

[e] There were 10 and 100 patients who received placebo and Mepro, respectively, in study MP2004, and who received Mepro in study MP2004X.

[f] In these crossover studies subjects received Mepro in more than one period of the study.

[g] The same subjects received digoxin, lithium, fluconazole, methotrexate, or warfarin alone and in combination with Mepro.

Source: Appendix Table EXP1.0.

Table AII1-6 Summary of the Number of Subjects by Data Sets

Data Sets	Placebo	Mepro	COX
Controlled Phase 2/3 studies	2200	5175	2225
All Phase 2/3 studies	2200	5410	2225
Phase 1 studies	71	373	0

Source: Appendix Table EXP1.1.

Table AII1-7 Number of Unique Subjects Exposed to Mepro by Data Sets

Data Sets	Unique Subjects
Controlled Phase 2/3 studies	5175
All Phase 2/3 studies	5210
Phase 1 studies	373
Total unique number of subjects exposed to Mepro	5583

Source: Appendix Table EXP1.3.

Table AII1-8 Estimated Number of Subjects in Ongoing Studies as of Data Cutoff Date of December 31, 2006

Study Number	Placebo[a]	M < 5 mg	M = 5 mg	Total M[a]	COX
MP2006	25	25	25	50	
MP2007		50		50	50
Total	25	75	25	100	50

M = Mepro.

[a] Subjects in Study MP2006 also receive etanercept 0.8 mg/kg/week.

Source: Appendix Table EXP1.4.

Table All1-9 Summary of Subjects by Dose and Data Set

	Placebo	M = 1.25 mg	M = 2.5 mg	M = 5 mg	M = 10 mg	M = 15 mg	M = 30 mg	Total Mepro	Other[a]	COX
Controlled Phase 2/3 studies	2200	0	25	2425	2400	325	0	5175	0	2225
All Phase 2/3 studies	2200	0	25	2540	2510	335	0	5410	0	2225
Phase 1 studies	71	18	30	134	108	24	59	373	95	0

M = Mepro.
[a] Other includes moxifloxacin, digoxin, lithium, fluconazole, methotrexate, and warfarin.
Source: Appendix Table EXP1.5.

Table All1-10 Exposure by Dose and Duration—Controlled Phase 2/3 Studies

Duration of Exposure (Weeks)	Placebo N = 2200	M ≤ 5 mg[a] N = 2450	M = 10 mg N = 2400	M = 15 mg N = 325	Total Mepro N = 5175	COX N = 2225
0 to < 1	38 (1.7%)	39 (1.6%)	36 (1.5%)	6 (1.8%)	81 (1.6%)	40 (1.8%)
≥ 1 to < 4	256 (11.6%)	114 (4.7%)	85 (3.5%)	13 (4.0%)	212 (4.1%)	195 (8.8%)
≥ 4 to < 12	301 (13.7%)	255 (10.4%)	242 (10.1%)	102 (31.4%)	599 (11.6%)	326 (14.7%)
≥ 12 to < 24	697 (31.7%)	624 (25.5%)	580 (24.2%)	204 (62.8%)	1408 (27.2%)	582 (26.2%)
≥ 24 to < 36	908 (41.3%)	1363 (55.6%)	1393 (58.0%)	0	2756 (53.3%)	1028 (46.2%)
≥ 36 to < 52	0	35 (1.4%)	40 (1.7%)	0	75 (1.4%)	36 (1.6%)
52	0	20 (0.8%)	24 (1.0%)	0	44 (0.9%)	18 (0.8%)

M = Mepro.
[a] Only 25 patients received < 5.0 mg of Mepro.
Source: Appendix Table EXP1.6.

Table AII1-11 **Exposure by Dose and Duration[a]—All Phase 2/3 Studies**

Duration of Exposure (Weeks)	Placebo N = 2200	M ≤ 5 mg[b] N = 2565	M = 10 mg N = 2510	M = 15 mg N = 335	Total Mepro N = 5410	COX N = 2225
0 to < 1	38 (1.7%)	37 (1.4%)	40 (1.6%)	7 (2.1%)	84 (1.6%)	40 (1.8%)
≥ 1 to < 4	256 (11.6%)	133 (5.2%)	127 (5.1%)	10 (3.0%)	270 (5.0%)	195 (8.8%)
≥ 4 to < 12	301 (13.7%)	331 (12.9%)	241 (9.6%)	105 (31.3%)	677 (12.5%)	326 (14.7%)
≥ 12 to < 24	697 (31.7%)	542 (21.1%)	520 (20.7%)	206 (61.5%)	1268 (23.4%)	582 (26.2%)
≥ 24 to < 36	908 (41.3%)	1410 (55.0%)	1458 (58.1%)	3 (0.9%)	2871 (53.1%)	1028 (46.2%)
≥ 36 to < 52	0	59 (2.3%)	66 (2.6%)	2 (0.6%)	127 (2.3%)	36 (1.6%)
≥ 52	0	53 (2.1%)	58 (2.3%)	2 (0.6%)	113 (2.1%)	18 (0.8%)

M = Mepro.

[a] For subjects who received placebo or COX in a short-term study and then received Mepro in a long-term extension study, Mepro exposure was calculated from the time the subject received the first dose of Mepro in the long-term extension study to the last dose of Mepro received. For subjects who continued to receive Mepro in a long-term extension study, exposure was calculated from the time the subject received the first dose of Mepro in the short-term study to the last dose of Mepro received in the long-term extension study.

[b] Only 25 patients received < 5 mg.

Source: Appendix Table EXP1.7.

In Phase 2/3 studies, the duration of Mepro treatment was between 24 and 52 weeks for the majority of patients. The most frequent Mepro doses administered were 5 mg and 10 mg. In all Phase 2/3 studies datasets, 2871 and 113 patients received Mepro for ≥ 24 weeks and ≥ 52 weeks, respectively, and 2029 subjects received Mepro for at least 6 months (Appendix EXP1.7A).

The Mepro dose group ≤ 5 mg in Phase 2/3 studies includes 25 patients who received Mepro 2.5 mg; the remainder received Mepro 5 mg. Because of the small number of patients who received 2.5 mg, this dose group was combined with the 5 mg group and essentially represents exposure to the 5-mg dose.

➡ **NOTE:** These values indicate that Mepro exposure meets the ICH minimum of 1500 subjects, including 300–600 subjects with ≥ 6 months' exposure and 100 subjects with ≥ 12 months' exposure.[8]

In Appendix Table EXP1.8 exposure by dose and duration of Phase 1 studies can be found. In Phase 1 studies, treatment duration was relatively short for most subjects and ranged from 1 day to 7 days. The most frequent Mepro dose given was 5 mg.

1.3.5 Person-Years Exposure

Person-years exposure (PYE) for completed studies is summarized in Table AII1-12 by data set.

Table AII1-12 **Person-Years Exposure (PYE) by Data Sets**

Data Sets	Placebo	Mepro	COX
Controlled Phase 2/3 studies	994.6	2730.1	1076.2
All Phase 2/3 studies	994.6	2933.2	1076.2
Phase 1 studies	1.0	3.3	0

Source: Appendix Table EXP1.9.

Mepro exposure was approximately 3 times the exposure of either placebo or COX.

1.4 Demographics and Other Baseline Characteristics

Demographic information and baseline weight and BMI are summarized in Appendices DEM1.1, DEM1.2, and DEM1.3 for controlled Phase 2/3 studies, all Phase 2/3 studies, and Phase 1 studies, respectively.

Table AII1-13 summarizes the demographics and baseline weight and BMI values in the controlled Phase 2/3 studies.

Table AII1-13 Summary of Demographic and Other Baseline Characteristics—Controlled Phase 2/3 Studies

Demographic Variable	Placebo N=2200	M≤5 mg N=2450	M=10 mg N=2400	M=15 mg N=325	Total M N=5175	COX N=2225
Gender						
Male	752 (34%)	735 (30%)	768 (32%)	94 (29%)	1597 (31%)	756 (34%)
Female	1448 (66%)	1715 (70%)	1632 (68%)	231 (71%)	3578 (69%)	1469 (66%)
Race						
Caucasian	1628 (74%)	1788 (73%)	1776 (74%)	224 (69%)	3788 (73%)	1691 (76%)
Black	396 (18%)	515 (21%)	480 (20%)	78 (24%)	1073 (21%)	423 (19%)
Asian	110 (5%)	98 (4%)	96 (4%)	7 (2%)	201 (4%)	89 (4%)
Other[a]	66 (3%)	49 (2%)	48 (2%)	16 (5%)	113 (2%)	22 (1%)
Age (years)						
Mean	43.8	46.0	45.1	40.5	45.4	45.1
SD	11.0	9.8	9.7	13.6	9.8	11.1
Median	44	46	45	41	45	45
Range	18–79	18–81	18–80	19–75	18–81	18–80
Age Category						
<40 years	770 (35%)	784 (32%)	816 (34%)	108 (33%)	1708 (33%)	801 (36%)
40–64 years	968 (44%)	1127 (46%)	1152 (48%)	153 (47%)	2432 (47%)	1001 (45%)
≥65 years	462 (21%)	539 (22%)	432 (18%)	64 (20%)	1035 (20%)	423 (19%)
Weight (kg)						
Mean	81.3	79.6	78.9	81.4	79.1	79.9
SD	19.2	18.2	18.5	19.1	18.6	18.8
Median	79.0	78.4	77.9	81.2	78.5	78.1
Range	43–137	44.2–140.3	45–135.7	44.5–138.7	44.2–140.3	43.7–140.6
BMI (kg/m²)						
Mean	27.8	27.9	27.2	27.5	27.7	26.8
SD	6.0	6.1	6.0	6.4	6.0	5.9
Median	27.1	27.0	26.9	27.4	27.3	26.1
Range	18.8–40.1	19.1–40.3	18.5–40	19–40.8	18.5–40.8	18.5–40.3

M = Mepro. SD = standard deviation.
[a] Includes Native Americans and Pacific Islanders.
Source: Appendix Table DEM1.1.

Demographics and other baseline characteristics were well matched across treatment groups. More females than males received study medication. Caucasians were the predominant race in all treatment groups. The majority of subjects in all treatment groups fell into the age categories of < 40 and 40–64 years with the mean age ranging from 40.5 years to 46.0.

The demographic profile, weight, and BMI were also similar across treatment groups for the all Phase 2/3 studies data set (Appendix DEM1.2).

➡ **NOTE:** Although there were no relevant differences among treatment groups, there was a disproportionate number of Caucasians compared to other racial groups. This observation may prompt a request from regulatory agencies to provide more safety information for the other racial groups. It is also interesting to look at the range of some other values listed in the table, for example BMI of > 40 kg/m². It can be argued that patients of this weight would not be suitable candidates for investigational trials due to the inherent risks associated with such excessive weight. Study protocols often exclude patients with very low or very high BMIs; nevertheless, such patients invariably end up in studies. Ongoing data review and edit checks are recommended. If this is done on a routine basis, then outliers like these would be identified earlier when corrective action is still feasible, e.g., sending a newsletter to investigators emphasizing the importance of following the protocol's exclusion criteria, withdrawing such patients from the study, etc.

In the Phase 1 population, there were no important differences in the demographic characteristics, weight, and BMI of the Mepro, placebo, and other groups. Subjects in all treatment groups were generally young (mean age 27–29 years old) and predominantly Caucasian males (Appendix DEM1.3).

In Appendices COEX1.1 and COEX1.2, the coexistent diseases at baseline, in controlled Phase 2/3 studies, and in all Phase 2/3 studies, respectively, are summarized. The most common coexistent illnesses (a rate of ≥ 5% in the total Mepro group in the controlled Phase 2/3 studies) were hypertension (7%) and Type II diabetes (5%).

Rates of these coexistent illnesses were similar across treatment groups (Appendix COEXI.1).

Similar results were found in all Phase 2/3 studies (Appendix COEX1.2).

In Appendix CONMED1.1 and Appendix CONMED1.2 the concomitant medication patients were taking at baseline in controlled Phase 2/3 studies and in all Phase 2/3 studies, respectively, are presented.

The most common concomitant medications (a rate of ≥ 5 % in the total Mepro group in the controlled Phase 2/3 studies) were acetaminophen (24%), proton pump inhibitors (12%), and laxatives (6%). The types and rates of common concomitant medication were similar across treatment groups (Appendix CONMED1.1). The all Phase 2/3 studies dataset showed similar findings (Appendix CONMED1.2).

➡ **NOTE:** In the sample results summarized previously, all treatment groups showed similar demographic and baseline characteristics. If, for instance, the Mepro group had a higher percentage of patients with coexistent hypertension compared to placebo and COX, and the safety findings showed a greater rate of strokes in the Mepro group, it would be difficult to determine whether this was due to the drug, due to the higher rate of hypertension in Mepro patients, or due to an interaction between the drug and patients with hypertension. This is an example of potential confounding; i.e., confusion regarding whether there is a drug effect or another reason for the observed difference. Similar demographics and baseline characteristics across treatment groups simplify the interpretation of safety findings, whereas imbalances make interpretation more difficult. Randomization minimizes the chance for any baseline imbalances.

1.5 Disposition

A summary of the disposition of subjects from controlled Phase 2/3 studies, all Phase 2/3 studies, and Phase 1 studies can be found in Appendix DISP1.1, Appendix DISP1.2, and Appendix DISP1.3, respectively.

If a subject was listed as discontinuing due to both an adverse event and lack of efficacy, the subject was

Table AII1-14 Summary of Subject Disposition—Controlled Phase 2/3 Studies

Patient Disposition	Placebo N = 2200	M ≤ 5 mg N = 2450	M = 10 mg N = 2400	M = 10 mg N = 325	Total M N = 5175	COX N = 2225
Completed	1023 (46.5%)	1624 (66.3%)	1713 (71.4%)	235 (72.3%)	3572 (69.0%)	1159 (52.1%)
Discontinued	1177 (53.5%)	826 (33.7%)	687 (28.6%)	90 (27.7%)	1603 (31.0%)	1066 (47.9%)
Lack of efficacy	1021 (46.4%)	632 (25.8%)	492 (20.5%)	50 (15.4%)	1174 (22.7%)	721 (32.4%)
Adverse event	90 (4.1%)	145 (5.9%)	170 (7.1%)	31 (9.5%)	346 (6.7%)	278 (12.5%)
Adverse event[a]	68 (3.1%)	140 (5.7%)	168 (7.0%)	31 (9.5%)	339 (6.6%)	267 (12.0%)
Disease progression[b]	22 (1.0%)	5 (0.2%)	2 (0.1%)	0	7 (0.1%)	11 (0.5%)
Lost to follow-up	22 (1.0%)	27 (1.1%)	0	6 (1.8%)	33 (0.6%)	45 (2.0%)
Other[c]	44 (2.0%)	22 (0.9%)	25 (1.0%)	3 (1.0%)	50 (1.0%)	22 (1.0%)

[a] Includes AEs not related to disease progression. M = Mepro

[b] Includes any rheumatoid arthritis-related disease; e.g., Disease progression, Worsening disease, Rheumatoid arthritis, Rheumatoid arthritis aggravated, Rheumatoid arthritis flare up events listed on the adverse event CRF that led to premature discontinuation.

[c] Other = withdrew informed consent, poor compliance, subject moved away, pregnancy.

Source: Appendix Table DISP1.1.

included in the adverse event category and was counted only once.

A summary of reasons for discontinuation in controlled Phase 2/3 studies is shown in Table AII1-14. It should be noted that if the investigator listed on the adverse event case report form, "Disease progression," "Worsening disease," "Rheumatoid arthritis," "Rheumatoid arthritis aggravated," or Rheumatoid arthritis flare up," and the event led to premature discontinuation from treatment, the event was included in the adverse event category.

All dose groups of Mepro had fewer discontinuations due to lack of efficacy compared to the placebo and COX treatment groups. The lower rate of discontinuations due to lack of efficacy appeared to be inversely related to the Mepro dose, with the lowest discontinuation rate (15.4%) observed at the highest Mepro dose (15 mg). The highest rate of adverse events (9.5%) that led to treatment discontinuation in the Mepro group was also seen in the 15-mg dose group. Although the rates of adverse events leading to discontinuation were greater in the Mepro group than in the placebo group, the rates were slightly lower than the rate noted in the COX group. The adverse events that led to premature discontinuation in Phase 2/3 studies are discussed further in Section 2.6.1.

Similar results were found for all Phase 2/3 studies (Appendix DISP1.2).

The majority of subjects participating in Phase 1 studies completed treatment. The rates due to discontinuation were similar in all treatment groups—3% Mepro, 2% placebo, and 2% other. One subject in the placebo group (1.4%), 1 subject in the other group (1.0%), and 3 Mepro subjects (0.8%) discontinued due to adverse events (see Section 2.6.1). All other discontinuations were due to withdrawal of consent (Appendix DISP1.3).

1.6 Summary of Exposure to Drug

As of the database cutoff date of December 31, 2006, a total of 5583 unique subjects received 1 or more doses of Mepro from 28 completed studies. In the majority of Phase 2/3 studies, patients received 5 mg or 10 mg of Mepro once daily for a duration of ≥ 24 weeks. A total of 2871 and 113 subjects received Mepro for ≥ 24 weeks and ≥ 52 weeks, respectively, and 2029 subjects received Mepro for at least 6 months. Exposure to Mepro in all Phase 2/3 studies was 2933.2 PYE and was approximately 3 times the exposure of either placebo (994.6) or COX (1076.2). In Phase 2/3 controlled studies, demographics and baseline characteristics were well matched across treatment groups. More females than males received study medication. Caucasians were the predominant race, and the mean age ranged from 40.5 to 46.0 years. More Mepro patients completed treatment (69.0%) compared to those who completed placebo (46.5%) and COX (52.1%) treatment. Discontinuations due to adverse events were 6.7% in the Mepro group compared to 4.1% and 12.5% in the placebo and COX groups, respectively, while discontinuations due to lack of efficacy were 22.7%, 46.4%, and 32.4% in the Mepro, placebo, and COX groups, respectively.

➡ **NOTE:** A summary of each section of the IAS as shown here and throughout this sample IAS is recommended. The IAS provides detailed information as illustrated in this and the others sections of the report. The story can get lost going through all the data. For these reasons, a brief summary synthesizing the key findings is very useful. These section summaries can also be used for the Safety Overview section of the Common Technical Document (CTD) used for drug registration.[1]

■ 2 Adverse Events

2.1 Overview of Adverse Events

An overview of adverse events including any subject who reported at least 1 AE, deaths, other SAEs, severe AEs, AEs related to treatment (as judged by the investigator), and AEs leading to discontinuation can be found in Appendices AE1.1, AE1.2, and AE1.3 for controlled Phase 2/3 studies, all Phase 2/3 studies, and Phase 1 studies, respectively.

Table AII2-1 is an overview of AEs from controlled Phase 2/3 studies. A higher rate of AE events overall—including serious (excluding deaths), severe, and related and AEs leading to discontinuation—was observed in the Mepro and COX groups compared to the placebo group.

In general the AE rates noted in the Mepro group, excluding deaths, appeared to be dose related. The rate of death was similar in the placebo and Mepro groups and slightly higher in the COX group. An additional Mepro patient died in an uncontrolled study (Appendix DEA1.2). No deaths were reported in Phase 1 studies and only 1 subject had an SAE. Deaths and other SAEs are discussed in Sections 2.4 and 2.5, respectively.

2.2 Common Adverse Events

A summary of AE rates for controlled Phase 2/3 studies, all Phase 2/3 studies, and Phase 1 studies grouped by MedDRA SOC and HLGT can be found in Appendices AE2.1, AE2.2, and AE2.3, respectively.

Table AII2-2 summarizes the SOCs and HLGTs from controlled Phase 2/3 studies, with rates ≥ 10 % in the total Mepro group.

The SOC and HLGT with the highest rates were *Gastrointestinal disorders* and *GI signs and symptoms*, respectively, observed in both the Mepro and COX groups. The rates in the Mepro groups appeared to be dose related. Similar results were seen in the all Phase 2/3 studies data set (Appendix AE2.2). In Phase 1 studies, the SOC with the highest rate was *General disorders and administration site conditions* (Appendix AE2.3) seen across all treatment groups.

AEs grouped by SOC and PTs can be found in Appendices AE3.1, AE3.2, and AE3.3 for controlled Phase 2/3 studies, all Phase 2/3 studies, and Phase 1 studies, respectively. AE rates ≥ 5% (in the total Mepro group)

Table AII2-1 **Overview of Adverse Events—Controlled Phase 2/3 Studies**

	Placebo N = 2200	M ≤ 5mg N = 2450	M = 10 mg N = 2400	M = 15 mg N = 325	Total M N = 5175	COX N = 2225
Subject with at least one AE	1366 (62.1%)	1774 (72.4%)	1805 (75.2%)	262 (80.6%)	3841 (74.2%)	1809 (81.3%)
Related adverse events[a]	618 (28.1%)	899 (36.7%)	910 (37.9%)	162 (49.8%)	1971 (38.1%)	1050 (47.2%)
Severe adverse events	200 (9.1%)	320 (13.1%)	382 (15.9%)	60 (18.5%)	762 (14.7%)	407 (18.3%)
Serious adverse events	178 (8.1%)	250 (10.2%)	356 (14.8%)	51 (15.7%)	657 (12.7%)	356 (16.0%)
Deaths	2 (0.09%)	3 (0.12%)	0	0	3 (0.06%)	7 (0.31%)
Adverse events leading to discontinuation	90 (4.1%)	145 (5.9%)	170 (7.1%)	31 (9.5%)	346 (6.7%)	278 (12.5%)

M = Mepro.
[a] As judged by the investigator.
Source: Appendix Table AE1.1.

Table AII2-2 Summary of Adverse Events by System Organ Class and High Level Group Term With Rates of ≥ 10%[a]—Controlled Phase 2/3 Studies

Adverse Event SOC/HLGT	Placebo N = 2200	M ≤ 5mg N = 2450	M = 10 mg N = 2400	M = 15 mg N = 325	Total M N = 5175	COX N = 2225
Any adverse event	1366 (62.1%)	1774 (72.4%)	1805 (75.2%)	262 (80.6%)	3841 (74.2%)	1809 (81.3%)
Gastrointestinal disorders (SOC)	555 (25.2%)	899 (36.7%)	929 (38.7%)	138 (42.5%)	1966 (38.0%)	1066 (47.9%)
Gastrointestinal signs and symptoms (HLGT)	464 (21.1%)	1183 (48.3%)	1202 (50.1%)	174 (53.5%)	2559 (49.4%)	1295 (58.2%)
General disorders and administration site conditions (SOC)	222 (10.0%)	313 (12.8%)	226 (9.4%)	30 (9.2%)	569 (11.0%)	223 (10.0%)
Infections and infestations (SOC)	266 (12.1%)	333 (13.6%)	276 (11.5%)	40 (12.3%)	649 (12.5%)	245 (11.0%)
Infections—pathogen unspecified (HLGT)	244 (11.1%)	275 (11.2%)	280 (11.7%)	30 (9.2%)	585 (11.3%)	220 (9.9%)
Nervous system disorders (SOC)	577 (26.2%)	411 (16.8%)	351 (14.6%)	40 (12.3%)	802 (15.5%)	353 (15.9%)
Neurological disorders (HLGT)	266 (12.1%)	331 (13.5%)	301 (12.5%)	40 (12.3%)	672 (13.0%)	260 (11.7%)

M = Mepro.
[a] Rate of ≥ 10% in the total Mepro group.
Source: Appendix Table AE2.1.

Table AII2-3 Summary of Adverse Events With a Rate of ≥ 5%[a]—Controlled Phase 2/3 Studies

	Placebo N = 2200	M ≤ 5 mg N = 2450	M = 10 mg N = 2400	M = 15 mg N = 325	Total M N = 5175	COX N = 2225
Any adverse event	1366 (62.1%)	1774 (72.4%)	1805 (75.2%)	262 (80.6%)	3841 (74.2%)	1809 (81.3%)
Dizziness	339 (15.4%)	358 (14.6%)	362 (15.1%)	43 (13.2%)	763 (14.7%)	334 (15.0%)
Epigastric discomfort	24 (1.1%)	164 (6.7%)	180 (7.5%)	29 (8.9%)	373 (7.2%)	200 (9.0%)
Nausea	68 (3.1%)	142 (5.8%)	170 (7.1%)	28 (8.6%)	340 (6.6%)	276 (12.4%)
Headache	539 (24.5%)	184 (7.5%)	134 (5.6%)	13 (4.0%)	331 (6.4%)	267 (12.0%)
Nasopharyngitis	143 (6.5%)	147 (6.0%)	106 (4.4%)	23 (7.1%)	276 (5.3%)	122 (5.5%)
Abdominal pain upper	66 (3.0%)	123 (5.0%)	180 (7.5%)	29 (8.9%)	332 (6.4%)	185 (8.3%)
Dyspepsia	44 (2.0%)	100 (4.1%)	142 (5.9%)	21 (6.5%)	263 (5.1%)	231 (10.4%)
Vomiting	64 (2.9%)	105 (4.3%)	132 (5.5%)	21 (6.5%)	258 (5.0%)	174 (7.8%)
PUBs[b]	1 (< 0.1%)	17 (0.7%)	41 (1.7%)	10 (3.1%)	68 (1.3%)	96 (4.3%)

M = Mepro; PUBs = perforations, ulcers, and bleeds.
[a] Rate of ≥ 5% in the total Mepro group.
[b] Although the rate of PUBs is < 5% in the total Mepro group, it was included because PUBs are known and important NSAID-related AEs, a Mepro dose-response was seen, the rate in the total Mepro and COX groups were twice placebo, and the rate was close to 5% in the COX group.
Source: Appendix Table AE3.1.

and comparative rates in the placebo and COX groups for controlled Phase 2/3 studies are shown in Table AII2-3.

The shaded AEs are the events considered to be common potential adverse reactions (ARs) to Mepro based on the criteria summarized in Section 1.2.2. Although the rates of PUBs in the total Mepro and COX groups were less than 5%, PUBs were also included as potential adverse reactions for the following reasons:

- PUBs are a known class effect of NSAIDs.
- The rates of PUBs for the Mepro and COX groups were greater than 2 times placebo.

- An evident dose effect in the Mepro group was seen.
- The rate in the COX group was close to 5%.

All the common potential adverse reactions were GI related, expected, and consistent with the known risk profile of NSAIDs. A dose relationship was noted across Mepro doses for all common potential adverse reactions. The same potential adverse reactions identified in the Mepro group were also seen in the COX group. At the recommended Mepro doses of 5-mg and 10-mg, the event rates of these potential adverse reactions were noted to be lower than in the COX group. The rate of PUBs in the COX group was more than twice the rate observed in the Mepro 5 mg and 10 mg dose groups.

➡ **NOTE:** The determination of common potential adverse reactions is of considerable importance in providing a focused and clinically meaningful summary of the data. Once identified, these events should be the ones discussed in the subsequent text. It makes *no sense* to write about events that are clearly not drug related, e.g., where the placebo rate is similar or greater than the rate in the investigational group. This distracts and confuses. Remember the goals are to identify what is drug related and to characterize those factors that add to or decrease the drug effect. Of course there is always a concern that something important will be missed. Don't worry; as long as the reviewers have access to all the data, e.g., appendix tables, and the methodology used for analysis is clear and transparent, the reviewers can do their own analyses of the data if they feel something important was left out or the analyses were done incorrectly. The table displays shown as in-text tables include the rate of any subject with 1 or more AEs providing the reviewer with an overview of all events; the remainder of the table is then devoted to the summary of the potential adverse reactions, which is the main focus of these tables.

In Appendix AE4.1, AE4.2, and AE4.3, AE rates per 100 PYE can be found for controlled Phase 2/3 studies, all Phase 2/3 studies, and Phase 1 studies, respectively.

Table AII2-4 summarizes the rates per 100 PYE for adverse events overall and for potential adverse reactions for controlled Phase 2/3 studies.

A dose response was seen in the Mepro group. At the recommended Mepro doses of 5 mg and 10 mg, the rates per 100 PYE for potential adverse reactions were less than those observed in the COX group. For PUBs, the COX group had a rate greater than 6.5 times and 2.5 times the 5-mg and 10-mg Mepro dose groups, respectively.

Table AII2-4 **Summary of Adverse Events Overall and Potential Adverse Reactions by 100 Person-Years Exposure—Controlled Phase 2/3 Studies**

	Placebo	M ≤ 5 mg	M = 10 mg	M = 15 mg	Total Mepro	COX
Person-year exposure	994.6	1308.3	1313.9	107.8	2730.1	1076.2
Any adverse event	137.3	135.6	137.4	243.0	140.7	168.1
Abdominal pain upper	6.6	9.4	13.7	26.9	12.2	17.2
Dyspepsia	4.4	7.6	10.8	19.5	9.6	21.5
Epigastric discomfort	2.4	12.5	13.7	26.9	13.7	18.6
Nausea	6.8	10.9	12.9	26.0	12.5	25.6
PUBs	0.1	1.3	3.1	9.3	2.5	8.9
Vomiting	6.4	8.0	10.0	19.5	9.5	16.2

M = Mepro; PUBs = perforations, ulcers, and bleeds.
Source: Appendix Table AE4.1.

Similar results were seen for the all Phase 2/3 studies data set (Appendix AE.4.2). AE rates by 100 PYE in the Phase 1 groups were difficult to interpret because the PYE for the Phase 1 studies was small due to the limited durations of these studies.

2.2.1 Summary of Adverse Events by Intensity

In Appendices AE5.1, AE5.2, and AE5.3, AEs by intensity are presented for the controlled Phase 2/3 studies, all Phase 2/3 studies, and Phase 1 studies, respectively. Table AII2-5 summarizes AEs by intensity for adverse events overall and for potential adverse reactions from controlled Phase 2/3 studies.

In the placebo group the majority of AEs overall were mild to moderate in intensity. There were more moderate to severe events seen in the Mepro and COX groups compared to placebo.

A similar pattern was seen in the all Phase 2/3 studies data set (Appendix AE5.2). The majority of events across treatment groups in the Phase 1 studies were listed as mild (Appendix AE5.3).

2.2.2 Summary of Adverse Events by Relationship to Study Medication (as Judged by the Investigator)

In Appendices AE6.1, AE6.2, and AE6.3, adverse events by relationship to study medication (as judged by the investigator) are presented for controlled Phase 2/3 studies, all Phase 2/3 studies, and Phase 1 studies, respectively.

In Table AII2-6, the relationship to study drug (as judged by the investigator) is presented for adverse events overall and for potential adverse reactions in controlled Phase 2/3 studies.

The rates for AEs overall and for the potential adverse reactions considered treatment related (as judged by the investigator) were greater in the Mepro and COX groups compared to placebo.

The results in all Phase 2/3 studies were similar (Appendix AE6.2).

The majority of events in Phase 1 studies were considered unrelated to treatment (Appendix AE6.3).

⮕ **NOTE:** In determining an AE's relationship to drug for common AEs, the best and most objective way of doing this is by utilizing the criteria for identification of potential adverse reactions described in the methods section (see Section 1.2.2). In the analysis of aggregate data, determining the relationship to treatment using the investigator's assessment is not as strong due to inconsistencies in investigator assessments. Nevertheless, for completeness, this type of analysis is included in clinical study reports and the IAS. The investigator's assessment of causality plays a more important role in the evaluation of individual events such as SAEs.

2.2.3 Summary of Adverse Events by Time to Onset and Time to Resolution

In Appendices AE7.1, AE7.2, and AE7.3 adverse events by time to onset can be found for controlled Phase 2/3 studies, all Phase 2/3 studies, and Phase 1 studies, respectively. A summary of adverse events by time to resolution for controlled Phase 2/3 studies, all Phase 2/3 studies, and Phase 1 studies can be found in Appendices AE8.1, AE8.2, and AE8.3, respectively.

Table AII2-7 summarizes the median time to onset and time to resolution for adverse events overall and for potential adverse reactions in controlled Phase 2/3 studies.

For those events considered to be potential adverse reactions, with the exception of PUBs, the median time to onset was shorter and time to resolution was longer for both the Mepro and COX treatment groups compared to placebo, but onset still occurred early, i.e., within the first month of treatment. For PUBs, however, the onset was later and the duration longer.

Time to onset by time interval was also analyzed for the potential adverse reactions for the controlled Phase 2/3 studies (Appendix AE7.1.1) and all Phase 2/3 studies (Appendix AE7.1.2).

In Table AII2-8, the time to onset of PUBs by time interval is summarized for controlled Phase 2/3 studies.

This analysis shows a different pattern in time to onset for Mepro compared to the COX group. For Mepro, the majority of PUBs occurred between 4 and 24 weeks, with no PUBs reported after 36 weeks. This pattern differed for COX where the onset of PUBs began between 4–12 weeks and the rate progressively increased over time.

⮕ **NOTE:** This type of analysis looks at the rates of events based on the number of subjects exposed to the drug over time. Note that only 18 COX subjects are exposed to study medication for 52 weeks; thus the rate of PUBs in the COX group is 5.6% (1/18) at week 52.

Table AII2-5 Summary of Adverse Events Overall and Potential Adverse Reactions by Intensity—Controlled Phase 2/3 Studies

	Placebo N = 2200 n/N (%)				Total Mepro N = 5175 n/N (%)				COX N = 2225 n/N (%)			
	Mild	Mod	Sev	Total	Mild	Mod	Sev	Total	Mild	Mod	Sev	Total
Any adverse event	811 (36.9%)	355 (16.1%)	200 (9.1%)	1366 (62.1%)	1629 (31.5%)	1450 (28.0%)	762 (14.7%)	3841 (74.2%)	623 (28.0%)	779 (35.0%)	407 (18.3%)	1809 (81.3%)
Abdominal pain upper	27 (1.2%)	27 (1.2%)	12 (0.5%)	66 (3.0%)	58 (1.1%)	166 (3.2%)	108 (2.1%)	332 (6.4%)	24 (1.1%)	50 (2.2%)	111 (5.0%)	185 (8.3%)
Dyspepsia	17 (0.8%)	11 (0.5%)	16 (0.7%)	44 (2.0%)	33 (0.6%)	72 (1.4%)	158 (3.1%)	263 (5.1%)	40 (1.8%)	85 (3.8%)	106 (4.8%)	231 (10.4%)
Epigastric discomfort	10 (0.5%)	7 (0.3%)	7 (0.3%)	24 (1.1%)	120 (2.3%)	183 (3.5%)	70 (1.4%)	373 (7.2%)	29 (1.3%)	111 (5.0%)	60 (2.7%)	200 (9.0%)
Nausea	25 (1.1%)	33 (1.5%)	10 (0.5%)	68 (3.1%)	133 (2.6%)	154 (3.0%)	53 (1.0%)	340 (6.6%)	76 (3.4%)	155 (7.0%)	45 (2.0%)	276 (12.4%)
PUBs	0	0	1 (<0.1%)	1 (<0.1%)	0	5 (0.1%)	63 (1.2%)	68 (1.3%)	0	3 (0.1%)	93 (4.2%)	96 (4.3%)
Vomiting	31 (1.4%)	29 (1.3%)	4 (0.2%)	64 (2.9%)	68 (1.3%)	140 (2.7%)	50 (1.0%)	258 (5.0%)	51 (2.3%)	101 (4.5%)	22 (1.0%)	174 (7.8%)

Mod = moderate; sev = severe; PUBs = perforations, ulcers, and bleeds.
Source: Appendix Table AE5.1.

Table AII2-6 Summary of Adverse Events Overall and Potential Adverse Reactions by Treatment Relationship[a]—Controlled Phase 2/3 Studies

	Placebo N=2200			Total Mepro N=5175			COX N=2225		
	NR	R	Total	NR	R	Total	NR	R	Total
Any adverse event	748 (34.0%)	618 (28.1%)	1366 (62.1%)	1870 (36.1%)	1971 (38.1%)	3841 (74.2%)	759 (34.1%)	1050 (47.2%)	1809 (81.3%)
Abdominal pain upper	29 (1.3%)	37 (1.7%)	66 (3.0%)	27 (0.5%)	305 (5.9%)	332 (6.4%)	29 (1.3%)	156 (7.0%)	185 (8.3%)
Dyspepsia	20 (0.9%)	24 (1.1%)	44 (2.0%)	19 (0.4%)	244 (4.7%)	263 (5.1%)	31 (1.4%)	200 (9.0%)	231 (10.4%)
Epigastric discomfort	0	24 (1.1%)	24 (1.1%)	62 (1.2%)	311 (6.0%)	373 (7.2%)	22 (1.0%)	178 (8.0%)	200 (9.0%)
Nausea	26 (1.2%)	42 (1.9%)	68 (3.1%)	72 (1.4%)	268 (5.2%)	340 (6.6%)	49 (2.2%)	227 (10.2%)	276 (12.4%)
PUBs	0	1 (< 0.1%)	1 (< 0.1%)	0	68 (1.3%)	68 (1.3%)	0	96 (4.3%)	96 (4.3%)
Vomiting	31 (1.4%)	33 (1.5%)	64 (2.9%)	52 (1.0%)	206 (4.0%)	258 (5.0%)	40 (1.8%)	134 (6.0%)	174 (7.8%)

NR = not related; R = related; PUBs = perforations, ulcers, and bleeds.
[a] As judged by the investigator.
Source: Appendix Table AE6.1.

Table AII2-7 Summary of Adverse Events Overall and Potential Adverse Reactions by Median Time to Onset and Resolution—Controlled Phase 2/3 Studies

	Placebo N = 2200	M ≤ 5 mg N = 2450	M = 10 mg N = 2400	M = 15 mg N = 325	Total M N = 5175	COX N = 2225
Any adverse event						
Median time to onset (days)	8.0	9.0	8.5	7.5	8.5	7.0
Median time to resolution (days)	3.0	4.0	4.5	5.5	4.5	5.5
Abdominal pain upper						
Median time to onset (days)	21.0	7.0	9.0	8.5	8.0	7.0
Median time to resolution (days)	3.5	5.0	6.0	7.0	5.5	9.0
Dyspepsia						
Median time to onset (days)	18.0	7.5	6.0	5.5	7.0	5.0
Median time to resolution (days)	2.5	7.0	7.0	8.0	7.0	8.5
Epigastric discomfort						
Median time to onset (days)	17.5	7.5	7.0	6.5	7.0	7.5
Median time to resolution (days)	4.0	8.0	8.0	8.5	8.0	8.5
Nausea						
Median time to onset (days)	15.0	7.0	6.0	6.0	6.5	5.5
Median time to resolution (days)	4.5	7.5	7.5	8.0	7.0	8.5
PUBs						
Median time to onset (days)	70.0	45.0	39.0	38.5	40.5	72.0
Median time to resolution (days)	9.5	11.0	12.0	11.5	11.5	18.5
Vomiting						
Median time to onset (days)	20.0	7.5	6.0	6.5	7.0	5.5
Median time to resolution (days)	2.0	3.0	3.5	4.0	3.5	5.0

M = Mepro; PUBs = perforations, ulcers, and bleeds.
Source: Appendix Tables AE7.1 and AE8.1.

2.2.4 Summary of Concomitant Medication

In Appendices CONMED2.1, CONMED2.2, and CONMED2.3, the concomitant medications (i.e., medication other than the study drug that was taken during the treatment period) are summarized for the controlled Phase 2/3 studies, all Phase 2/3 studies, and the Phase 1 studies, respectively.

Table AII2-9 summarizes the most common (i.e., used by ≥ 5% of the subjects) concomitant medication across treatment groups in the controlled Phase 2/3 studies.

The most common concomitant medication taken was acetaminophen with no relevant difference in rates seen across treatment groups. H$_2$-receptor antagonists and antacids were the other common concomitant medications taken. Usage rates were higher in the Mepro and COX groups compared to placebo. In the Mepro group this was correlated with dose, i.e., higher usage rates with higher Mepro doses. Higher usage rates of H$_2$-receptor antagonists and antacids were noted in the COX group compared to the Mepro 5-mg and 10-mg groups. These findings are consistent with the higher rate of GI-related events seen in the COX group compared to the 5-mg and 10-mg Mepro groups.

2.3 Summary of Adverse Events by Subgroup

The following subgroup analyses were done, and the results are presented in Section 5.

- Gender
- Age
- Race
- Geographic region
- Renal function
- Hepatic function

Table AII2-8 Summary of PUBs by Time to Onset and Time Interval—Controlled Phase 2/3 Studies

Duration of Exposure	Placebo N = 2200	M ≤ 5 mg N = 2450	M = 10 mg N = 2400	M = 15 mg N = 325	Total Mepro N = 5175	COX N = 2225
0 to < 1	2200	2450	2400	325	5175	2225
	0	0	0	0	0	0
≥ 1 to < 4	2162	2411	2364	319	5094	2185
	0	0	0	0	0	0
≥ 4 to < 12	1906	2297	2279	306	4882	1990
	0	8 (0.4%)	22 (1.0%)	9 (2.9%)	39 (0.8%)	28 (1.4%)
≥ 12 to < 24	1605	2042	2037	204	4283	1664
	1 (0.1%)	7 (0.3%)	18 (0.9%)	1 (0.5%)	26 (0.6%)	35 (2.1%)
> 24 to < 36	908	1418	1457	0	2875	1082
	0	2 (0.1%)	1 (0.1%)	0	3 (0.1%)	30 (2.8%)
≥ 36 to < 52	0	55	64	0	119	54
	0	0	0	0	0	2 (3.7%)
52	0	20	20	0	40	18
	0	0	0	0	0	1 (5.6%)

M = Mepro; PUBs = perforations, ulcers, and bleeds.
Source: Appendix Table AE7.1.1.

Table AII2-9 Summary of Concomitant Medication in ≥ 5% of Patients—Controlled Phase 2/3 Studies

	Placebo N = 2200	M ≤ 5 mg N = 2450	M = 10 mg N = 2400	M = 10 mg N = 325	Total M N = 5175	COX N = 2225
Acetaminophen	1132 (51.5%)	1176 (48.0%)	1104 (46.0%)	146 (44.9%)	2426 (46.9%)	1068 (48.0%)
H₂-receptor antagonists	202 (9.2%)	510 (20.8%)	583 (24.3%)	91 (28.0%)	1184 (22.9%)	661 (29.7%)
Antacids	107 (4.9%)	250 (10.2%)	295 (12.3%)	51 (15.7%)	596 (11.5%)	412 (18.5%)

M = Mepro.
Source: Appendix Table CONMED2.1.

Table AII2-10 Summary of Deaths—All Phase 2/3 Studies

Treatment Group	Total Number of Patients	Total Number of Deaths	Mortality Rate	Person-Years Exposure (PYE)	Mortality per 100 PYE
Placebo	2200	2	0.09%	994.6	0.20
Mepro	5410	4	0.07%	2933.2	0.14
COX	2225	7	0.31%	1076.2	0.65

Source: Appendix Table DEA1.2.

2.4 Deaths

Deaths were captured up to 30 days after treatment. Crude mortality rates and mortality rates per 100 PYE can be found in Appendix DEA1.1 and DEA1.2, for controlled Phase 2/3 studies and all Phase 2/3 studies, respectively. Listings of all deaths can be found in Appendix DEALIST1.1. Narratives of patients who died are located in Appendix DEANAR1.1. No deaths were reported in the Phase 1 studies.

Table AII2-10 is a summary of deaths that occurred in all Phase 2/3 studies by crude rate and rate per 100 PYE. A listing of these events is shown in Table AII2-11.

Table AII2-11 Listing of Deaths—All Phase 2/3 Studies

Study No.	Patient No.	Age/Gender/Race	Dose	Exposure to Study Medication (Days)	Reported AE Term	MedDRA PT	Relationship to Study Medication
Placebo							
MP2004	2004-0054	65/male/Caucasian	0	70	Acute myocardial infarction	Acute myocardial infarction	Unlikely
MP3002	3002-0102	36/female/Black	0	8	Auto accident	Road traffic accident	None
Mepro							
MP2001	2001-0004	24/female/Caucasian	5 mg	4	Gunshot	Gunshot wound	None
MP2004X	2004X-0023	72/female/Caucasian	10 mg	302	Septic shock	Septic shock	Unlikely
MP3002	3002-0876	71/male/Black	5 mg	259	MI	Myocardial infarction	Unlikely
MP3003	3003-0443	64/female/Caucasian	5 mg	330[a]	Suicide	Completed suicide	Unlikely
COX							
MP2003	2003-0098	75/male/Caucasian	25 mg	42[b]	Sudden death	Sudden death	Unlikely
MP3001	3001-0649	80/female/Caucasian	25 mg	79	Bleeding stomach ulcer; cardiac arrest	Gastric ulcer haemorrhage; cardiac arrest	Probable
MP3001	3001-0018	66/male/Black	25 mg	150[c]	Ruptured aortic aneurysm	Aortic aneurysm rupture	None
MP3001	3001-0110	34/male/Black	25 mg	42	Car accident	Road traffic accident	None
MP3001	3001-0329	79/female/Asian	25 mg	93	Ischemic stroke	Cerebrovascular accident	Unlikely
MP3003	3003-0066	73/male/Caucasian	25 mg	290	Myocardial infarction	Myocardial infarction	Unlikely
MP3003	3003-0761	69/female/Black	25 mg	116	Diabetic coma; staph wound infection	Diabetic coma; wound infection staphylococcal	Unlikely

[a] Died 28 days after last dose of study medication.
[b] Died 30 days after last dose of study medication.
[c] Died 25 days after the last dose of study medication.
Source: Appendix DEALIST1.1.

The crude mortality rate and mortality per 100 PYE (although low) were greatest for the COX treatment group (0.31% and 0.65/100 PYE, respectively). The lowest crude mortality rate and mortality rate per 100 PYE were observed in the Mepro group (0.07% and 0.14/100 PYE, respectively).

Three of the deaths—1 in the Mepro group (suicide, Patient 3003-0443, study MP3003) and 2 deaths in the COX group (sudden death, Patient 2003-098, study MP2003; and ruptured aortic aneurysm, Patient 3001-0018, study MP3001) occurred 28, 30, and 25 days after the last dose of study medication, respectively. Only 1 death was considered related to study medication as judged by the investigator, and it occurred in the COX group. The full narrative of this event can be found in Appendix DEANAR1.0; a brief narrative of the event follows.

An 80-year-old Caucasian female (Patient 3001-0649, study MP3001) was brought to the emergency room after she vomited large quantities (approximately 1 liter) of bright red material. In the emergency room, she was confused, diaphoretic, with a blood pressure of 60/30 mmHg and a pulse of 160 beats per minute. An intravenous line was started, and she received large volumes of 0.9% normal saline solution. She was typed and cross-matched for packed red blood cells and other blood work was pending. Before emergency endoscopy could be done, the patient had a cardiac arrest. All attempts at resuscitation failed, and she was pronounced dead at 5:43 PM on May 2, 2006—10 minutes after arriving in the emergency room. She received COX 25 mg for 79 days before the onset of these events. She was on no other medication. There was no history of alcohol use and she had no prior history of ulcers or gastrointestinal complaints. An autopsy showed a gastric ulcer 1.0 cm in diameter with erosion of the gastroduodenal artery. The investigator judged the gastric ulcer and hemorrhage and subsequent cardiac arrest as probably related to study medication.

➡ **NOTE:** The all Phase 2/3 studies data set rather than the controlled Phase 2/3 studies data set was selected for in-text discussion of deaths, other SAEs, and other significant events. This ensures that events that occurred in the uncontrolled studies are also included and discussed in the text where appropriate. In this section and the sections that follow, a top-down approach is taken, i.e., going from group results to individual patients. First, the crude rate/rate per 100 PYE is presented, followed by a listing of subjects (if not too long), and then narratives are presented. When referring to a patient in the text, it is important to provide the patient ID number and study number so the reviewer can locate more patient information if desired. For electronic submissions this is usually hyperlinked, making it even easier to access. Brief, in-text narratives for events of interest, i.e., deaths, other SAEs, and other significant AEs considered related to treatment (as judged by either the investigator or the sponsor) should also be included in the text unless the volume would preclude this. Patients who received placebo or active control should also be discussed in the text for comparison purposes.

2.5 Other SAEs

In Appendix tables SAE1.1, SAE1.2, and SAE1.3, the crude rates and rates per PYE 100 for SAEs are presented for the controlled Phase 2/3 studies, all Phase 2/3 studies, and Phase 1 studies, respectively.

Table AII2-12 is a summary of the crude rates and rates per 100 PYE for SAEs from all Phase 2/3 studies.

The rate of SAEs in all Phase 2/3 studies was higher in the Mepro group (13.5%) than in the placebo (8.1%) group, but it was the highest in the COX group (16.0%). A similar pattern was seen when rates were calculated by 100 PYE. The findings in the controlled Phase 2/3 studies data set (Appendix SAE1.1) were similar. There was only 1 SAE reported in Phase 1 studies.

In Appendix tables SAE2.1, SAE2.2, and SAE2.3, SAEs are summarized by MedDRA PT and SOC, for subjects in controlled Phase 2/3 studies, all Phase 2/3 studies, and Phase 1 studies, respectively. In Appendices SAELIST1.1 (all Phase 2/3 studies) and SAELIST1.2 (Phase 1 studies), listings of all subjects with SAEs can be found. Narratives of all subjects with SAEs can be found in Appendices SAENAR1.1 and SAENAR1.2 for all Phase 2/3 studies and Phase 1 studies, respectively.

The majority of SAEs were considered unrelated to study medication (as judged by the investigator). PUBs were the SAEs most commonly considered treatment related and are discussed further in Section 2.7.1. Only 10 SAEs (excluding PUBs) were considered drug related

Table AII2-12 Summary of Serious Adverse Events—All Phase 2/3 Studies

Treatment Group	Total Number of Patients	Number of Patients With SAEs	Crude SAE Rate	Person–Years Exposure (PYE)	SAEs per 100 PYE
Placebo	2200	178	8.1%	994.6	17.9
Mepro	5410	730	13.5%	2933.2	24.9
COX	2225	356	16.0%	1076.2	33.1

SAE = serious adverse event.
Source: Appendix Table SAE1.2.

(as judged by the investigator); 3 (0.06%) occurred in the Mepro group, 3(0.14%) in the placebo group, and 4 (0.18%) in the COX group. A listing of these SAEs is found in Table AII2-13.

Only 1 nonrelated SAE was reported in a Phase 1 study (Subject 1004-003, study MP 1004). This subject had emergency bronchoscopy to remove a foreign body (chicken bone) that he inadvertently aspirated. He was admitted to the hospital overnight for observation, recovered without any sequelae, and continued participation in the study.

➡ **NOTE:** This is an example of telling the story, i.e., focusing the text on the information considered to be of the greatest relevance, i.e., treatment-related SAEs in this case. If there are SAEs that the sponsor considers treatment related or worthy of mention, these should be included in the text as well. Remember, don't worry about leaving something important out of the text. As long as you state where the complete information can be found, i.e., the appendix number, the reviewer can pick and choose which events he or she is interested in.

Even though the SAE from the Phase 1 study mentioned above was not treatment related, the reviewer might still be curious and want to know what this event was. Because this was easily done with a minimum number of words, a brief description of the event was included. If there were many unrelated SAEs, in-text descriptions of these events would not be recommended.

Complete narratives of these events can be found in Appendix SAENAR1.0. Brief narratives presented by treatment group are presented next.

Mepro

■ Patient 2003X-0601 from study MP2003X, a 48-year-old Caucasian male, was brought to the emergency room by police after they found him talking loudly to himself and rapidly pacing back and forth at a bus stop. Subsequent history obtained by his wife revealed that for the last month, the patient hardly slept except for 1 or 2 hours each night; talked incessantly about a get-rich scheme that couldn't fail; and impulsively bought $1000 worth of merchandise over the internet. According to his wife, his behavior started to change at about the same time he was laid off work due to company downsizing—about 2 months before this event. There was no history of drugs or alcohol abuse and no previous psychiatric history. Subsequent drug screens were negative for alcohol and drugs. Study medication (Mepro 10 mg) was discontinued after 116 days of treatment. He was admitted to the psychiatric ward with a diagnosis of acute mania. He was treated with lithium and zolpidem, and had an uneventful and full recovery. The investigator accessed this event as possibly related to study medication. This case is discussed further in Section 2.7.11.

■ Patient 3002-0867 from study MP3002, a 34-year-old Asian female, was admitted to the hospital with the diagnosis of Stevens-Johnson syndrome (SJS). On the day of admission, she was found to have facial swelling, blisters ranging in size of 2–3 cm in her mouth and conjunctiva, and

Table AII2-13 Listing of Treatment-Related Serious Adverse Events (Excluding PUBs)[a]—All Phase 2/3 Studies

Study No./Patient Number	Age/Gender/Race	Dose	Exposure to Study Medication (Days)	Reported AE term	MedDRA PT	Premature D/C	Outcome
Placebo							
MP2001/2001-0023	58/male/Caucasian	0	34	Severe diarrhea; dehydration	Diarrhea; dehydration	No	Recovered
MP2002/2002-0016	47/female/Black	0	16	Depression; suicidal thoughts	Depression; suicide ideation	Yes	Ongoing
MP3002/3002-1901	63/female/Caucasian	0	114	Memory problems	Memory impairment	Yes	Ongoing
Mepro							
MP2003X/2003X-0601	48/male/Caucasian	10 mg	116	Mania	Mania	Yes	Recovered
MP3002/3002-0867	34/female/Asian	5 mg	97	Stevens-Johnson syndrome	Stevens-Johnson syndrome	Yes	Recovered
MP3003/3003-0535	62/male/Caucasian	10 mg	7	Nausea and vomiting	Nausea; vomiting	Yes	Recovered
COX							
MP2003/2003-0017	47/male/Black	25 mg	5	Nausea and vomiting; dehydration	Nausea; vomiting; dehydration	Yes	Recovered
MP3001/3001-0518	80/female/Black	25 mg	79	Leg swelling, congestive heart failure	Oedema peripheral; congestive heart failure	Yes	Recovered with sequelae
MP3001/3001-0761	41/female/Caucasian	25 mg	128	Depression	Depression	Yes	Ongoing
MP3003/3003-0535	62/male/Black	25 mg	275	TIA, hypertension	Transient ischemic attack; hypertension	Yes	Recovered

[a] As judged by the investigator.
Source: Appendix SAELIST1.1.

large blisters ranging in size from 10-20 cm on her arms, legs, abdomen, chest, and back. She also had a fever of 38.9°C (102°F), blood pressure of 88/57 mmHg, and pulse of 120 bpm. Study medication (Mepro 5 mg) was discontinued (after 97 days of exposure). She was given supportive care that included intravenous fluid replacement and medication for pain control. When her blisters ruptured, the dead skin was debrided and dressed with sterile dressings. She had a slow but complete recovery and was discharged from the hospital 3 weeks after admission. Seven days before her hospitalization, she was started on penicillin for treatment of strep throat and was taking the antibiotic at the time her symptoms began. Subsequent blood testing revealed she carried the B*1502 allele of HLA-B. The investigator considered this event to be possibly related to study medication (Mepro 5 mg). This case is discussed further in Section 2.7.10.1.

- Patient 3003-0535 from study MP3003, a 62-year-old Caucasian male, was admitted to the hospital with severe nausea and vomiting 7 days after starting Mepro 10 mg. His nausea and vomiting began within a day of starting Mepro and became progressively worse until his hospitalization for severe dehydration. Treatment included stopping study medication (after 7 days of treatment), intravenous fluids, and prochlorperazine given intramuscularly. He recovered fully and was discharged 48 hours later. The investigator considered these events to be probably related to study medication.

Placebo

- Patient 2001-0023 from study MP2001, a 58-year-old Caucasian male, was hospitalized for severe diarrhea and dehydration on day 34 of treatment (placebo). Onset of diarrhea was sudden and severe with the patient reporting approximately 5 liters of watery diarrhea within 2 hours of onset. In the emergency room, the subject was febrile (38.3°C), hypotensive (BP 90/60 mmHg), and tachycardic (108 bpm). He was hospitalized for intravenous fluid replacement and observation. His stool was cultured and investigated for ova and parasites, but no causative agent was found. Within 48 hours he was afebrile, with normal blood pressure and pulse. His diarrhea had also resolved. Study medication was stopped for 2 days while he was hospitalized,

and it was restarted after discharge without any further episodes of diarrhea reported. The investigator assessed these events as possibly related to study medication (placebo).

- Patient 2002-0016 from study MP2002, a 47-year-old Black female, was hospitalized for suicidal thoughts and depression 16 days after starting study medication (placebo). Ten years earlier, the patient had a 2-week period of feeling depressed after her mother suddenly died. She was seen by a psychiatrist and received antidepressant therapy for 4 months and fully recovered. Five days after starting study medication, she started to feel low. No precipitating events such as job loss or divorce were identified. Study medication was discontinued after 16 days of treatment. She was admitted into the psychiatric ward, placed on suicide precautions, and started on fluoxetine treatment. The events were still ongoing after the last follow-up call. The investigator assessed these events to be possibly related to study medication (placebo).

- Patient 3002-1901 from study MP3002, a 63-year-old Caucasian female, developed progressive memory problems over a 3-month period. She was evaluated by her family physician and found to have significant memory loss. Study medication (placebo) was stopped after 114 days of treatment, and she was scheduled for a neurological evaluation. The event was ongoing at time of the last follow-up call. The investigator considered the patient's memory loss to be possibly related to study medication (placebo).

COX

- Patient MP2003-0017 from study MP2003, a 47-year-old Black male, developed nausea and vomiting 5 days after starting study medication (COX 25 mg). He was instructed to stop his study medication, but the nausea and vomiting persisted and he went to the emergency room 2 days later. His blood pressure was 96/60 mmHg, pulse 104 bpm, and his skin was dry with poor skin turgor. His blood urea nitrogen level was elevated (42 mg/dl; normal range = 7–18 mg/dl). He was given intravenous fluid and electrolyte replacement and prochlorperazine intramuscularly for nausea. Three days later, he was discharged from the hospital fully recovered. The investigator considered these events to be probably related to study medication (COX 25 mg).

- Patient 3001-0518 from study MP3001, an 80-year-old Black female receiving amlodipine 5 mg daily and metformin 500 mg twice daily for treatment of hypertension and diabetes, respectively, noticed progressive swelling of her legs approximately 60 days after study medication (COX 25 mg) was started. Nineteen days later, she developed acute shortness of breath and was hospitalized for congestive heart failure. Her study medication was stopped after 79 days of treatment. She was treated with furosemide and digoxin and gradually improved. She was discharged 7 days later much improved but with some residual mild shortness of breath. The investigator considered the leg swelling and congestive heart failure to be probably related to study medication (COX 25 mg).

- Patient 3001-0761 from study MP 3001, a 41-year-old Caucasian female, was admitted to the psychiatric ward for depression after 128 days of receiving study medication. Her husband said over the previous 2 weeks, his wife became increasingly withdrawn, crying often, and uninterested in eating. She refused to get out of bed, eat, or bathe. The paramedics were called when the patient's husband found her completely withdrawn and the patient wouldn't talk to him or leave her bed. He said he was not aware of any suicidal thoughts or actions. He denied any obvious triggers for her depression, e.g., work problems, family illness, etc., and said that up until then, their marriage was good. Her study medication was stopped when she was admitted to the psychiatric ward and she was started on paroxetine. Her depression was still ongoing during a follow-up call 2 weeks later. The investigator considered this event to be possibly related to study medication (COX 25 mg).

- Patient 3003-0535 from study MP 3003, a 62-year-old Black male, was hospitalized for a transient ischemic attack and hypertension after 275 days on study medication (COX 25 mg). The subject had a 10-year history of hypertension that at time of entry into the study was adequately controlled with lisinopril 20 mg/day. At study start, the patient's blood pressure was normal (118/77 mmHg); however the dose of lisinopril had to be increased to 40 mg/day after 3 months in the study due to increasing blood pressure values (BP 149/104 mmHg, study day 90). On the day of

his hospitalization he awoke with severe left-sided weakness and numbness. In the emergency room, his blood pressure was 175/118 mmHg. Marked left-sided weakness with decreased sensation to pinprick was noted on neurological exam. Funduscopic examination revealed flat optic disks with AV nicking, but no hemorrhages or exudates were noted. A cardiac echo revealed no evidence of left ventricular hypertrophy or thrombus. An emergency CAT and MRI scan were normal. By the time his scans were completed, his left-sided weakness and decreased sensation resolved completely, and his blood pressure decreased to 147/98 mmHg. His study medication was discontinued and he was admitted to the hospital for treatment of his hypertension and further testing and observation. While in the hospital, hydrochlorothiazide 25 mg was added to his antihypertensive medication. He was discharged 48 hours later with no neurological deficits, a normal blood pressure (119/78) mmHg, and follow-up instructions to see his physician in 2 days. The investigator assessed the hypertension and transient ischemic attack to be probably and possibly related to study medication (COX 25 mg), respectively.

➡ **NOTE:** It is important to provide details of events that occurred in other treatment groups. Cases that occur in the placebo group help the reviewer to understand the background noise of an event, i.e., the types of conditions the study population experiences that are not drug related. Events in the active control group allow the reviewer to better understand class effect AEs. Events that occur in the active control group give the reviewer a sense of whether the events in the investigational group appear to be the same, less common/severe, or more common/severe than what is known for the drug class. However, caution should be used in making such assessments because these assessments are retrospective and the events of interest can be few in number. The best way to show superiority to an active control is to do a prospective, randomized, controlled study, which is not always feasible.

2.6 Other Significant Adverse Events

2.6.1 Adverse Events Leading to Discontinuation

In Appendix tables AEDC1.1, AEDC1.2, and AEDC1.3, the AEs leading to discontinuation are summarized for controlled Phase 2/3 studies, all Phase 2/3 studies, and Phase 1 studies, respectively. Narratives of subjects who discontinued treatment due to an AE can be found in Appendix AEDCNAR1.1 (Phase 2/3 studies) and Appendix AEDCNAR1.2 (Phase 1 studies).

Table AII2-14 is a summary of adverse events overall and potential adverse reactions that led to premature discontinuation in controlled Phase 2/3 studies.

The rates of discontinuations due to AEs overall were higher in the Mepro and COX groups compared to placebo. The discontinuation rate in the Mepro group for potential adverse drug reactions was dose related and generally lower at the 5 mg and 10 mg doses compared to the COX group. All patients with PUBs discontinued treatment prematurely.

Similar results were found in the all Phase 2/3 studies data set (Appendix AEDC1.2).

In Phase 1 studies, 3 subjects receiving the highest Mepro dose of 30 mg in study MP1004 discontinued treatment due to an AE (0.8%); all were GI-related nausea (Subject 1004-20), vomiting (Subject 1004-24), and dyspepsia (Subject 1004-26). One subject (1.1%) (Subject 1013-3, study MP1013) discontinued due to nausea while taking digoxin. One subject (1.4%) in the placebo group

(Subject 1003-2, study MP1003) discontinued due to dizziness.

2.6.2 Other Significant Adverse Events

The rates of anemia-related events were higher in the Mepro and COX groups compared to placebo. This was expected and is discussed further in Section 2.7.5. There were 5 cases of nonserious photosensitivity-related events observed in patients exposed to Mepro. These cases are discussed further in Section 2.7.10.2.

2.7 Analysis of Adverse Events by Organ System or Syndrome

The following risks are associated with NSAIDs and will be discussed in this section.[9]

- PUBs
- Cardiovascular and cerebrovascular thrombotic events
- Hypertension
- Congestive heart failure and edema
- Hematologic effects
- Renal effects
- Hepatic effects
- Anaphylaxis and anaphylactoid reactions
- Preexistent asthma
- Skin reactions

In addition to these events, mania will also be discussed.

Table AII2-14 **Summary of Adverse Events Overall and Potential Adverse Reactions Leading to Discontinuation—Controlled Phase 2/3 Studies**

	Placebo N = 2200	M ≤ 5 mg N = 2450	M = 10 mg N = 2400	M = 15 mg N = 325	Total M N = 5175	COX N = 2225
Any adverse event	90 (4.1%)	145 (5.9%)	170 (7.1%)	31 (9.5%)	346 (6.7%)	278 (12.5%)
Abdominal pain upper	0	10 (0.4%)	18 (0.8%)	3 (0.9%)	31 (0.6%)	22 (1.0%)
Dyspepsia	0	15 (0.6%)	27 (1.1%)	4 (1.2%)	46 (0.9%)	34 (1.5%)
Epigastric discomfort	2 (0.1%)	12 (0.5%)	21 (0.9%)	2 (0.6%)	35 (0.7%)	47 (2.1%)
Nausea	3 (0.1%)	10 (0.4%)	23 (1.0%)	7 (2.2%)	40 (0.8%)	33 (1.5%)
PUBs	1 (< 0.1%)	17 (0.7%)	41 (1.7%)	10 (3.1%)	68 (1.3%)	96 (4.3%)
Vomiting	2 (0.1%)	7 (0.3%)	18 (0.8%)	4 (1.2%)	29 (0.6%)	20 (0.9%)

M = Mepro. PUBs = perforations, ulcers, and bleeds.
Source: Appendix Table AEDC1.1.

➡ **NOTE:** It is important to remember in preparing this section that each investigational drug is different. Determination of what should be included in this section is based on many factors, including theoretical risks based on the pharmacology of the drug, drug class, and any unexpected or unusual findings in the IAS.

For each of these conditions, the following methodology was used:

The entire safety database was searched (i.e., all Phase 1, 2, and 3 studies) using a MedDRA Standardised Query (SMQ) if one was available. If an existing SMQ was modified (mSMQ), the terms added or deleted terms were listed. If there was no SMQ available, an HLGT or HLT was used, or an AHQ was developed. Rates were calculated according to the conventions summarized in Section 1.2.2.

Listings of any subject who had 1 or more events included in an SMQ, mSMQ, HLGT, HLT or AHQ were provided. The listing included the following:

- Patient ID, study number
- Age, gender, and race
- Study medication and dose
- AE—both the verbatim and MedDRA Preferred Term
- AE onset date and resolution dates including study days
- Whether the AE was serious or not
- Whether the AE led to premature discontinuation
- The intensity of the AE
- Relationship to treatment (as judged by the investigator)
- Outcome of the event

- Any other concurrent AEs reported, including onset and resolution dates and study days
- All concomitant medication including treatment dates

2.7.1 PUBs

An AHQ for PUBs was created and included PTs from the HLGTs *Gastrointestinal haemorrhages NEC* and *Gastrointestinal ulceration and perforation*. In Appendices PUBs1.1 and PUBs1.2 the crude rate and rate per 100 PYE are summarized for controlled Phase 2/3 studies and all Phase 2/3 studies, respectively. There were no reports of PUBs in Phase I studies. A listing of all patients who had 1 or more events included in the PUBs AHQ can be found in Appendix PUBList.1.1. Narratives of these events are located in Appendix PUBNAR1.1.

PUBs are included as one of the common potential adverse drug reactions summarized in detail in Section 2.2 for the controlled Phase 2/3 studies dataset. This dataset was used because it was the best data set to use for comparison purposes of common events. The all Phase 2/3 studies data set was used to summarize PUBs in this section of the IAS to ensure all PUBs were accounted for and includes an additional patient from an uncontrolled study.

Table AII2-15 shows the crude rate of PUBs and rate per 100 PYE for all Phase 2/3 studies.

All PUBs were categorized as SAEs, and study medication was permanently withdrawn from all patients. The 1 patient in the placebo group who developed a PUB (Patient 3002-012, study MP3002) developed hematemesis after drinking a 6-pack of beer. Only 1 patient died; all of the remaining patients recovered. The patient who died (Patient 3001-0649, study MP3001) received COX 25 mg and is discussed in Section 2.4, "Deaths."

As discussed in the "Common Adverse Events" section, the rate of PUBs in the Mepro group was dose related.

Table AII2-15 **Summary of PUBs—All Phase 2/3 Studies**

Treatment Group	Total Number of Patients	Number of Patients With PUBs	Crude Rate of PUBs	Person-Years Exposure (PYE)	PUBs per 100 PYE
Placebo	2200	1	0.05%	994.6	0.1
Mepro	5410	69	1.3%	2933.2	2.4
COX	2225	96	4.3%	1076.2	8.9

M = Mepro; PUBs = perforations, ulcers, and bleeds.
Source: Appendix Table PUBs1.2.

The rate of PUBs was greatest in the 15-mg Mepro dose group and was similar to the rate seen in the COX group. The rates of PUBs for the 5-mg and 10-mg Mepro dose groups (the recommended doses) were lower. Although PUBs were dose related, females showed no greater risk than males even though females have 40–50% greater plasma levels than males given the same dose (see Section 5.1.1.1). Also of interest, the rate of PUBs was similar between the elderly and nonelderly (see Section 5.1.1.2).

The pattern of onset for PUBs as shown in Table AII2-8 was different in the Mepro group compared to the COX groups. For Mepro, the majority of PUBs occurred between 4 and 24 weeks, with no PUBs reported after 36 weeks. This pattern differed for COX, where the onset of PUBs began between 4 and 12 weeks and the rate progressively increased over time. It is unknown at this time whether the pattern seen with Mepro thus far will be different with more and longer exposures.

> ➡ **NOTE:** The pattern of onset for PUBs observed with Mepro would be advantageous compared to the pattern seen with COX— if this finding was real. If this were the true pattern, the risk for PUBs would be limited to within the first 6 months of Mepro treatment. Because exposure was not long enough to show this with any degree of confidence, this is purely conjecture. To determine whether the risk for PUBs is less than other NSAIDs and decreases over time, a prospective, randomized, long-term active control study adequately powered (has enough patients to show a treatment group difference) would have to be conducted.

2.7.2 Cardiovascular and Cerebrovascular Thrombotic Events

The SMQs used to search for cardiovascular and cerebrovascular thrombotic (CV/CV) events included the SMQs *Myocardial infarction* and *Ischemic cerebrovascular conditions.*

In Appendix CVS1.1 and CVS1.2 the crude rates and rates per 100 PYE are shown for controlled Phase 2/3 studies and all Phase 2/3 studies, respectively. There were no reports of CV/CV events reported in Phase I studies. A listing of all patients who had 1 or more events included in these SMQs can be found in Appendix CVSLIST1.1. Narratives of all serious cases or those that led to be premature termination are located in Appendix CVSNAR1.1.

Table AII2-16 is a summary of the crude rate and rate per 100 PYE for CV/CV thrombotic events reported in all Phase 2/3 studies.

All these events were serious and resulted in premature withdrawal from study medication. Four of these events resulted in death (1 placebo subject, 1 Mepro subject, and 2 COX subjects). There was also 1 sudden death reported in the COX group (see Table AII2-11), but this occurred 30 days after the last dose of COX. None of these events was considered related to treatment as judged by the investigator. Although the rates were low in all treatment groups, the rates were noted to be similar in the placebo and Mepro groups, but slightly greater in the COX group.

> ➡ **NOTE:** These results are interesting and suggest that perhaps Mepro does not have the same cardiovascular/cerebrovascular risks as COX and other NSAIDs. This however is a hypothesis and would have to be proven with a proper study; e.g., a prospective,

---

Table AII2-16 Summary of Cardiovascular and Cerebrovascular Thrombotic Events— All Phase 2/3 Studies

Treatment Group	Total Number of Patients	Number of Patients With CV/CV Thrombotic Events	Crude Rate of CV/CV Thrombotic Events	Person-Years Exposure (PYE)	CV/CV Thrombotic Events per 100 PYE
Placebo	2200	2	0.09%	994.6	0.2
Mepro	5410	3	0.06%	2933.2	0.1
COX	2225	7	0.31%	1076.2	0.7

CV/CV = cardiovascular and cerebrovascular.
Source: Appendix Table CVS1.2.

randomized, long-term, active control study adequately powered (i.e., the sample size would need to be large enough and exposures long enough) to show a meaningful difference between Mepro and another NSAID.

2.7.3 Hypertension

The *Hypertension* SMQ was used to search for hypertension-related terms. In Appendices HYP1.1 and HYP1.2 the crude rates and rates per 100 PYE are summarized for the controlled Phase 2/3 studies and all Phase 2/3 studies, respectively. There were no reports of hypertension in Phase I studies.

A listing of all patients in Phase 2/3 studies who had 1 or more events included in the *Hypertension* SMQ can be found in Appendix HYPLIST.1.1. Narratives of all serious cases or those that led to premature discontinuation patients are located in Appendix HYPNAR1.1.

Table AII2-17 summarizes the crude rate and rate per 100 PYE for hypertension-related events in all Phase 2/3 studies.

The rates were similar between the Mepro and placebo groups and higher in the COX group. Similar trends were also seen in the mean change, categorical shift, and clinically significant change blood pressure analyses summarized in Section 4.1.1.

2.7.4 Congestive Heart Failure and Edema

The SMQ used to search for subjects with congestive heart failure (CHF)-related events was *Cardiac failure*. In Appendices CHF1.1, and CHF1.2, the crude rates and rates per 100 PYE for CHF-related events are shown for the controlled Phase 2/3 studies and all Phase 2/3 studies, respectively. There were no reports of CHF-related events in Phase I studies. A listing of all patients who had 1 or more events included in the CHF SMQ can be found in Appendix CHFLIST.1.1 for Phase 2/3 studies. A narrative of serious events or those that led to premature termination can be found in Appendix CHFNAR1.1.

Table AII2-18 is a summary of the crude rate and rate per 100 PYE of CHF-related events in all Phase 2/3 studies.

There were very few CHF events reported across treatment groups (4 total). All these events were serious and led to discontinuation. Only 1 case of CHF reported in a patient who received COX (Patient 3001-0518 from study MP3001) was considered related to treatment. A brief narrative can be found in Section 2.5.

Table AII2-17 **Summary of Hypertension Events—All Phase 2/3 Studies**

Treatment Group	Total Number of Patients	Number of Patients With Hypertension Events	Crude Rate of Hypertension Events	Person-Years Exposure (PYE)	Hypertension Events per 100 PYE
Placebo	2200	64	2.9%	994.6	6.4
Mepro	5410	173	3.2%	2933.2	5.9
COX	2225	129	5.8%	1076.2	12.0

Source: Appendix Table HYP1.2.

Table AII2-18 **Summary of Congestive Heart Failure—Related Events—All Phase 2/3 Studies**

Treatment Group	Total Number of Patients	Number of Patients With CHF-Related Events	Crude Rate of CHF-Related Events	Person-Years Exposure (PYE)	CHF-Related Events per 100 PYE
Placebo	2200	1	0.05%	994.6	0.1
Mepro	5410	1	0.02%	2933.2	< 0.1
COX	2225	2	0.09%	1076.2	0.2

CHF = congestive heart failure.
Source: Appendix Table CHF1.2.

The AHQ used to search for edema-related events included the following PTs: *Generalized oedema, Oedema, Oedema peripheral*, and *Pitting oedema*. Appendices EDM1.1, EDM1.2, and EDM1.3 summarize the crude rate and rate per 100 PYE for edema-related events in controlled Phase 2/3 studies, all Phase 2/3 studies, and Phase 1 studies, respectively. A listing of all subjects with 1 or more events included in the AHQ is located in Appendix EDMLIST1.1 and in Appendix EDMLIST1.2 for subjects in Phase 2/3 studies and Phase 1 studies, respectively. Narratives of serious events or those that led to premature discontinuation can be found in Appendix EDMNAR1.1.

Table AII2-19 summarizes the crude rate and rate per 100 PYE of edema-related events in all Phase 2/3 studies.

The rate of edema-related events was similar between the placebo and Mepro groups. In the COX group, the rate of these events, although not high, was approximately 3 times greater. The majority of these events across all treatment groups were considered unrelated to treatment. Only 1 of these events was serious, led to premature discontinuation of study medication, and was considered related to treatment. This event occurred in the same COX-treated patient who had CHF (Patient 3001-0518 from study MP3001), which was discussed previously.

Edema-related events were reported in 1 placebo subject (1.4%), 2 Mepro subjects (0.5%), and 1 subject in the other group (1.1%) in Phase 1 studies. None of these events were serious, led to discontinuation, or were considered related to treatment (see Appendix EDMList1.2).

2.7.5 Hematologic Effects

The *Erythropenia* SMQ was used to search for cases of anemia-related events. In Appendix ANEM1.1, ANEM1.2, and ANEM1.3, the crude rate and rate per 100 PYE are shown for anemia-related AEs for controlled Phase 2/3 studies, all Phase 2/3 studies, and Phase 1 studies, respectively. A listing of all patients in Phase 2/3 studies and Phase 1 studies with 1 or more of the events included in the SMQ can be found in Appendix ANEMLIST1.1 and ANEMLIST1.2, respectively. Narratives of events that were serious or led to premature discontinuation are located in Appendix ANEMNAR1.1.

Table AII2-20 summarizes the crude rate and rate per 100 PYE of anemia-related events in all Phase 2/3 studies.

Rates of anemia-related events were higher in the Mepro and COX groups compared to placebo, with the highest rate seen in the COX group. Similar trends were seen in the mean change, categorical shift, and clinically

---

Table AII2-19 **Summary of Edema-Related Events—All Phase 2/3 Studies**

Treatment Group	Total Number of Patients	Number of Patients With Edema-Related Events	Crude Rate of Edema-Related Events	Person-Years Exposure (PYE)	Edema-Related Events per 100 PYE
Placebo	2200	10	0.5%	994.6	1.0
Mepro	5410	22	0.4%	2933.2	0.8
COX	2225	31	1.4%	1076.2	2.9

Source: Appendix Table EDM1.2.

Table AII2-20 **Summary of Anemia-Related Events—All Phase 2/3 Studies**

Treatment Group	Total Number of Patients	Number of Patients With Anemia-Related Events	Crude Rate of Anemia-Related Events	Person-Years Exposure (PYE)	Anemia-Related Events per 100 PYE
Placebo	2200	11	0.5%	994.6	1.1
Mepro	5410	104	1.9%	2933.2	3.5
COX	2225	129	5.8%	1076.2	12.0

Source: Appendix Table ANEM1.2.

significant change analyses for hemoglobin summarized in Section 3.1. The only serious cases of anemia were those that were associated with PUBs and occurred in < 0.1%, 1.0%, and 3.4% in the placebo, Mepro, and COX treatment groups, respectively. These were the only anemia-related events that resulted in premature termination of treatment.

The rates of anemia-related events were similar among the placebo (5.6%), Mepro (5.9%), and other (5.5%) groups in Phase 1 studies. None of these events were serious, led to premature termination of treatment, or were considered drug related. Most of these events were due to multiple blood draws. A platelet function AHQ was created to search for events suggestive of potential platelet dysfunction and included the following PTs: *Platelet adhesiveness decreased*, *Platelet aggregation decreased*, and *Bleeding time prolonged*. No subjects in any treatment groups in Phase 1 or Phase 2/3 studies were identified in the search.

2.7.6 Renal Effects

The *Acute renal failure* SMQ was used to search for cases of acute renal failure. In Appendix ARF1.1 and ARF1.2 the crude rates and rates per 100 PYE for acute renal failure are presented for controlled Phase 2/3 studies and all Phase 2/3 studies, respectively. A listing of all patients who had 1 or more events included in the *Acute renal failure* SMQ can be found in Appendix ARFLIST1.1. No subject in Phase 1 studies was identified in the search.

Only 2 patients were identified in the search—1 Mepro patient (Patient 3002-0016, study MP3002) who reported proteinuria and 1 COX patient (Patient 3003-0225, study MP3003) with an increased blood creatinine. Both of these events were not serious and did not lead to discontinuation of treatment. There were no reports of acute renal failure. A trend however toward increases in creatinine and BUN was observed in the mean change, categorical shift, and clinically significant change analyses discussed in Section 3.2.2.

2.7.7 Hepatic Effects

The *Possible drug related hepatic disorders comprehensive search* SMQ was used to search for cases of possible drug-induced hepatic events. In Appendix HEP1.1, HEP1.2, and HEP1.3, the crude rates and rates per 100 PYE are shown for hepatic-related events in controlled Phase 2/3 studies, all Phase 2/3 studies, and Phase 1 studies, respectively. A listing of all subjects with 1 or more events included in the SMQ can be found in Appendices HEPLIST1.1 and HEPLIST1.2 for subjects in Phase 2/3 studies and Phase 1 studies, respectively. Narratives of patients who had serious events or discontinued treatment prematurely due to these events can be found in Appendix HEPNAR1.1. No subject in Phase 1 studies had a serious event or an event that led to premature termination.

Table AII2-21 summarizes the crude rates and rates per 100 PYE for hepatic-related events in all Phase 2/3 studies.

The crude rates for Mepro and COX were greater than those noted for placebo, although the COX rate was approximately twice the rate noted for Mepro. The rates per 100 PYE were similar between the placebo and Mepro groups and less than the COX group. In the analysis of liver function tests (see Section 3.2.1), there was also a small trend toward increases in ALT and AST values observed in both the Mepro and COX groups, but the trend appeared greater in the COX group. There was 1 serious case that led to premature discontinuation. Patient 3003-0205 in study MP 3003, who received Mepro 5 mg, developed high levels of ALT, AST, and elevated total bilirubin, and alkaline phosphatase values that were due to gallstones and considered unrelated to Mepro treatment. There were no cases of Hy's Law or any cases suggestive of drug-induced liver injury in any treatment group. A more comprehensive analysis of liver function tests can be found in Section 3.2.1.

Table AII2-21 **Summary of Hepatic-Related Events—All Phase 2/3 Studies**

Treatment Group	Total Number of Patients	Number of Patients With Hepatic-Related Events	Crude Rate of Hepatic-Related Events	Person-Years Exposure (PYE)	Hepatic-Related Events per 100 PYE
Placebo	2200	14	0.6%	994.6	1.4
Mepro	5410	57	1.1%	2933.2	1.9
COX	2225	53	2.4%	1076.2	4.9

Source: Appendix Table HEP1.2.

NOTE: To get the full picture of potential drug-related findings, other safety findings, if applicable, have to be mentioned as well. For example, for the evaluation of hypertension-related AEs, the results from blood pressure analyses also have to be taken into account. Similarly, hematological effects, renal effects, and hepatic effects require a review of the results from analyses of relevant laboratory tests. This is fundamental to an integrated review of the data. Showing similar trends with different analyses of the data, e.g., similar findings in AEs and the analysis of mean changes, categorical changes, and clinically significant changes, provides more weight that a finding is drug related. How this is best done is your decision. In the examples shown, the details of the results of different but related analyses are provided in different sections of the IAS, but a brief summary of the results is provided here, so the story is not interrupted and the reviewer is not left hanging for the results until she reaches the other sections of the IAS.

2.7.8 Anaphylaxis and Anaphylactoid Reactions

The following SMQs were used to identify subjects with hypersensitivity-related events: *Anaphylactic reactions* and *Angioedema*. In Appendices ANA1.1, ANA1.2, and ANA1.3 the crude rates and rates per 100 PYE are summarized for controlled Phase 2/3 studies, all Phase 2/3 studies, and Phase 1 studies, respectively. Any subject who had 1 or more of these events in either SMQ was counted in the rate for hypersensitivity-related events. If the subject experienced the same PT more than once or experienced more than 1 PT in either SMQ, the subject was counted only once. Listings of these events can be found in Appendix ANALIST1.1 and ANALIST1.2 for Phase 2/3 studies and Phase 1 studies, respectively.

Table AII2-22 summarizes the crude rates and rates per 100 PYE for hypersensitivity-related events in all Phase 2/3 studies.

There were no reported cases of anaphylaxis or anaphylactoid reactions reported in any treatment group in either Phase 2/3 or Phase 1 studies. The search revealed only nonspecific terms, e.g., dyspnea, cough, sneezing, etc. The rates of these events were similar across treatment groups. Rates were also similar in Phase 1 studies—1.4% in the placebo group, 1.1% in the Mepro group, and 1.1% in the other group (Appendix ANA1.3). None of these nonspecific events was serious or led to premature discontinuation. The majority of events across treatment groups were considered unrelated to treatment.

2.7.9 Preexistent Asthma

The *Asthma/bronchospasm* SMQ was used to search for cases of asthma-related AEs. In Appendices ASMA1.1, ASMA1.2, and ASMA1.3 the crude rates and rates per 100 PYE can be found for controlled Phase 2/3 studies, all Phase 2/3 studies, and Phase 1 studies, respectively. A listing of all subjects with 1 or more events included in the SMQ can be found in Appendix ASMAList.1.1 for Phase 2/3 studies and Appendix ASMAList1.2 for Phase 1 studies.

Table AII2-23 summarizes the crude rate and rate per 100 PYE for asthma-related-related events for all Phase 2/3 studies.

The rates of asthma-related events were similar across treatment groups for all Phase 2/3 studies. No differences

Table AII2-22 Summary of Hypersensitivity-Related Adverse Events—All Phase 2/3 Studies

Treatment Group	Total Number of Patients	Number of Patients With Hypersensitivity-Related Events	Crude Rate of Hypersensitivity-Related Events	Person-Years Exposure (PYE)	Hypersensitivity-Related Events per 100 PYE
Placebo	2200	33	1.5%	994.6	3.3
Mepro	5410	70	1.3%	2933.2	2.4
COX	2225	31	1.4%	1076.2	2.9

Source: Appendix Table ANA1.2.

Table AII2-23 **Summary of Asthma-Related Adverse Events—All Phase 2/3 Studies**

Treatment Group	Total Number of Patients	Number of Patients With Asthma-Related Events	Crude Rate of Asthma-Related Events	Person-Years Exposure (PYE)	Asthma-Related Events (PYE)
Placebo	2200	16	0.7%	994.6	1.6
Mepro	5410	27	0.5%	2933.2	0.9
COX	2225	11	0.5%	1076.2	1.0

Source: Appendix Table ASMA1.2.

Table AII2-24 **Summary of Photosensitivity-Related Adverse Events—All Phase 2/3 Studies**

Treatment Group	Total Number of Patients	Number of Patients With Photosensitivity-Related Events	Crude Rate of Photosensitivity-Related Events	Person-Years Exposure (PYE)	Photosensitivity-Related Events per 100 PYE
Placebo	2200	0	0	994.6	0
Mepro	5410	5	0.1%	2933.2	0.2
COX	2225	0	0	1076.2	0

Source: Appendix Table PHOTO1.2.

in rates were seen in Phase 1 studies (1.4% placebo; 1.3% Mepro; 1.1% other). None of the asthma-related AEs was serious or led to premature termination. The majority of these events were considered unrelated to treatment.

2.7.10 Skin Reactions

In this section, the following 2 types of skin reactions are discussed:

- Severe cutaneous adverse reactions
- Photosensitivity skin reactions

2.7.10.1 Severe Cutaneous Adverse Reactions

The *Severe cutaneous adverse reactions* SMQ was used to search for cases of severe skin reactions, e.g., erythema multiforme, SJS, and toxic epidermal necrolysis. There was only 1 report of a severe skin reaction that occurred in a Phase 2/3 study. A listing of this event can be found in Appendix SKINLIST1.1 and the narrative in Appendix SKINAR1.1.

SJS was reported in a 34-year-old Asian female (Patient 3002-0867 from study MP3002) who received Mepro 5 mg. She tested positive for the gene B*1502 allele of HLA-B—the gene associated with the development of SJS in subjects exposed to carbamazepine and phenytoin.[10] A narrative of this case is provided in Section 2.5. Attribution to Mepro could not be ruled out but the case

was confounded by the concomitant use of penicillin prior to the onset of the event. It is unclear based on this single case whether the event was more likely due to penicillin alone, Mepro alone, or an interaction between penicillin and Mepro. Whether there is an increased risk of SJS in people with the B*1502 allele of HLA-B gene and exposure to Mepro is also unknown at this time.

2.7.10.2 Photosensitivity-Related Skin Reactions

The HLT *Photosensitivity skin reactions* was used to identify cases of photosensitivity-related skin reactions. In Appendices PHOTO1.1 and PHOTO1.2 the crude rates and rates per 100 PYE are presented for controlled Phase 2/3 studies and all Phase 2/3 studies, respectively. There were no reports of photosensitivity-related events in Phase 1 studies. A listing of all patients with 1 or more events included in the HLT can be found in Appendix PHOTOLIST1.1 for patients in Phase 2/3 studies.

Table AII2-24 summarizes the crude rate and rate per 100 PYE for photosensitivity-related events for all Phase 2/3 studies.

There were 5 reports of photosensitivity-related events, and all occurred in the Mepro group. Table AII2-25 is a listing of these events.

None of the events was serious and only 1 patient discontinued from treatment. Three of the 5 events were considered treatment related. Of note, all these events

Table AII2-25	**Patients With Photosensitivity Reactions—All Phase 2/3 Studies**						
Study No./Patient Number	Age/Gender/ Race	Dose	Exposure to Study Medication (Days)	Reported AE Term	MedDRA PT	Premature Discontinuation/ Intensity/ Serious	Relationship to Study Medication/ Outcome
MP2003X/ 2003X-0099	48/male/ Caucasian	10 mg	163 days	Rash after exposure to the sun	Photosensitivity allergic reaction	No/ moderate/ no	Possible/ recovered
MP2004X/ 2004X-0037	64/female/ Caucasian	10 mg	93 days	Red itchy bumps after exposure to sunlight	Photosensitivity, allergic reaction	No/ mild/no	Possible/ recovered
MP3001/ 3001-0723	27/male/ Caucasian	5 mg	104 days	Red rash and blisters from sun	Photosensitivity, allergic reaction	No/moderate/ no	Unlikely/ recovered
MP3002/ 3002-0603	34/female/ Caucasian	10 mg	123 days	Sensitive red patches from sun	Photo-dermatosis	No/mild/ no	Unlikely/ recovered
MP3003/ 3003-1004	41/female/ Caucasian	5 mg	214 days	Blisters in sun-exposed areas	Photosensitivity, allergic reaction	Yes/ moderate/no	Probable/ recovered

Source: Appendix PHOTOLIST1.1.

occurred in Caucasians after exposure to Mepro for 3 months or more.

2.7.11 Mania

The safety database was searched to identify any subject reporting 1 or more events included in the HLGT *Manic and bipolar mood disorders and disturbances.* Appendices MAN1.1 and MAN1.2 summarize the crude rates and rates per 100 PYE for controlled Phase 2/3 studies and all Phase 2/3 studies, respectively. There were no reports of mania-related events in Phase 1 studies. Only 1 patient in the Phase 2/3 studies was identified in the search. A listing of this case and a narrative can be found in Appendices MANLIST1.1 and MANNAR1.1, respectively.

This case (Patient 2003X-0601 from study MP2003X) was summarized in the "Other SAEs" section (Section 2.5). The patient's mania occurred around the time he was laid off from his job. Whether this was a factor in the onset of his mania cannot be determined. Based on the details of this case, attribution to Mepro cannot be ruled out.

Review of the PTs in the SOC psychiatric disorders revealed no relevant rate differences across treatment groups in the controlled Phase 2/3 studies, all Phase 2/3 studies, or the Phase 1 studies (see Appendices AE3.1, AE3.2, and AE3.3, respectively), indicating no obvious trends in the occurrence of other psychiatric events.

2.8 Summary of Adverse Events

The common adverse events considered drug related were GI-related events—upper abdominal pain, dyspepsia, epigastric pain, nausea, PUBs, and vomiting, and they were dose related. These findings are consistent with the known risk profile of NSAIDs. At the recommended Mepro doses of 5 mg and 10 mg, the rates of these events were less than those seen in the Mepro 15 mg and COX groups. The pattern of onset for PUBs was also different in the Mepro group compared to the COX group. For Mepro, the majority of PUBs occurred between 4 and 24 weeks, with no PUBs reported after 36 weeks. This pattern differed for COX, where the onset of PUBs began between 4–12 weeks and the rate progressively increased over time. Whether or not the risk for PUBs after Mepro exposure is limited to the first 36 weeks cannot be determined at this time due to the limited number and duration of exposures. The risk for anemia- and hepatic-related events was greater in the Mepro and COX groups compared to placebo, but a slightly greater trend was seen in the COX group. No trend toward hypertension or renal dysfunction was observed with Mepro, but a small trend in the COX group could not be ruled out. There were no reports of drug-related hepatotoxicity or anaphylaxis in any treatment group. There were no relevant differences in the rates of asthma or CHF seen across treatment groups; however, a small trend toward increases in edema-related events could not be ruled out in the COX group. There was no difference in the rate of cardiovascular and cerebrovascular thrombotic events in the Mepro and placebo groups, but the rate of these events in the COX group, although small, was more than fourfold greater compared to the other treatment groups. One case of SJS was reported in an Asian female who tested positive for the B*1502 allele of HLA-B, a gene associated with an increased risk for Stevens-Johnson syndrome in subjects exposed to phenytoin and carbamazepine. The case was further confounded by the concomitant use of penicillin, a drug associated with the development of SJS. However, based on the available case information, attribution to Mepro cannot be entirely ruled out. Nonserious photosensitivity reactions were observed in 5 patients who received Mepro. All were Caucasian and received Mepro for 3 or more months. One patient discontinued treatment; all cases resolved even with continued treatment in the 4 patients who remained on treatment. One case of mania was reported. Attribution to Mepro cannot be ruled out at this time. No other trends in psychiatric-related events were identified.

■ 3 Clinical Laboratory Evaluations

> ➡ **NOTE:** There are a number of software tools that are currently available or are under development that assist in creating user-friendly graphic data displays and help the reviewer drill down to individual or subsets of data of interest. The sample text that follows focuses on how clinical laboratory data should be handled regardless of how the data are displayed and should be relevant whether tables, graphs, or figures are used.

3.1 Hematology

In Appendices MHEMA1.1, CASHEMA1.1, and CSCHEMA1.1, mean change from baseline, categorical shifts, and clinically significant changes for hematology values, respectively, can be found for controlled Phase 2/3 studies. In Appendices MHEMA1.2, CASHEMA1.2, and CSCHEMA1.3, mean change from baseline, categorical shifts, and clinically significant changes for hematology values, respectively, can be found for all Phase 2/3 studies.

In Appendices MHEM1.3, CASHEM1.3, and CSCHEM1.3, mean change from baseline, categorical shifts, and clinically significant changes for hematology values, respectively, can be found for Phase 1 studies.

> ➡ **NOTE:** Although it is tedious to list all the appendices where the source data can be found, it is a necessary evil so that the reviewer can confirm what was written in the text and review more detailed information if necessary. In electronic reports, hyperlinks to the appendices provide easy access to the appendices.

The following SMQs were selected to identify subjects with hematology-related events: *Agranulocytosis, Cytopenia and hematopoietic disorders affecting more than 1 type of blood cell, Erythropenia, Leukopenia, Thrombocytopenia, Haemolytic disorders*; and *Haemorrhages*. For the *Agranulocytosis* SMQ, only the narrow terms were used in calculating the rate. Rates of these events can be found in Appendix AESEARCH1.1 (controlled Phase 2/3 studies), Appendix AESEARCH1.2 (all Phase 2/3 studies), and Appendix AESEARCH1.3 (Phase 1 studies). Listing of subjects included in these SMQs can be found in AESEARCHLIST1.1 (controlled Phase 2/3 studies and all Phase 2/3 studies) and AESEARCHLIST1.2 (Phase 1 studies).

3.1.1 White Blood Cells and Platelets

For the controlled Phase 2/3 studies, no relevant differences across treatment groups for WBCs (including WBC differential counts) and platelets were observed in the mean change, categorical shift, and clinical significant change analyses for WBC and platelets. No difference in rates across treatment groups were seen for the SMQs, *Agranulocytosis, Cytopenias and haematopoietic disorders affecting more than 1 type of blood cell, Leukopenia*, and *Thrombocytopenia*. Furthermore, there were no treatment-related serious AEs or AEs that led to premature discontinuation. Similar results were seen in the all Phase 2/3 studies. No adverse trends in WBCs or platelets were seen in Phase 1 studies.

3.1.2 Red Blood Cells

A dashboard summary of changes in Hb values across treatment groups is provided in Table AII3-1 for controlled Phase 2/3 studies. Also included are the rates of patients with 1 or more AEs included in the SMQs *Erythropenia, Haemolytic disorders*, and *Haemorrhages*. Only Hb results are shown in the table since Hct and RBC results showed similar trends.

Table AII3-1 Dashboard Summary of Hemoglobin and Anemia-Related Adverse Events—Controlled Phase 2/3 Studies

	Placebo	M ≤ 5 mg	M = 10 mg	M = 15 mg	Total M	COX
Hb (g/L)						
N	2100	2315	2290	300	4905	2095
Baseline mean	144.3	144.7	144.3	145.2	144.5	144.4
Mean change[a]	−0.1	−0.5	−0.8	−1.5	−0.7	−2.4
N	2100	2315	2290	300	4905	2095
H/N to L	109 (5.2%)	167 (7.2%)	202 (8.8%)	30 (10.0%)	399 (8.1%)	465 (22.2%)
N	1987	2183	2145	287	4615	1906
Clinically significant decreases	10 (0.5%)	17 (0.8%)	25 (1.2%)	5 (1.7%)	47 (1.0%)	63 (3.3%)
Anemia-Related Adverse Events						
N	2200	2450	2400	325	5175	2225
Erythropenia (SMQ)	11 (0.5%)	37 (1.5%)	50 (2.1%)	9 (2.8%)	96 (1.9%)	129 (5.8%)
Haemolytic disorders (SMQ)	1 (< 0.1%)	0	1 (< 0.1%)	0	1 (< 0.1%)	0
Haemorrhages (SMQ)	5 (0.2%)	24 (1.0%)	52 (2.2%)	11 (3.4%)	87 (1.7%)	103 (4.6%)

M = Mepro; N = number of subjects; H = above normal; N = normal; L = below normal; SMQ = Standardised MedDRA Query.

[a] Change from baseline to the worst (i.e., most extreme) treatment value.

Source: Appendix Tables MHEMA1.1, CASHEMA1.1, CSCHEMA1.1, and AESEARCH1.1.

➡ NOTE: Notice that the *N*s (i.e., the number of subjects included in the analyses) are different for some of these analyses. For the AE analysis, all subjects who received 1 or more doses of study drug were included, whereas for the clinically significant change analysis, only subjects who had a normal baseline value and at least 1 treatment value were included in the clinically significant change analysis.

A downward trend in Hb values in the Mepro and COX groups compared to placebo was noted in the mean change, categorical shift, and clinically significant change analyses. Changes in the Mepro group appeared to be dose related. Although a decreased trend in Hb was seen for both the Mepro and COX groups, the changes in the COX group were approximately twofold greater than in the total Mepro group. Consistent with these findings was the greater rate of anemia-related events in the Mepro and COX groups, compared to placebo. Most of the hemorrhages seen were gastrointestinal. One patient who received COX died from a gastrointestinal hemorrhage (Patient 3001-0649, study MP3001). This patient is discussed in Section 2.4, and PUBs and anemia are discussed in Sections 2.7.1 and 2.7.5, respectively.

Similar findings were observed for the all-Phase 2/3 studies data set. No treatment group differences in Hb or anemia-related AEs were noted in Phase 1 studies.

3.2 Clinical Chemistry

In Appendices MCHEM1.1, CASCHEM1.1, and CSCCHEM1.1, mean change from baseline, categorical shifts, and clinically significant changes for clinical chemistry parameters (excluding LFTs), respectively, can be found for controlled Phase 2/3 studies. In Appendices MCHEM1.2, CASCHEM1.2, and CSCCHEM1.2, mean change from baseline, categorical shifts, and clinically significant changes for clinical chemistry parameters (excluding LFTs), respectively, can be found for all Phase 2/3 studies. In Appendices MCHEM1.3, CASCHEM1.3, and CSCCHEM1.3, mean change from baseline, categorical shifts, and clinically significant changes for clinical chemistry parameters (LFTs), respectively, can be found for Phase 1 studies.

The results of the analysis of liver function tests (LFTs) based on the FDA drug-induced liver injury (DILI) guidance document[3] can be found in Appendices LFT1.1, LFT1.2, and LFT1.3 for controlled Phase 2/3 Studies, all Phase 2/3 studies, and Phase 1 studies, respectively.

Rates of events included in the following SMQs can be found in Appendices AESEARCH1.1 (controlled Phase 2/3 studies and all Phase 2/3 studies) and AESEARCH1.2 (Phase 1 studies): *Possible drug related hepatic-disorders—comprehensive search, Acute renal failure, Hyperglycaemia/new onset diabetes mellitus, Rhabdomyolysis/myopathy* and *Dyslipidaemia.*

Listings of subjects included in these SMQs can be found in Appendices AESEARCHLIST1.1 (controlled Phase 2/3 studies and all Phase 2/3 studies) and AESEARCHLIST1.2 (Phase 1 studies). Narratives of lab-related AEs that were serious or led to premature termination can be found in Appendix SAENAR1.1 and AEDCNAR1.1, respectively, for Phase 2/3 studies. No Phase 1 study subject had a serious lab-related AE or a lab-related AE that led to discontinuation.

3.2.1 Hepatic Profile

Table AII3-2 is a dashboard summary of the LFT analysis for controlled Phase 2/3 studies.

A small upward trend in ALT and AST values in both the Mepro and COX groups compared to placebo was observed. The rate of AEs from the SMQ *Possible drug related hepatic-disorders—comprehensive search* was also slightly higher in the Mepro and COX groups, compared to placebo. No cases meeting the criteria for Hy's Law

Table AII3-2 **Dashboard Summary of Liver Function Tests and Liver-Related Adverse Events—Controlled Phase 2/3 Studies**

	Placebo	M ≤ 5 mg	M = 10 mg	M = 15 mg	Total M	COX
Liver Function Tests						
ALT						
N	1915	2208	2187	261	4656	1988
≥ 3 × ULN	21 (1.1%)	66 (3.0%)	92 (4.2%)	14 (5.4%)	172 (3.7%)	157 (7.9%)
≥ 5 × ULN	2 (0.1%)	7 (0.3%)	7 (0.3%)	2 (0.8%)	16 (< 0.3%)	12 (0.6%)
≥ 10 × ULN	0	1 (< 0.1%)	0	0	1 (< 0.1%)	0
≥ 20 × ULN	0	0	0	0	0	0
AST						
N	1898	2190	2165	252	4607	1963
≥ 3 × ULN	28 (1.5%)	61 (2.8%)	95 (4.4%)	13 (5.2%)	169 (3.7%)	167 (8.5%)
≥ 5 × ULN	4 (0.2%)	11 (0.5%)	6 (0.3%)	2 (0.8%)	19 (0.4%)	10 (0.5%)
≥ 10 × ULN	0	1 (< 0.1%)	0	0	1 (< 0.1%)	0
≥ 20 × ULN	0	0	0	0	0	0
ALT and AST						
N	1898	2190	2165	252	4607	1963
≥ 3 × ULN	18 (0.9%)	50 (2.3%)	73 (3.4%)	3 (1.2%)	126 (2.7%)	120 (6.1%)
≥ 5 × ULN	1 (< 0.1%)	2 (0.1%)	1 (< 0.1%)	0	3 (< 0.1%)	3 (0.2%)
≥ 10 × ULN	0	1 (< 0.1%)	0	0	1 (< 0.1%)	0
≥ 20 × ULN	0	0	0	0	0	0
Total bilirubin						
N	2100	2315	2290	300	4905	2095
N to H	23 (1.1%)	23 (1.0%)	18 (0.8%)	3 (1.0%)	44 (0.9%)	21 (1.0%)
> 2 × ULN	10 (0.5%)	9 (0.4%)	9 (0.4%)	2 (0.7%)	20 (0.4%)	10 (0.5%)
ALP						
N	1996	2187	2175	282	4644	1981
> 1.5 ULN	44 (2.2%)	52 (2.4%)	44 (2.0%)	7 (2.5%)	103 (2.2%)	40 (2.0%)
N	1905	2196	2173	259	4628	1976
ALT > 3 × ULN + TBL > 1.5 × ULN	0	0	0	0	0	0
ALT > 3 × ULN + TBL > 2 × ULN	0	1 (< 0.1%)	0	0	1 (< 0.1%)	0
N	1890	2182	2148	251	4581	1950
AST > 3 × ULN + TBL > 1.5 × ULN	0	0	0	0	0	0
AST > 3 × ULN + TBL > 2 × ULN	0	1 (< 0.1%)	0	0	1 (< 0.1%)	0

Continues

Table AII3-2 Dashboard Summary of Liver Function Tests and Liver-Related Adverse Events—Controlled Phase 2/3 Studies, Continued

N	1902	2190	2169	258	4617	1971
Hy's Law						
ALT > 3 × ULN + ALP < 2 × ULN + TBL ≥ 2 × ULN	0	0	0	0	0	0
N	1888	2181	2147	250	4578	1948
Hy's Law						
AST > 3 × ULN + ALP < 2 × ULN + TBL ≥ 2 × ULN	0	0	0	0	0	0
Liver-Related Adverse events						
N	2200	2450	2400	325	5175	2225
ALT or AST > 3 × ULN + Nausea, Vomiting, Anorexia, Abdominal pain or Fatigue[a]	0	1 (< 0.1%)	0	0	1 (< 0.1%)	0
Possible drug related hepatic-disorders—comprehensive search (SMQ)	14 (0.6%)	27 (1.1%)	24 (1.0%)	4 (1.2%)	55 (1.1%)	53 (2.4%)

M = Mepro; *N* = number of subjects; ULN = upper limit of normal; N = normal; H = above normal; SMQ = Standardised MedDRA Query.

[a] To be included, the AEs had to occur within +/− 14 days of ALT/AST values > 3 × ULN.

Source: Appendix Tables LFT1.1 and AESEARCH1.1.

were identified. The findings in Table AII3-2 shaded in gray were of concern, and further investigation revealed that all these values were from the same patient (Patient 3003-0205, study MP3003). Table AII3-3 is a listing summarizing the patient's key findings.

This patient, a 43-year-old Caucasian female, developed severe right upper-quadrant pain associated with nausea and vomiting after 56 days of receiving Mepro 5 mg. She was discontinued from study medication and hospitalized. Subsequent workup revealed her pain and abnormal liver functions tests were due to gallstones. She had laparoscopic removal of her gallbladder and had a full and uneventful recovery. None of her reported adverse events or abnormal liver functions tests were considered drug related.

➡ **NOTE:** The type of listing shown in Table AII3-3 is very useful and reviewer friendly. It provides a snapshot view of key information all located in one place. Displaying the data by visit allows the reviewer to identify useful data patterns, e.g., an isolated finding versus a trend. Listings of concurrent AEs and concomitant medication can provide insight into the event itself, e.g., alternative reasons for the event. It is also important to display lab tests that are related to each other to see if changes are also noted in these other parameters. These are all factors that determine the weight of evidence for or against a causal relationship to the drug. Other examples of data listings are provided in Part 1 and Part 2 of the book.

The results from the LFT analysis for the all Phase 2/3 studies data set (Appendix LFT1.2) were similar to the findings in the controlled Phase 2/3 studies dataset.

The only findings in Phase 1 studies were mild (< 2 × ULN) and transient increases in ALT and AST values with similar rates seen across all treatment groups.

No cases that met the criteria for Hy's Law were identified in any treatment group in any study.

3.2.2 Renal Profile

Table AII3-4 is a dashboard summary of mean changes, categorical shifts, and clinically significant changes for creatinine, BUN, and albumin from controlled Phase 2/3 studies. Rates of events included in the SMQ *Acute renal failure* are also shown.

No differences in mean changes, categorical shifts, and clinically significant changes were seen between the placebo and Mepro treatment groups. A small but

Table AII3-3 **Listing of Liver Function Tests for Patient 3003-0205 (Study MP3003)**

Study Day	ALT U/L	AST U/L	ALP U/L	TBL μmol/L	Adverse Events	Concomitant Medications
0 (baseline)	25	20	110	7.2	None	None
28	32	28	108	7.1	None	None
56 (PT, final)	673[a] (H)	641[a] (H)	330[b] (H)	40[b] (H)	Abdominal pain upper, nausea, vomiting	None
91 (35 days after the last dose)	35	24	102	8.2	Cholelithiasis	Acetaminophen

PT = premature termination; H = above normal.

[a] > 10 × ULN.

[b] > 2 × ULN.

Source: LFTLIST1.1.

Table AII3-4 **Dashboard Summary of Renal Profile and Renal-Related Adverse Events—Controlled Phase 2/3 Studies**

	Placebo	M ≤ 5 mg	M = 10 mg	M = 15 mg	Total M	COX
Creatinine (μmol/L)						
N	2100	2315	2290	300	4905	2095
Baseline mean	76.5	77.0	76.9	77.2	77.0	76.4
Mean change[a]	1.2	1.3	1.3	1.0	1.3	2.7
N	2100	2315	2290	300	4905	2095
L/N to H	105 (5.0%)	109 (4.7%)	112 (4.9%)	12 (4.0%)	233 (4.8%)	151 (7.2%)
N	2001	2221	2181	275	4677	1979
Clinically significant increases	14 (0.7%)	11 (0.5%)	15 (0.7%)	2 (0.7%)	28 (0.6%)	24 (1.2%)
BUN (mmol/L)						
N	2100	2315	2290	300	4905	2095
Baseline mean	4.5	4.5	4.6	4.4	4.6	4.4
Mean change[a]	−0.2	−0.2	−0.5	0.0	−0.4	0.8
N	2100	2315	2290	300	4905	2095
L/N to H	151 (7.2%)	160 (6.9%)	149 (6.5%)	23 (7.7)%	332 (6.8%)	230 (11.0%)
N	1982	2209	2156	280	4645	2001
Clinically significant decreases	14 (0.7%)	11 (0.5%)	13 (0.6%)	2 (0.7)%	26 (0.6%)	20 (1.0%)
Albumin g/L						
N	2100	2315	2290	300	4905	2095
Baseline mean	38.5	39.0	38.7	38.2	38.8	38.6
Mean change[a]	0.7	0.7	0.1	0.3	0.4	0.5
N	2100	2315	2290	300	4905	2095
H/N to L	25 (1.2%)	30 (1.3%)	25 (1.1%)	3 (1.0%)	58 (1.2%)	25 (1.2%)
N	2093	2306	2284	297	4887	2091
Clinically significant decreases	4 (0.2%)	5 (0.2%)	0	0	5 (0.1%)	4 (0.2%)
N	2200	2450	2400	325	5175	2225
Acute renal failure (SMQ)	0	0	1 (< 0.1%)	0	1 (< 0.1%)	1 (< 0.1%)

M = Mepro; N = number of subjects; BUN = blood urea nitrogen; L = below normal; N = normal; H = above normal; SMQ = Standardised MedDRA Query.

[a] Change from baseline to the worst (i.e., most extreme) treatment value.

Source: Appendix tables MCHEM1.1, CASCHEM1.1, CSCCHEM1.1, and AESEARCH1.1.

consistent trend toward increases in creatinine and BUN values was observed in the COX group. Two patients had adverse events included in the *Acute renal failure* SMQ. *Proteinuria* was reported in 1 Mepro (10 mg) patient (Patient 3002-0016, study MP3002); and *Increased blood creatinine* was reported in a COX patient (Patient 3003-0225, study MP3003). Both of these events were not serious and considered unrelated to treatment.

The findings in the all Phase 2/3 studies data set were similar to the controlled Phase 2/3 studies data set; and no additional patients with events in the *Acute renal failure* SMQ were identified.

In Phase 1 studies there were no treatment group differences noted in the results of the renal analyses; and no subject reported any events included in the *Acute renal failure* SMQ.

3.2.3 Metabolic and Muscle Profile

For controlled 2/3 studies, all Phase 2/3 studies and Phase 1 study data sets, no relevant differences across treatment groups in mean changes, categorical shifts, and clinically significant changes were observed for metabolic- and muscle-related parameters. No treatment group differences were seen in the rates for the SMQs *Hyperglycaemia/new onset diabetes mellitus* and *Rhabdomyolysis/myopathy* in the controlled- and all Phase 2/3 studies data sets. None of the events identified were serious or led to premature discontinuation. No subject in the Phase 1 study reported any of the events included in these SMQs.

There were no subjects with the diagnosis of rhabdomyolysis reported in any treatment group or in any study.

3.2.4 Lipid Profile

Mean changes, categorical shifts, clinically significant changes, and lipid-related adverse events showed no relevant differences across treatment groups in the controlled Phase 2/3 studies, all Phase 2/3 studies, or Phase 1 studies data sets. None of the events included in the *Dyslipidaemia* SMQ were serious or led to discontinuation.

3.3 Urinalysis

In Appendices CSUA1.1, CSUA1.2, and CSUA1.3, clinically significant urinalysis changes can be found for controlled Phase 2/3 studies, all Phase 2/3 studies, and Phase 1 studies, respectively. Listings of subjects with clinically significant changes can be found in UALIST1.1 and UALIST1.2 for Phase 2/3 studies and Phase 1 studies, respectively.

Urinalysis results revealed no treatment group differences in the controlled Phase 2/3 studies, all Phase 2/3 studies, or Phase 1 studies data sets.

NOTE: Because this sample IAS is simplified, dashboard displays of the WBC and platelet analyses, metabolic and muscle profile, lipid profile, and urinalysis were not shown in the text. For an ISS and SCS (assuming the number of pages for the SCS are not exceeded),[1] summary tables of the data are still presented in the text of the report even though the data may not show any treatment group differences.

3.4 Summary of Clinical Laboratory Evaluations

A downward trend in RBC-related lab values and an upward trend in ALT and AST values were observed in both the Mepro and COX groups. These were not unexpected and are known NSAID-related effects. Although the changes were small, the increases in ALT/AST and the decreases in RBC parameters were greater in the COX group compared to Mepro. Small but consistent trends toward increases in creatinine and BUN values were also noted in the COX group compared to the Mepro and placebo groups. There were no subjects in any treatment group with changes in liver function tests that met Hy's Law criteria.

4 Vital Signs, Physical Findings, and Other Observations Related to Safety

4.1 Vital Signs

4.1.1 Blood Pressure

4.1.1.1 Systolic Blood Pressure

Appendices MSBP1.1, MSBP1.2, and MSBP1.3 provide the mean changes in supine systolic blood pressure for the controlled Phase 2/3 studies, all Phase 2/3 studies, and the Phase 1 studies, respectively. Appendices MSBP2.1, MSBP2.2, and MSBP2.3 provide the mean changes in standing systolic blood pressure for the controlled Phase 2/3 studies, all Phase 2/3 studies, and the Phase 1 studies, respectively.

A summary of categorical shifts in supine SBP can be found in Appendix CASSBP1.1 (controlled Phase 2/3 studies), Appendix CASSBP1.2 (all Phase 2/3 studies), and Appendix CASSBP1.3 (Phase 1 studies). Summaries of categorical shifts in standing SBP can be found in Appendix CASSBP2.1 (controlled Phase 2/3 studies), Appendix CASSBP2.2 (all Phase 2/3 studies), and Appendix CASSBP2.3 (Phase 1 studies).

In Appendices CSCSBP1.1, CSCSBP1.2, and CSCSBP1.3, the rates of clinically significant changes in supine systolic blood pressure are summarized for the controlled Phase 2/3 studies, all Phase 2/3 studies, and the Phase 1 studies, respectively. In Appendices CSCSBP2.1, CSCSBP2.2, and CSCSBP2.3, the rates of clinically significant changes in standing systolic blood pressure are presented for the controlled Phase 2/3 studies, all Phase 2/3 studies, and the Phase 1 studies, respectively.

A listing of subjects with 1 or more clinically significant systolic blood pressure changes during treatment can be found in Appendices CSLISTSBP1.1 and CSLISTSBP1.2 for Phase 2/3 studies and Phase 1 studies, respectively. Listings include all baseline, treatment, and posttreatment values for these subjects.

4.1.1.2 Diastolic Blood Pressure

In Appendices MDBP1.1, MDBP1.2, and MDBP1.3, mean changes in supine diastolic blood pressure are summarized for the controlled Phase 2/3 studies, all Phase 2/3 studies, and the Phase 1 studies, respectively. In Appendices MDBP2.1, MDBP2.2, and MDBP2.3, mean changes in standing diastolic blood pressure are presented for the controlled Phase 2/3 studies, all Phase 2/3 studies, and the Phase 1 studies, respectively.

The results of the categorical shift analysis for supine DBP can be found in Appendix CASDBP1.1 (controlled Phase 2/3 studies), Appendix CASDBP1.2 (all Phase 2/3 studies), and Appendix CASDBP1.3 (Phase 1 studies). The results of the categorical shift analysis for standing DBP can be found in Appendix CASDBP2.1 (controlled Phase 2/3 studies), Appendix CASDBP2.2 (all Phase 2/3 studies), and Appendix CASDBP2.3 (Phase 1 studies).

In Appendices CSCDBP1.1, CSCDBP1.2, and CSCDBP1.3, the rates of clinically significant changes in supine diastolic blood pressure are presented for the controlled Phase 2/3 studies, all Phase 2/3 studies, and the Phase 1 studies, respectively. In Appendices CSCDBP2.1, CSCDBP2.2, and CSCDBP2.3, the rates of clinically significant changes in standing diastolic blood pressure can be found for the controlled Phase 2/3 studies, all Phase 2/3 studies, and the Phase 1 studies, respectively.

A listing of subjects with 1 or more clinically significant diastolic blood pressure changes during treatment can be found in Appendices CSCLISTDBP1.1 and CSCLISTDBP1.2 for Phase 2/3 studies and Phase 1 studies, respectively. Listings include all baseline, treatment, and posttreatment values for these subjects.

4.1.1.3 Orthostatic Blood Pressure

The rates of subjects with orthostatic blood pressure changes can be found in Appendices OBP1.1, OBP1.2, and OBP1.3 for controlled Phase 2/3 studies, all Phase 2/3 studies, and Phase 1 studies, respectively. A listing of subjects with orthostatic blood pressure changes can be found in Appendices OBPLIST1.1 and OBPLIST1.2 for Phase 2/3 studies and Phase 1 studies, respectively. Listings include all baseline, treatment, and posttreatment values for these subjects.

Because of MedDRA's convention of using PTs for signs/symptoms and other PTs for diagnoses for terms that are often used interchangeably in practice, a combined term was used in the calculation of the rate for hypertension and hypotension. This was to ensure the rates of these events would not be underestimated. The PTs for hypertension included *Accelerated hypertension, Blood pressure ambulatory increased, Blood pressure diastolic increased, Blood pressure increased, Blood pressure systolic increased, Diastolic hypertension, Essential hypertension, Hypertensive crisis, Hypertensive emergency, Labile hypertension, Malignant hypertension, Prehypertension,* and *Systolic hypertension.* The PTs for hypotension included *Blood pressure ambulatory decreased, Blood pressure decreased, Blood pressure diastolic decreased, Blood pressure systolic decreased, Diastolic hypotension, Hypotension,* and *Orthostatic hypotension.*

➡ **NOTE:** *Combined term* is our own terminology; use whatever term you want as long as you clearly define it. As indicated, combined terms are sometimes required to avoid underestimating rates for certain findings that can be described by more than 1 PT. The use of combined terms is recommended for inclusion *in the text only.* We recommend that the AE tables located in the appendices summarize rates by individual PTs rather than combining them as we did here. In this way, the reviewer can easily see how the combined rates discussed in the text were derived.

Table AII4-1 is a dashboard summary of the analysis of supine blood pressure and includes mean changes, categorical shifts, clinically significant blood pressure changes, and blood pressure-related adverse events for controlled Phase 2/3 studies.

Mean changes in supine systolic and diastolic blood pressure were small and similar between the placebo and the Mepro treatment groups. The COX treatment group showed the greatest mean blood pressure changes (systolic +2.4 mmHg; diastolic +1.0 mmHg). In the categorical shift analysis, there was a greater rate of subjects who

Table AII4-1 Dashboard Summary of Supine Blood Pressure Changes—Controlled Phase 2/3 Studies

	Placebo	M ≤ 5 mg	M = 10 mg	M = 15 mg	Total M	COX
N	2122	2392	2305	305	5002	2124
SBP—Supine (mmHg)						
Baseline mean	122.3	122.7	122.3	122.2	122.5	122.4
Mean change[a]	−0.1	−0.1	0.0	0.5	0.0	2.4
H/N to L	70 (3.3%)	77 (3.2%)	71 (3.1%)	9 (3.0%)	151 (3.0%)	23 (1.1%)
L/N to H	323 (15.2%)	354 (14.8%)	341 (14.8%)	47 (15.4%)	742 (14.8%)	474 (22.3%)
Clinically significant:						
Decreases	1 (< 0.1%)	0	1 (< 0.1%)	0	2 (< 0.1%)	0
Increases	6 (0.3%)	5 (0.2%)	9 (0.4%)	1 (0.3%)	15 (0.3%)	25 (1.2%)
DBP—Supine (mmHg)						
Baseline mean	77.7	78.2	77.6	77.4	77.9	78.0
Mean change[a]	0.5	0.6	0.4	0.2	0.5	1.0
H/N to L	11 (0.5%)	10 (0.4%)	15 (0.7%)	1 (0.3%)	26 (0.5%)	2 (0.1%)
L/N to H	108 (5.1%)	120 (5.0%)	111 (4.8%)	15 (4.9%)	246 (4.9%)	181 (8.5%)
Clinically significant:						
Decreases	2 (0.1%)	1 (< 0.1%)	0	0	1 (< 0.1%)	0
Increases	2 (0.1%)	3 (0.1%)	2 (0.1%)	0	5 (0.1%)	17 (0.8%)
Orthostatic Blood Pressure Changes						
Orthostatic blood pressure changes	11 (0.5%)	13 (0.5%)	12 (0.5%)	1 (0.3%)	26 (0.5%)	9 (0.4%)
Blood Pressure–Related Adverse Events						
N	2200	2450	2400	325	5175	2225
Hypertension*	64 (2.9%)	76 (3.1%)	74 (3.1%)	10 (3.1%)	160 (3.1%)	129 (5.8%)
Hypotension**	11 (0.5%)	15 (0.6%)	14 (0.6%)	1 (0.3%)%	30 (0.6%)	4 (0.2%)
Syncope	1 (< 0.1%)	0	2 (0.1%)	0	2 (< 0.1%)	1 (< 0.1%)

M = Mepro; N = number of subjects; H = above normal; N = normal; L = below normal.

* Hypertension includes the PTs: *Accelerated hypertension, Blood pressure ambulatory increased, Blood pressure diastolic increased, Blood pressure increased, Blood pressure systolic increased, Diastolic hypertension, Essential hypertension, Hypertensive crisis, Hypertensive emergency, Labile hypertension, Malignant hypertension, Prehypertension,* and *Systolic hypertension.*

** Hypotension includes the PTs: *Blood pressure ambulatory decreased, Blood pressure decreased, Blood pressure diastolic decreased, Blood pressure systolic decreased, Diastolic hypotension, Hypotension,* and *Orthostatic hypotension.*

[a]Change from baseline to the worst (i.e., most extreme) treatment value.

Source: Appendix Tables MSBP1.1, CASSBP1.1, CSCSBP1.1, MDBP1.1, CASDBP1.1, CSCDBP1.1, OBP1.1, and AE3.1.

had systolic and diastolic blood pressure values that shifted to above normal values during the treatment period in the COX group compared to the Mepro and placebo groups. A similar pattern was seen for clinically significant systolic and diastolic blood pressure increases. In addition, the rate of hypertension reported as an AE was also greater in the COX group compared to both the placebo and the Mepro treatment groups. In 1 patient in the COX group (Patient 3003-0535, study MP3003), hypertension associated with a transient ischemic attack was reported. These events were serious and led to premature termination. Further details of this case are discussed in Section 2.5.

There were a total of 4 cases of syncope reported in controlled Phase 2/3 studies—1 in the Placebo group, 2 in the Mepro group, and 1 in the COX group. A listing of these events is shown in Table AII4-2.

None of the syncopal episodes were considered treatment related, and with 1 exception (placebo Patient 3002-0023, study 3002 where the reason for the syncope was unknown) appeared to be secondary to other nondrug-related conditions. No additional syncopal cases were reported in the uncontrolled studies.

In the Phase 1 studies, no blood pressure trends were noted in any of the treatment groups. Syncope was reported

Table AII4-2   Summary of Patients With Syncope—All Phase 2/3 Studies

Study No./ Patient No.	Age/Gender/ Race	Dose	Exposure to Study Medication (Days)	Reported AE Term	MedDRA PT	Serious/WD/ Related (as Judged by the Investigator)	Outcome
Placebo							
MP3002/ 3002-0023	51/female/ Black	0	28	Brief syncopal episode—no known reason	Syncope	No/no/no	Recovered
Mepro							
MP2001/ 2001-0012	42/male/ Black	10 mg	16	Dehydration; Gastroenteritis; Syncope	Dehydration; Gastroenteritis; Syncope	Yes/no/no	Recovered
MP3003/ 3003-1014	74/female/ Caucasian	10 mg	53	Heat stroke; Syncope	Heat stroke; Syncope	Yes/yes/no	Unknown
COX							
MP3003/ 3003-0649	28/male/ Caucasian	25 mg	7	Fainted after giving blood	Syncope	No/no/no	Recovered

WD = withdrawal.
Source: SYNCLIST1.1.

in 1 subject (Subject 1002-0003, study MP1002) in the placebo group and 1 subject in the Mepro group (Subject 1009-0002, study MP 1009). Both events occurred during the time blood was drawn and were considered secondary to a vasovagal response to the fear of needles. Both subjects completely recovered.

➡ **NOTE:** Syncope can be quite benign; e.g., it might result from fear from seeing a needle, or in the other extreme, it might be due to a life-threatening ventricular arrhythmia. For these reasons, all cases of syncope should be reviewed to determine cause and discussed in the text as illustrated—even for cases that are not drug related. This is an example of preemptive strike, i.e., addressing an issue before it is raised.

4.1.2 Heart Rate

In Appendices MHR1.1, MHR1.2, and MHR1.3, the mean changes in supine HR are summarized for the controlled Phase 2/3 studies, all Phase 2/3 studies, and the Phase 1 studies, respectively. In Appendices MHR2.1, MHR2.2, and MHR2.3, the mean changes in standing HR are shown for the controlled Phase 2/3 studies, all Phase 2/3 studies, and the Phase 1 studies, respectively.

The results of the categorical shift analysis for supine HR can be found in Appendix CASHR1.1 (controlled Phase 2/3 studies), Appendix CASHR1.2 (all Phase 2/3 studies), and Appendix CASHR1.3 (Phase 1 studies). The results of the categorical shift analysis for standing HR can be found in Appendix CASHR2.1 (controlled Phase 2/3 studies), Appendix CASHR2.2 (all Phase 2/3 studies), and Appendix CASHR2.3 (Phase 1 studies).

In Appendices CSCHR1.1, CSCHR1.2, and CSCHR1.3, the rates of clinically significant changes in supine heart rate are summarized for the controlled Phase 2/3 studies, all Phase 2/3 studies, and the Phase 1 studies, respectively. In Appendices CSCHR2.1, CSCHR2.2, and CSCHR2.3, the rates of clinically significant changes in standing heart rate are presented for the controlled Phase 2/3 studies, all Phase 2/3 studies, and the Phase 1 studies, respectively.

A listing of subjects with 1 or more clinically significant heart rate changes during treatment can be found in Appendices CSLISTHR1.1 and CSLISTHR1.2 for Phase 2/3 studies and Phase 1 studies, respectively. The listing includes all baseline, treatment, and posttreatment values for these subjects.

Combined terms were used in the calculation of rates for tachycardia and bradycardia. For tachycardia, the PTs *Sinus tachycardia, Tachycardia, and Heart rate increased*

were combined; for bradycardia the PTs *Bradycardia, Sinus bradycardia,* and *Heart rate decreased* were combined.

Mean changes, categorical shifts, clinically significant changes in heart rate, and heart rate-related adverse events showed no relevant differences among the placebo, Mepro, or COX treatment groups in the controlled Phase 2/3 studies and all Phase 2.3 studies. No heart rate differences across treatment groups were noted in the Phase 1 studies. There were no serious heart rate-related AEs or HR-related AEs that led to premature termination reported in any study.

➡ **NOTE:** Normally a summary table of heart rate changes similar in format to Table AII4-1 should be included in the text of an ISS/SCS. Because this sample IAS is simplified, the table display of heart rate changes was not shown in the text.

4.1.3 Temperature

In Appendices MTEMP1.1, MTEMP1.2, and MTEMP1.3, mean changes in temperature are summarized for the controlled Phase 2/3 studies, all Phase 2/3 studies, and the Phase 1 studies, respectively.

The results of the categorical shift analysis for temperature can be found in Appendix CASTEMP1.1 (controlled Phase 2/3 studies), Appendix CASTEMP1.2 (all Phase 2/3 studies), and Appendix CASTEMP1.3 (Phase 1 studies).

The rates of clinically significant changes in temperature can be found in Appendix CSCTEMP1.1 (controlled Phase 2/3 studies), Appendix CSCTEMP1.2 (all Phase 2/3 studies), and Appendix CSCTEMP1.3 (Phase 1 studies).

A listing of subjects with 1 or more clinically significant changes in temperature during treatment can be found in Appendices CSLISTTEMP1.1 and CSLIST-TEMP1.2 for Phase 2/3 studies and Phase 1 studies, respectively. The listing includes all baseline, treatment, and posttreatment values for these subjects.

A combined term was used in calculation of the rate of pyrexia and includes the PTs *Pyrexia* and *Body temperature increased*.

Table AII4-3 is a dashboard summary of temperature changes in controlled Phase 2/3 studies.

Mean changes and categorical shifts showed a small trend toward decreases in temperature in the Mepro and COX groups compared to placebo. Consistent with these findings were the lower rate of AEs related to increased temperature. These findings were not unexpected and were consistent with the antipyretic effects of NSAIDs. None of the temperature-related AEs were serious or led to premature termination.

Table AII4-3 Dashboard Summary of Temperature Changes—Controlled Phase 2/3 Studies

	Placebo	M ≤ 5 mg	M = 10 mg	M = 15 mg	Total M	COX
N	2122	2392	2305	305	5002	2124
Temperature °C						
Baseline mean	36.8	36.9	36.8	36.8	36.8	37.0
Mean change[a]	0.0	−0.1	−0.3	−0.2	−0.2	−0.1
H/N to L	7 (0.3%)	24 (1.0%)	35 (1.5%)	5 (1.6%)	64 (1.3%)	19 (0.9%)
L/N to H	6 (0.3%)	12 (0.5%)	7 (0.3%)	1 (0.3%)	20 (0.4%)	11 (0.5%)
Clinically significant:						
Decreases	0	0	0	0	0	0
Increases	1 (<0.1%)	0	1 (<0.1%)	0	1 (<0.1%)	1 (<0.1%)
Temperature-Related Adverse Events						
N	2200	2450	2400	325	5175	2225
Pyrexia*	57 (2.6%)	27 (1.1%)	22 (0.9%)	3 (0.9%)	52 (1.0%)	31 (1.4%)

M = Mepro; N = number of subjects; H = above normal; N = normal; L = below normal.
* Pyrexia includes the PTs: *Pyrexia* and *Body temperature increased.*
[a] Change from baseline to worst (i.e., most extreme) treatment value.
Source: Appendix Tables MTEMP1.1, CASTEMP1.1, CSCTEMP1.1, and AE3.1.

Similar findings were observed in all Phase 2/3 studies.

In the Phase 1 studies, no difference in temperature changes was noted across treatment groups.

4.2 Body Weight and Body Mass Index

In Appendices MBW1.1, MBW1.2, and MBW1.3, mean changes in body weight are summarized for the controlled Phase 2/3 studies, all Phase 2/3 studies, and the Phase 1 studies, respectively. In Appendices MBMI1.1, MBMI1.2, and MBMI1.3, mean changes in BMI are shown for the controlled Phase 2/3 studies, all Phase 2/3 studies, and the Phase 1 studies, respectively.

In Appendices CSCBW1.1, CSCBW1.2, and CSCBW1.3, the rates of clinically significant changes in body weight are summarized for the controlled Phase 2/3 studies, all Phase 2/3 studies, and the Phase 1 studies, respectively. In Appendices CSCBMI1.1, CSCBMI1.2, and CSCBMI1.3, the rates of clinically significant changes in BMI can be found for the controlled Phase 2/3 studies, all Phase 2/3 studies, and the Phase 1 studies, respectively.

A listing of subjects with 1 or more clinically significant changes in body weight during treatment can be found in Appendices CSLISTBW1.1 and CSLISTBW1.2 for Phase 2/3 studies and Phase 1 studies, respectively. A listing of subjects with 1 or more clinically significant changes in BMI during treatment can be found in Appendices CSLISTBMI1.1 and CSLISTBMI1.2 for Phase 2/3 studies and Phase 1 studies, respectively. These listings include all baseline, treatment, and posttreatment values for these subjects.

A combined term was used for weight increased and included the PTs *Abnormal weight gain* and *Weight increased*. A combined term was also used for weight decreased and included the PTs *Abnormal loss of weight* and *Weight decreased*.

Table AII4-4 is a dashboard summary of changes in body weight and BMI in controlled Phase 2/3 studies.

No relevant differences in body weight or body mass index were noted between the placebo and Mepro treatment groups with respect to mean changes, clinically significant changes, or weight-related adverse events. In the COX group, an upward trend in weight and BMI was observed.

Table AII4-4 **Dashboard Summary of Changes in Body Weight and Body Mass Index—Controlled Phase 2/3 Studies**

N	Placebo 2122	M ≤ 5 mg 2392	M = 10 mg 2305	M = 15 mg 305	Total M 5002	COX 2124
BW (kg)						
Baseline mean	79.9	78.8	78.4	79.8	78.6	79.0
Mean change[a]	0.5	0.3	0.6	0.5	0.5	1.8
Clinically significant:						
Increases	176 (8.3%)	196 (8.2%)	182 (7.9%)	24 (7.9%)	402 (8.0%)	278 (13.1%)
Decreases	13 (0.6%)	10 (0.4%)	14 (0.6%)	0	24 (0.5%)	4 (0.2%)
BMI (kg/m²)						
Baseline mean	27.4	27.6	27.0	27.1	27.3	26.8
Mean change[a]	0.5	0.6	0.4	0.2	0.5	1.0
Clinically significant:						
Increases	23 (1.1%)	29 (1.2%)	25 (1.1%)	4 (1.3%)	58 (1.2%)	36 (1.7%)
Decreases	9 (0.4%)	7 (0.3%)	7 (0.3%)	0	14 (0.3%)	0
Weight-Related Adverse Events						
N	2200	2450	2400	325	5175	2225
Weight increased*	33 (1.5%)	37 (1.5%)	50 (2.1%)	9 (2.8%)	96 (1.9%)	129 (5.8%)
Weight decreased**	8 (0.4%)	9 (0.4%)	12 (0.5%)	1 (0.3%)	22 (0.4%)	2 (0.1%)

M = Mepro.

[a] Change from baseline to worst (i.e., most extreme) treatment value.

* Weight increased includes the PTs: *Abnormal weight gain* and *Weight increased*.

** Weight decreased includes the PTs: *Abnormal loss of weight* and *Weight decreased*.

Source: Appendix Tables MBW1.1, CSCBW1.1, MBMI1.1, CSCBMI1.1, and AE3.

4.3 12-Lead Electrocardiograms

4.3.1 ECG Parameters (Excluding QTc)

4.3.1.1 Heart Rate

In Appendices MECGHR1.1, MECGHR1.2, and MECGHR1.3, mean changes in heart rate are summarized for the controlled Phase 2/3 studies, all Phase 2/3 studies, and the Phase 1 studies, respectively.

The results of the categorical shift analysis for HR can be found in Appendix CASECGHR1.1 (controlled Phase 2/3 studies), Appendix CASECGHR1.2 (all Phase 2/3 studies), and Appendix CASECGHR1.3 (Phase 1 studies).

In Appendices CSCECGHR1.1, CSCECGHR1.2, and CSCECGHR1.3, the rates of clinically significant changes in HR are provided for the controlled Phase 2/3 studies, all Phase 2/3 studies, and the Phase 1 studies, respectively.

A listing of subjects with clinically significant changes in HR during treatment can be found in Appendices CSLISTECGHR1.1 and CSLISTECGHR1.2 for Phase 2/3 studies and Phase 1 studies, respectively. These listings include all baseline, treatment, and posttreatment values.

No differences were seen across treatment groups for heart rate in the analysis of mean change, categorical shifts, and clinically significant changes, in controlled Phase 2/3 studies, all Phase 2/3 studies, and Phase 1 studies. These findings were consistent with the analysis of heart rate (obtained as a vital sign measurement) summarized in Section 4.1.2. No heart rate–related events that were serious or led to discontinuation were reported in any treatment group (see Section 4.1.2).

> **NOTE:** HR data come from 2 different sources, as a vital sign measurement and from an ECG tracing. If there is a true drug effect on heart rate, similar trends should be seen in both the vital signs and ECG analyses of heart rate.

4.3.1.2 PR Interval

In Appendices MPR1.1, MPR1.2, and MPR1.3, mean changes in PR interval are summarized for the controlled Phase 2/3 studies, all Phase 2/3 studies, and the Phase 1 studies, respectively.

The results of the categorical shift analysis for PR interval can be found in Appendix CASPR1.1 (controlled Phase 2/3 studies), Appendix CASPR1.2 (all Phase 2/3 studies), and Appendix CASPR1.3 (Phase 1 studies).

In Appendices CSCPR1.1, CSCPR1.2, and CSCPR1.3, the rates of clinically significant changes in PR interval can be found for the controlled Phase 2/3 studies, all Phase 2/3 studies, and the Phase 1 studies, respectively.

A listing of subjects with clinically significant changes in PR interval during treatment can be found in Appendices CSCLISTPR1.1 and CSCLISTPR1.2 for Phase 2/3 studies and Phase 1 studies, respectively. These listings include all baseline, treatment, and posttreatment values for these subjects.

A combined term was used for atrioventricular block and includes the following PTs: *Atrioventricular block, Atrioventricular block complete, Atrioventricular block first, Atrioventricular block second, AV dissociation,* and *Electrocardiogram PR prolongation.* A combined term was also used for atrioventricular conduction time shortened and includes the PTs: *Atrioventricular conduction time shortened* and *Electrocardiogram PR shortened.*

Table AII4-5 is a dashboard summary of PR changes in controlled Phase 2/3 studies.

There were no treatment group differences noted for any of the analyses evaluating changes in PR interval. None of the PR-related AEs was serious or led to premature discontinuation. Similar findings were seen in all Phase 2/3 studies and Phase 1 studies.

> **NOTE:** Because this is a simplified IAS, a dashboard display is shown only for the PR interval and not for changes in HR or QRS complex. Even if there are no treatment group differences as shown in Table AII4-5, it is good to summarize the findings of HR and QRS in a dashboard display anyway so the reviewer doesn't think you are overlooking or hiding any important information that should be discussed. What to include is a judgment call. Clearly any treatment differences should be shown and discussed in the text. Also, if the drug is part of a class with known ECG changes, the relevant ECG parameters should be discussed in the text. The amount of detail provided in the text is also dependent on whether you are writing the ISS or the SCS. The SCS has page limitations so the text should be succinct, whereas in the ISS, a more detailed analysis is required.[1,2]

4.3.1.3 QRS Complex

In Appendices MQRS1.1, MQRS1.2, and MQRS1.3, mean changes in the QRS complex are shown for the controlled Phase 2/3 studies, all Phase 2/3 studies, and the Phase 1 studies, respectively.

Table AII4-5 **Dashboard Summary of Changes in the PR Interval—Controlled Phase 2/3 Studies**

	Placebo	M ≤ 5mg	M = 10 mg	M = 15 mg	Total M	COX
Mean changes						
PR interval (ms)						
N	2005	2254	2195	270	4719	2024
Baseline mean	161.4	159.8	160.4	159.0	160.1	160.8
Mean change[a]	0.9	0.8	0.9	0.9	0.9	0.8
N	2005	2254	2195	270	4719	2024
L/N to H	24 (1.2%)	23 (1.0%)	24 (1.1%)	2 (0.7%)	49 (1.0%)	20 (1.0%)
H/N to L	6 (0.3%)	7 (0.3%)	2 (0.1%)	3 (0.4%)	12 (0.3%)	4 (0.2%)
N	1956	2201	2134	265	4600	1998
Clinically significant:						
Increases	4 (0.2%)	4 (0.2%)	9 (0.4%)	0	13 (0.3%)	6 (0.3%)
Decreases	0	0	0	0	0	1 (< 0.1%)
PR-Related Adverse Events						
N	2200	2450	2400	325	5175	2225
Atrioventricular block*	7 (0.3%)	10 (0.4%)	5 (0.2%)	1 (0.3%)	16 (0.3%)	9 (0.4%)
Atrioventricular conduction time shortened**	0	0	0	0	0	0

M = Mepro; N = number of subjects; L = below normal; N = normal; H = above normal; ms = milliseconds

[a] Change from baseline to worst (i.e., most extreme) treatment value.

* Atrioventricular block included the PTs: *Atrioventricular block, Atrioventricular block complete, Atrioventricular block first, Atrioventricular block second, AV dissociation,* and *Electrocardiogram PR prolongation.*

** Atrioventricular conduction time shortened includes the PTs: *Atrioventricular conduction time shortened* and *Electrocardiogram PR shortened.*

Source: Appendix Tables MPR1.1, CASPR1.2, CSCPR1.2, and AE3.1.

The results of the categorical shifts for QRS complex can be found in Appendix CASQRS1.1 (controlled Phase 2/3 studies), Appendix CASQRS1.2 (all Phase 2/3 studies), and Appendix CASQRS1.3 (Phase 1 studies).

In Appendices CSCQRS1.1, CSCQRS1.2, and CSCQRS1.3, the rates of clinically significant changes in QRS complex can be found for the controlled Phase 2/3 studies, all Phase 2/3 studies, and the Phase 1 studies, respectively.

The rates of clinically significant changes in QRS can be found in Appendix CSQRS1.1 (controlled Phase 2/3 studies), Appendix CSQRS1.2 (all Phase 2/3 studies), and Appendix CSQRS1.3 (Phase 1 studies).

A listing of subjects with clinically significant changes in QRS complex during treatment can be found in Appendices CSCLISTQRS1.1 and CSCLISTQRS1.2 for Phase 2/3 studies and Phase 1 studies, respectively. These listings include all baseline, treatment, and posttreatment values for these subjects.

Mean changes, categorical shifts, and clinically significant changes in the QRS complex showed no relevant differences across treatment groups in controlled Phase 2/3 studies, all Phase 2/3 studies, and Phase 1 studies. There were no treatment-related serious QRS-related events or events that led to discontinuation in any treatment group or study reported.

4.3.2 QTc
4.3.2.1 Nonclinical QTc Evaluation
An extensive nonclinical evaluation of the QTc interval was done in accordance with the guidance, *The Nonclinical Evaluation of the Potential for Delayed Ventricular Repolarization (QT Interval Prolongation) by Human Pharmaceuticals S7B.*[11] In Appendix NCOVR1.0 the results of these evaluations can be found. No potential for QTc prolongation was identified in these nonclinical studies.

4.3.2.2 Thorough QT/QTc Study

A thorough QT/QTc study was conducted to determine Mepro's affect on the QTc interval in humans. Study MP1010 was a multiple-dose placebo and active-controlled study evaluating the QTc interval in a total of 105 healthy subjects. Subjects received Mepro 30 mg (35 subjects), placebo (35 subjects), or moxifloxacin 400 mg (35 subjects) for 7 days. The results of this study showed a mean difference in QTc values of 2 milliseconds after exposure to Mepro 30 mg (compared to placebo), and a 5-milliseconds mean difference after moxifloxacin exposure (compared to placebo). No treatment group differences in the rates of categorical/clinically significant shifts as described in Section 1.2.4.2.2.2 were seen. The results indicated that exposure to Mepro was not associated with prolongation of the QT/QTc interval. The study report and complete results can be found in Appendix CSR1010.

4.3.2.3 Clinical Studies

In Appendices MQTCB1.1, MQTCB1.2, and MQTCB1.3, mean changes in QTc using the Bazett correction formula for the controlled Phase 2/3 studies, all Phase 2/3 studies, and the Phase 1 studies, respectively, can be found. In Appendices MQTCF1.1, MQTCF1.2, and MQTCF1.3, mean changes in QTc using the Fridericia correction formula can be found for the controlled Phase 2/3 studies, all Phase 2/3 studies, and the Phase 1 studies, respectively.

The results of the categorical/clinically significant shift analysis for QTc (using the Bazett correction formula) can be found in Appendix CASQTCB1.1 (controlled Phase 2/3 studies), Appendix CASQTCB1.2 (all Phase 2/3 studies), and Appendix CASQTCB1.3 (Phase 1 studies). The results of the categorical/clinically significant shift analysis for QTc (using the Fridericia correction formula) can be found in Appendix CASQTCF1.1 (controlled Phase 2/3 studies), Appendix CASQTCF1.2 (all Phase 2/3 studies), and Appendix CASQTCF1.3 (Phase 1 studies).

A listing of subjects with categorical/clinically significant QTc shifts (using the Bazett correction formula) can be found in Appendices CSCLISTQTCB1.1 and CSCLISTQTCB1.2 for Phase 2/3 studies and Phase 1 studies, respectively. A listing of subjects with categorical/clinically significant QTc shifts (using the Fridericia correction formula) during treatment can be found in Appendices CSCLISTQTCF1.1 and CSCLISTQTCF1.2 for Phase 2/3 studies and Phase 1 studies, respectively.

Table AII4-6 is a dashboard summary of QTc changes in controlled Phase 2/3 studies using the Bazett's correction formula.

Mean changes from baseline were small and similar among the placebo, Mepro, and COX groups. There were no clinically relevant differences observed in the rates of categorical/clinical shifts among the placebo, Mepro, and COX groups. Only 1 patient (Patient 3002-0112, study MP3002), a 54-year-old female who received Mepro 10 mg, had a QTc value at study day 28 that was > 500 milliseconds (504 milliseconds). Her values were above normal range both pretreatment and posttreatment. She remained asymptomatic with no syncopal or ventricular-related arrhythmias reported. The investigator did not consider this finding to be treatment related.

A summary of her QTc values is shown in Table AII4-7.

Review of the *Torsades de pointes/QT prolongation* SMQ showed similar rates across treatment groups. Review of the individual events in this SMQ revealed that all but one event in a COX subject (who died suddenly 30 days after the last dose of drug—see Table AII2-11) were all due to syncope with no evidence of prolongation of the QTc interval in any of these subjects. Two cases of syncope were also reported in Phase 1 studies, 1 in a placebo subject, and the other in a subject who received Mepro; both events were thought to be vasovagal episodes. All reported cases of syncope are discussed in Section 4.1.1.

There were no reports of TdP, or ventricular fibrillation reported for any subject in any Phase 2/3 or Phase 1 study.

There were no clinically important differences in results when the Fridericia correction formula was used.

4.4 Summary of Vital Signs, Physical Findings, and Other Observations Related to Safety

There were no treatment differences in blood pressure, heart rate, body weight, or BMI in the Mepro group, compared to placebo. An upward trend in blood pressure, body weight, and BMI, however, was seen in the COX group. A small trend toward temperature decreases was identified in the Mepro and COX groups, compared to placebo. This was not unexpected and was consistent with the antipyretic effect of both drugs.

Nonclinical evaluations and a thorough QT/QTc showed no evidence of QT/QTc prolongation after Mepro exposure. The data from routine ECG monitoring in Phase 2/3 and Phase 1 studies also showed no evidence of QT/QTc prolongation with Mepro treatment. Review of other ECG parameters—heart rate, PR interval, and QRS complex showed no clinically relevant changes after Mepro exposure compared to the other treatment groups.

Table AII4-6 **Dashboard Summary of Changes in QTc-Controlled Phase 2/3 Studies**

	Placebo	M ≤ 5 mg	M = 10 mg	M = 15 mg	Total M	COX
			Mean Change[a]			
QTc ms (Bazett)						
N	2005	2254	2195	270	4719	2024
Baseline Mean	403.2	403.1	401.1	402.9	402.1	403.8
Mean Change[a]	0.9	0.8	0.9	0.4	0.9	0.8
			Categorical/Clinically Significant Shifts (Normal Baseline Values)			
N	1910	2105	1991	249	4345	1901
QTc (B) > 450	29 (1.5%)	21 (1.0%)	24 (1.2%)	4 (1.6%)	49 (1.1%)	25 (1.3%)
QTc (B) > 480	10 (0.5%)	8 (0.4%)	8 (0.4%)	1 (0.4%)	17 (0.4%)	6 (0.3%)
QTc (B) > 500	0	0	0	0	0	0
QTc(B) > 30	27 (1.4%)	32 (1.5%)	24 (1.2%)	4 (1.6%)	60 (1.4%)	27 (1.4%)
QTc(B) > 60	4 (0.2%)	6 (0.3%)	4 (0.2 %)	2 (0.8%)	12 (0.3%)	6 (0.3%)
			Categorical/Clinically Significant Shifts (Abnormal Baseline Values)			
N	95	149	204	21	374	123
QTc (B) > 450	9 (9.5%)	13 (8.7%)	18 (8.8%)	0	31 (8.3%)	10 (8.1%)
QTc (B) > 480	2 (2.1%)	3 (2.0%)	3 (1.5%)	0	6 (1.6%)	2 (1.6%)
QTc (B) > 500	0	1 (0.7%)	0	0	1 (0.3%)	0
QTc(B) > 30	5 (5.3%)	8 (5.4%)	10 (4.9%)	1 (4.8%)	19 (5.1%)	7 (5.7%)
QTc(B) > 60	1 (1.1%)	2 (1.3%)	2 (1.0%)	0	4 (1.1%)	1 (0.8%)
			Torsades de Pointes/QT Prolongation-Related AEs			
N	2200	2450	2400	325	5175	2225
Torsades de pointes/QT prolongation (SMQ)	1 (< 0.1%)	0	2 (0.1%)	0	2 (< 0.1%)	2 (0.1%)*

M = Mepro; B = Bazett; SMQ = Standardised MedDRA Query.

[a] Change from baseline to the worst (i.e., most extreme) treatment value.

* Includes one subject with sudden death 30 days after the last dose of study medication.

Source: Appendix Tables MQTCB1.1, CASQTCB1.1, and AESEARCH1.1.

Table AII4-7 **Summary of QTc Values for Patient 3002-0112, Study MP3002**

Study Day	QTc (B) ms	Adverse Events	Concomitant Medications
0 (baseline)	490 ms (H)	None	None
28	504 ms (H, CS)	None	None
56	480 ms (H)	None	None
84 (last day of treatment)	490 ms (H)	None	None
91 (7 days after the last dose)	495 ms (H)	None	None

B = Bazett. ms = millisecond; H = above normal; CS = Clinically significant change.

Source: Appendix CSCLISTQTCB1.1.

■ 5 Safety in Special Groups and Situations

5.1 Interactions

The following is a brief summary of Mepro's pharmacology profile in normal, healthy volunteers. Complete information can be found in the "Clinical Pharmacology Overview Report" located in Appendix CLINPHAR-MOV1.0.

- Mepro is completely (> 99%) absorbed after oral administration and is approximately 99.4% protein bound.

- No difference in apparent volumes of distribution after intravenous and oral administration are observed. Mepro crosses the blood-brain barrier.

- Peak concentration is generally attained within 1.4–1.5 hours.

- Half-life is approximately 24 hours.

- Pharmacokinetic properties show linearity across the dose range of 1.25 mg to 15 mg/day.

- Mepro is almost completely metabolized in the liver to 3 inactive metabolites (the major metabolite is 6'-carboxy-meproamine) via the P450 2C9 pathway.

- These inactive metabolites are excreted in the urine; very little Mepro (< 1%) is excreted unchanged in the urine.

- The residual effect of the drug is approximately 7 days after the last dose is taken.

5.1.1 Drug-Demographic Interactions
5.1.1.1 Gender

5.1.1.1.1 Study MP1009   A pharmacokinetic (PK) study (study MP1009) was conducted in 12 male and 12 female healthy volunteers who received a single dose of Mepro 5 mg. Results showed females had a 52% greater C_{max} compared to males. The complete report can be found in Appendix CSR1009.

5.1.1.1.2 Population Pharmacokinetics   A total of 300 blood samples were obtained at steady state from subjects exposed to Mepro in study MP3001. Of these samples, 200 were obtained from females and 100 from males. Results showed approximately 40% higher Mepro plasma levels in females compared to males (see Appendix CSR3001 for complete results).

5.1.1.1.3 Subgroup Analysis   A subgroup analysis of adverse events by gender for AEs ≥ 1% was done for females versus males from controlled Phase 2/3 studies (see Appendix AEGEN1.1). In Table AII5-1, the AE rate and the attributable risk ratio (ARR) by gender are summarized for the common potential adverse reactions described in Section 2.2.

Both the rates and ARRs of potential adverse reactions were greater in females than males in both the Mepro and COX groups compared to placebo with the exception of PUBs in females exposed to Mepro. A greater risk in females was expected since the common potential adverse drug reactions described in Section 2.2 were all dose related and females have 40–50% greater plasma Mepro levels compared to males given the same dose. For

Table AII5-1 Adverse Event Rates and Attributable Risks in Females versus Males for Potential Adverse Drug Reactions—Controlled Phase 2/3 Studies

	Placebo	Total M	COX
N, Females	1448	3578	1469
N, Males	752	1597	756
Abdominal Pain Upper			
Females	43 (3.0%)	247 (6.9%)	147 (10.0%)
Males	23 (3.1%)	85 (5.3%)	38 (5.0%)
AR_F		3.9%	7.0%
AR_M		2.2%	1.9%
AR_F/AR_{M^*}		1.8	3.7
Dyspepsia			
Females	30 (2.1%)	207 (5.8%)	178 (12.1%)
Males	14 (1.9%)	56 (3.5%)	53 (7.0%)

Continues

Table AII5-1 Adverse Event Rates and Attributable Risks in Females versus Males for Potential Adverse Drug Reactions—Controlled Phase 2/3 Studies, Continued

AR_F		3.7%	10.0%
AR_M		1.6%	5.1%
AR_F/AR_{M^*}		2.3	2.0
Epigastric Discomfort			
Females	16 (1.1%)	286 (8.0%)	155 (10.6%)
Males	8 (1.1%)	87 (5.4%)	45 (6.0%)
AR_F		6.9%	9.5%
AR_M		4.3%	4.9%
AR_F/AR_{M^*}		1.6	1.9
Nausea			
Females	44 (3.0%)	260 (7.3%)	222 (15.1%)
Males	24 (3.2%)	80 (5.0%)	54 (7.1%)
AR_F		4.3%	12.1%
AR_M		1.8%	3.9%
AR_F/AR_{M^*}		2.4	3.1
PUBs			
Females	0	48 (1.3)	76 (5.2%)
Males	1 (0.1%)	20 (1.3)	20 (2.6%)
AR_F		1.3%	5.2%
AR_M		1.2%	2.5%
AR_F/AR_{M^*}		1.1	2.1
Vomiting			
Females	46 (3.2%)	211 (5.9%)	140 (9.5%)
Males	18 (2.4%)	47 (2.9%)	34 (4.5%)
AR_F		2.7%	6.3%
AR_M		0.5%	2.1%
AR_F/AR_{M^*}		5.4	3.0

M = Mepro; AR = attributable risk; PUBs = perforations, ulcers, and bleeds; AR = attributable risk; * = attributable risk ratio (ARR).

Source: Appendix Table AEGEN1.1.

this reason a greater risk of PUBs in females was expected but not seen. There are insufficient data at this time to determine if this finding is real. More and longer Mepro exposures are required before any conclusions can be made.

Based on this PK profile, it is recommended that females start Mepro at the lowest effective dose.

5.1.1.2 Age
5.1.1.2.1 Study MP1006 Study MP1006 evaluated the effect of age on PK profiles in 12 elderly subjects ($\geq$ 65 years old) and 12 nonelderly subjects (< 65 years old) given a single dose of Mepro 5 mg. The study showed no clinically important differences in PK profiles between the 2 age groups when matched for gender. The complete clinical study report can be found in Appendix CSR1006.

5.1.1.2.2 Study MP 1007 Study MP1007 was a placebo-controlled, single-dose study evaluating the PK profiles of Mepro 2.5 mg (12 subjects), Mepro 5 mg (12 subjects), and Mepro 10 mg (12 subjects) and placebo (6 subjects) in 12–16-year-olds. The PK profile was linear over the 3 different Mepro doses. When the dose was normalized to 0.07–0.14 mg/kg/day (the recommended adult dose of 5–10 mg in a 70-kg person), the PK profiles of subjects 12–16 years old were similar to those in adults. The complete study report can be found in Appendix CSR1007.

5.1.1.2.3 Population Pharmacokinetics In the 300 blood samples obtained from Mepro patients in study MP3001, 240 were from patients < 65 years, and the remaining 60 samples were from patients $\geq$ 65 years old. Although higher plasma concentrations were seen in elderly females compared to elderly males, higher plasma concentrations were also seen in nonelderly females compared to nonelderly males, indicating the difference in plasma levels was gender based rather than age based (see Appendix CSR3001).

5.1.1.2.4 Subgroup Analysis

A subgroup analysis of AEs by age for controlled Phase 2/3 studies was done, and the results can be found in Appendix AEAGE1.1. The results showed no difference in the AE rate or ARR in the elderly versus nonelderly for the AEs considered to be potential adverse drug reactions including PUBs in the Mepro group, whereas in the COX group a trend toward greater risk in the elderly compared to the nonelderly was seen. It should be noted, however, that historically, the elderly are at greater risk of developing PUBs with NSAID use. There are insufficient data at this time to determine if the risk for PUBs in the elderly is any different with Mepro use compared to other NSAIDs.

5.1.1.3 Race
5.1.1.3.1 Population Pharmacokinetics

The blood samples from study MP3001 obtained for PK analyses included samples from 222 Caucasians, 63 Blacks, 9 Asians, and 6 Native Americans exposed to Mepro. There were no relevant differences in Mepro plasma levels seen in Caucasians versus Blacks. There were too few blood samples from Asians and Native Americans to make any conclusions of the data for these racial groups (see Appendix CSR3001 for the complete study report).

5.1.1.3.2 Subgroup Analysis

A subgroup analysis of adverse events by race can be found in Appendix AERACE1.1 for controlled Phase 2/3 studies. No clinically relevant difference in the rate or ARR was noted between Caucasians and Blacks for the common potential AEs in either the Mepro or COX treatment groups. There were too few Asians and other racial groups to make any meaningful conclusions from the data in these racial groups.

5.1.1.3.3 Skin Reactions

Five cases of photosensitivity reactions occurred in Caucasians only (see Section 2.7.10.2). One case of SJS was reported in an Asian female who tested positive for the B*1502 allele of HLA-B, a gene associated with an increased risk for Stevens-Johnson syndrome in subjects exposed to phenytoin and carbamazepine. This case was further confounded by the concomitant use of penicillin, a drug associated with the development of SJS. However, based on the available case information, attribution to Mepro cannot be entirely ruled out (see Section 2.7.10.1). Otherwise, no important differences were seen in the AE profile based on race.

5.1.2 Drug-Disease Interactions
5.1.2.1 Renal Impairment

Study MP1012 evaluated the PK profile of 6 subjects with normal renal function given a single 5 mg dose of Mepro compared to 6 subjects with mild-to-moderate renal impairment given a single dose of Mepro 5 mg. No clinically important differences in PK profiles were identified based on renal function. The complete study report can be found in Appendix CSR1012.

Based on the results of this study, no dose adjustment is necessary for subjects with mild-to-moderate renal impairment. Patients with severe renal impairment were not studied.

5.1.2.2 Hepatic Impairment

Study MP1011 evaluated the hepatic effects on the PK profile of 6 subjects with normal hepatic function given a single 5-mg dose of Mepro, compared to 6 subjects with mild-to-moderate hepatic impairment given a single dose of Mepro 5 mg. Mean total plasma concentrations were approximately 50% greater in subjects with mild-to-moderate hepatic impairment compared to normal subjects. The complete study report can be found in Appendix CSR1011.

Based on the results of this study, Mepro 5 mg (the lowest recommended dose) is advised for subjects with mild-to moderate hepatic impairment along with routine monitoring. Mepro is not recommended for subjects with severe hepatic impairment.

5.1.3 Drug-Drug Interactions
5.1.3.1 Lithium

Study MP1014 evaluated the PK parameters in 12 subjects given lithium 600 mg alone 3 times daily for 7 days and then concomitantly with Mepro 10 mg for 7 days. Mean steady-state plasma concentration of lithium increased 20% with concomitant Mepro administration. The complete study report can be found in Appendix CSR1014.

Based on these results, patients receiving lithium treatment should be closely monitored when Mepro is introduced and withdrawn.

5.1.3.2 Fluconazole

Study MP1015 was a 3-period crossover drug interaction study in 12 subjects evaluating the PK effects of fluconazole and Mepro after a single dose of fluconazole 150 mg, a single dose of Mepro 10 mg, and a single dose of fluconazole 150 mg given in combination with a single dose of Mepro 10 mg. The results of the study showed a 1.5 times increase in Mepro plasma concentrations and no clinically relevant changes in the PK profile of fluconazole. This was not unexpected and considered to be due to fluconazole's competitive inhibition of Mepro metabolism via the P-450 2C9 pathway. The complete study results can be found in Appendix CSR1015.

Based on the results of this study, the lowest recommended dose (5-mg dose) of Mepro is advised if fluconazole treatment is given concomitantly.

5.1.3.3 Digoxin

Study MP1013 evaluated the PK parameters of 12 subjects given digoxin 0.25 mg once daily for 7 days alone and then given in combination with Mepro 10 mg daily for an additional 7 days. There were no relevant changes in the PK profile of digoxin with concomitant Mepro administration. The full clinical study report can be found in Appendix CSR1013.

5.1.3.4 Warfarin

Study MP1017 evaluated the PK and PD effects (as measured by the international normalized ratio) of 12 subjects given warfarin 5 mg when given alone once daily for 7 days, and then in combination with Mepro 10 mg for 7 days. The PK profile of warfarin was essentially unchanged, and no relevant changes in international normalized ratio values were seen with concomitant Mepro administration. The complete clinical study report can be found in Appendix CSR1017.

5.1.3.5 Methotrexate

Study MP1016 evaluated the PK effects in 12 subjects given a single dose of methotrexate 7.5 mg alone and then in combination with a single dose of Mepro 10 mg. The PK profile of methotrexate was essentially unchanged with concomitant administration of Mepro. The complete clinical study report can be found in Appendix CSR1016.

5.1.4 Effect of Food

Study MP1005 was a single-dose crossover study in 12 subjects evaluating the PK properties of Mepro 5 mg given in the fasting state and when given with food. There were no significant differences in PK parameters with and without food. The complete study report can be found in Appendix CSR1005.

5.1.5 Geographic Regions
5.1.5.1 Population Pharmacokinetics

Of the 300 samples obtained from study MP3001, 178 were from North America and 122 were from Europe. Comparison of plasma levels between geographic regions showed no differences between regions (see Appendix CSR3001).

5.1.5.2 Subgroup Analysis

Appendix AEGEO1.1 and Appendix AEGEO1.2 present a summary of AEs from controlled Phase 2/3 studies from North American sites and European sites, respectively.

In general, the rates of AEs overall and those considered potential adverse drug reactions were lower across all treatment groups in Europe compared to those in North America. The rates of these events were also lower in the placebo group in Europe compared to the rates in the placebo group in North America. The differences in AE rates between placebo, Mepro, and COX were similar regardless of geographic location. This was consistent with the ARR results, which showed no regional differences for the common potential adverse drug reactions.

5.2 Pregnancy and Lactation

5.2.1 Summary of Nonclinical Findings

Relative exposure ratios were used in an attempt to correlate the findings in animals to those in humans by comparing the dose causing a reproductive toxic effect in animals to the therapeutic dose in humans, normalized to the doses causing a response common to both animals and humans. Once calculated, relative drug exposure ratios were classified as follows[12]:

- ≤ 10—increased concern
- > 10 and < 25—no change in concern
- ≥ 25—decreased concern

In Appendix NONCLINOV1.0, complete information on genotoxicity and animal reproductive and developmental studies can be found. The following is a summary of the clinically relevant findings from these nonclinical studies.

5.2.1.1 Mutagenesis, Impairment of Fertility

Mepro was not mutagenic in an Ames test. It was not clastogenic in a chromosome aberration assay in Chinese hamster ovaries or in an in vivo test in mice bone marrow.

Mepro did not impair male and female fertility in rats at oral doses of up to 50 mg/kg/day (relative exposure ratio of approximately 35).

5.2.1.2 Teratogenic Effects

An increased incidence of ventricular septal defect of the heart, a rare event, was seen at Mepro oral doses of > 85 mg/kg/day (relative exposure ratio of approximately 60); and embryo lethality at oral doses of 45 mg/kg/day (relative exposure ratio approximately 30) when rabbits were treated through organogenesis. A dose-dependent increase in skeletal abnormalities including fused ribs and misshapen vertebrae was observed at Mepro oral doses of ≥ 60 mg/kg/day (relative exposure ratio > 40) in rats treated through organogenesis.

5.2.1.3 Nonteratogenic Effects

Mepro caused preimplantation and postimplantation losses and reduced live births and neonatal survival at oral doses of >55 mg/kg/day (relative exposure ratio of approximately >40) when rats were treated through the late gestation and lactation period. These changes were expected with inhibition of prostaglandin synthesis and were not considered the result of permanent alterations of female reproductive function. Nonsteroidal anti-inflammatory drugs as a class are known to induce closure of the ductus arteriosus, but this has not been studied in Mepro clinical trials.[9]

Mepro was also observed to cross the placenta barrier in rats.

5.2.1.4 Labor and Delivery

Mepro produced no evidence of delayed labor or parturition in rats treated with oral doses of up to 42 mg/kg/day (relative exposure ratio of 30).

> **NOTE:** Although delayed labor or parturition in rats was not seen in rats exposed to Mepro, NSAIDs as a class have been shown to cause such delays and as such labeling will typically include the class effects seen.

5.2.1.5 Lactation

Mepro is excreted in the milk of lactating rats at concentrations 1.5 times greater than those found in plasma.

5.2.2 Pregnancy Reports and Outcomes from Clinical Studies

Six patients became pregnant during the clinical development program. Of these 6 pregnancies, 3 occurred in patients randomized to Mepro, 2 received placebo, and 1 received COX. In addition, 2 female partners of male patients participating in clinical trials also became pregnant. One of these male patients received Mepro, and the other received COX. Table AII5-2 provides a listing of these pregnancies.

Brief narratives of these pregnancies follow (complete narratives can be found in Appendix PREGNAR1.1).

Patient 2003-0089 (study MP2003), a 25-year-old Caucasian female, was randomized to Mepro 5 mg and had a positive pregnancy test result at visit 4. She was discontinued from the study after receiving 30 days of treatment. She was taking birth control pills during the study, but inadvertently missed 7 days of her pills without using an alternative birth control method. Her last menstrual period (LMP) was August 11, 2006. Estimated fetal exposure was 18 days. This was her first pregnancy and she elected to have an abortion.

Table AII5-2 Pregnancy Outcomes During Clinical Development

Study No./ Patient No.	Age/Race	Treatment Group/ Drug Exposure	Estimated Fetal Exposure	Outcome
MP2003/ 2003-0089	25/Caucasian	Mepro 5 mg/ 30 days	18 days	Elective abortion
MP2003X/ 2003X-0506	32/Black	Mepro 10 mg/ 270 days	84 days	Normal birth
MP3002/ 3002-0618	31/Caucasian	Mepro 5 mg/ 101 days	28 days	Premature delivery; infant survived, no abnormalities reported
MP3002/ 3002-0061	26/Asian	Placebo/ 70 days	22 days	Normal birth
MP3002/ 3002-0024	36/Black	Placebo/ 80 days	45 days	Stillbirth
MP3003/ 3003-0098	18/Caucasian	COX/ 55 days	28 days	Spontaneous abortion
MP3002/ 3002-0725*	28/Unknown	Mepro 10 mg/ 116 days**	180 days	Normal birth
MP3001/3001-0519*	Unknown/ unknown	COX/ 146 days**	Unknown	Lost to follow-up

* Female partner of male patient.

** Dose and duration of study drug received by male patient.

Source: PREGLIST1.1.

Patient 2003X-0506 (study MP2003X), a 32-year-old Black female, received Mepro 10 mg in study MP2003 and continued receiving Mepro 10 mg in the long-term extension study (study MP2003X) for a total of 270 days of treatment. She was using a diaphragm and a spermicide for birth control protection. She always had irregular periods (her LMP was December 2, 2005), but she decided to take a home pregnancy test after not having a period for 2.5 months. The test was positive and she was instructed to stop study medication immediately. Estimated fetal exposure was 84 days. This was her second pregnancy, which resulted in the birth of a normal term female infant (her first pregnancy resulted in the delivery of a normal term male infant). The baby showed normal growth and development at her 1-month visit to the pediatrician.

Patient 3002-0618 (study MP3002), a 31-year-old Caucasian female, received Mepro 5 mg. Birth control was achieved by her husband's use of a condom and her use of a spermicidal jelly. However, on 1 occasion the condom ruptured and she became pregnant. She was discontinued from the study on study day 101. Her LMP was October 12, 2006. Estimated fetal exposure was 28 days. She went into premature labor at gestational week 34 and delivered a female infant who was normal except for a low birth weight of 2.4 kg (5.25 lbs). Subsequent follow-up 1 month after delivery indicated normal infant weight, length, and development. This was the patient's third pregnancy. Her first pregnancy ended in a spontaneous abortion. She delivered a normal term male during her second pregnancy. Her medical history was noncontributory, and she was taking no concomitant medications other than prenatal vitamins during her pregnancy.

Patient 3002-0061 (study MP3002), a 26-year-old Asian female, was randomized to placebo. After 70 days in the study, she had a positive pregnancy test during her visit 10 evaluation. The pregnancy test was repeated, the second test was also positive, and the patient was discontinued from the study. Her LMP was June 15, 2005, and fetal exposure was estimated to be 22 days. Her birth control method was the use of a diaphragm and spermicidal jelly, but on several occasions she had unprotected sex. She had an uneventful pregnancy and gave birth to a normal male. This was her second pregnancy (her first pregnancy resulted in the birth of another normal term male infant). One month after delivery, the baby was in the 80th percent range for both weight and height. Development was reported to be normal.

Patient 3002-0024 (study MP3002), a 36-year-old Black female, was randomized to the placebo group. She missed her period, and a subsequent pregnancy test revealed she was pregnant. She was discontinued from the trial on study day 80. LMP was February 1, 2005, and estimated fetal exposure was 45 days. Her birth control method was condom/spermicidal jelly, but on 1 occasion about 2 weeks after her last period, leakage from the condom was noted. She had an uneventful pregnancy but delivered a stillborn infant (female) at term. The patient had no history of diabetes, hypertension, use of recreational drugs, or other risk factors, and her only concomitant medication was multivitamins. Gross inspection of the baby, placenta, and umbilical cord revealed no obvious abnormalities. The patient refused an autopsy for the infant. This was the patient's fourth pregnancy. She delivered a normal term female and male after her first and second pregnancies, respectively, and had an elective abortion following her third pregnancy.

Patient 3003-0098 (study MP3003), an 18-year-old Caucasian female randomized to COX, had a positive pregnancy test during her visit 4 evaluation and was discontinued from the study on study day 55. Estimated fetal exposure was 28 days. She had a spontaneous abortion 7 days later. Her birth control methods were use of condoms and spermicidal jelly, but on several occasions she had unprotected sex. This was her first pregnancy. She admitted to smoking 1 marijuana joint around the estimated time of her conception (even though this was not permitted in the study). Otherwise her medical history was unremarkable.

The following are narratives of the female partners of 2 male patients who participated in the clinical development program.

The female partner of Patient 3002-0725 (study MP3002, randomized to Mepro 10 mg) was found to be 2 months pregnant on her partner's study day 116. Her LMP was March 5, 2005. No birth control methods were used 3 months prior to the reported pregnancy. The female partner delivered a normal term male. This was her first pregnancy.

The female partner of Patient 3001-0519 (study MP3001, randomized to COX 25 mg) was reported to have become pregnant while her male partner participated in the study. He was randomized to COX and received treatment for an estimated 146 days. He missed his next scheduled visit and was contacted by the study coordinator. He told the coordinator that his girlfriend was pregnant and he was dropping out of the study and hung up before the study coordinator could get additional information about the pregnancy. All subsequent attempts at contacting the patient were unsuccessful and he was considered lost to follow-up.

➡ **NOTE:** It is important to obtain complete and detailed information on each pregnancy. If a female partner of a study patient becomes pregnant, information of her pregnancy should also be sought to rule out any adverse effects on her partner's reproductive capability. If the drug was marketed in another country(ries), a summary of all relevant postmarketing information on pregnancy, labor and delivery, lactation, and development and growth of the infant should also be included in this section of the IAS.

In view of the known effects of NSAIDs on the fetal cardiovascular system (risk of closure of the ductus arteriosus), use in the last trimester of pregnancy should be avoided. The onset of labor may be delayed and the duration increased with an increased bleeding tendency in both mother and child. Mepro should not be used during the first 2 trimesters of pregnancy or labor unless the potential benefit to the patient outweighs the potential risk to the fetus.[9] The potential risk to the lactating mother and nursing infant cannot be determined at this time.

➡ **NOTE:** Any postmarketing information regarding pregnancy and lactation should be summarized in this section. For drugs that belong to a drug class, class labeling for pregnancy and lactation is typically used.

5.3 Overdose

5.3.1 Overdose Cases From Clinical Trials
Mepro overdose information is limited, with only 2 overdoses reported in clinical trials to date. These cases are briefly described here; full narratives can be found in Appendix ODNAR1.1.

A 64-year-old Black female (Patient 3002-0104, study MP3002) randomized to Mepro 5 mg, on study day 40 accidentally took 3 tablets of study drug (total Mepro dose 15 mg). She wasn't wearing her glasses and mistakenly took her study drug rather than her antihypertensive medication. She called the investigator, who told her to go to the emergency room if she developed any severe gastrointestinal pains or bleeding or any other worrisome symptoms. She was also instructed not to take study medication for the next 2 days. She developed some mild dyspepsia 24 hours later and took 2 teaspoons of Maalox (a mixture of aluminum hydroxide and magnesium hydroxide) that resolved her dyspepsia the same day. She reported no other symptoms, continued on study drug, and completed the study without any other complaints.

A 34-year-old Caucasian male (Patient 3001-0211, study MP3001) randomized to Mepro 10 mg, was found by his girlfriend to be unconscious and lying on the floor of his apartment on study day 18. Next to him was an empty bottle of Ambien (zolpidem) 10 mg. The quantity listed on the bottle was 30 tablets and was filled the same day so it was assumed the patient took all 30 tablets. Empty strips of blister-wrapped study medication that had contained 30 doses of study medication were also found at his side. Paramedics were called and he was taken to the emergency room, where he was found to be unresponsive with a respiratory rate of 6 respirations/minute (normal rate = 12–20 rpm) and tachycardic with a heart rate of 120 beats/min. Blood and urine samples were obtained for a drug screen, complete blood count, electrolytes, liver function tests, glucose, BUN, and creatinine. An IV was started, and he was given Narcan (naloxone) in case he also overdosed on narcotics. He was intubated and put on a respirator, and a nasogastric tube was placed. His stomach was lavaged until his stomach contents were clear. He was then given activated charcoal via the nasogastric tube. A rectal exam revealed no blood in his stool. The patient's girlfriend informed the emergency room staff that the patient was recently fired from his job and he was very depressed. The last time she saw or spoke to him was 8 hours before calling the paramedics. The patient was admitted to the intensive care unit for treatment and observation. Within 24 hours, the patient was awake and able to breathe on his own, and he was taken off the respirator. ALT values (200 U/L—normal range 5–40 U/L) and AST values (220 U/L—normal range 5–35 U/L) were transiently elevated but normalized within 48 hours. Bilirubin values remained within normal limits. Two days after admission to the intensive care unit, he was medically stable, was transferred to the psychiatric ward, and put on suicide precautions. He told the staff he had taken 30 tablets of zolpidem and 12 tablets of study medication (120 mg Mepro) before losing consciousness. The patient was treated for his depression with Prozac (fluoxetine) and received psychiatric counseling. He was discharged from the hospital 2 weeks later, fully recovered from the effects of his overdose. His last dose of study medication was on day 18. The investigator did not consider the patient's depression to be due to Mepro.

> ➡ **NOTE:** If the drug is marketed in another country(ies), all postmarketing cases of overdose/misuse should be summarized in this section.

5.3.2 Management of Overdose

No specific information is available regarding the treatment of Mepro overdose, and there is no known antidote. In cases of overdose, routine supportive and symptomatic care is recommended. Gastric lavage, administration of activated charcoal, and use of an osmotic cathartic may be indicated depending on the time and extent of the overdose, but this has not been prospectively studied. Forced diuresis, alkalinization of urine, hemodialysis, or hemoperfusion may not be useful due to Mepro's high protein binding.

5.4 Drug Abuse

5.4.1 Nonclinical Data

In nonclinical studies, there was no evidence that Mepro had any effect on mood or was a central nervous system stimulant/depressant. In a rat study (nonclinical study M2012), Mepro administration did not show any increased sensitivity to the rewarding effects of electrical stimulation of the ventral segmental area of the brain, this was in contrast to the administration of amphetamine and cocaine, which showed significantly increased sensitivity for both drugs (see Appendix NONCLINOV1.0).

5.4.2 Clinical Data

No signal for drug abuse was identified in nonclinical studies; therefore no specific clinical abuse studies were performed. Nevertheless, adverse events often associated with potential abuse from controlled Phase 2/3 studies were reviewed, and a summary of these events is shown in Table AII5-3.

Table AII5-3 **Summary of Potential Abuse Adverse Events—Controlled Phase 2/3 Studies**

Adverse Event Preferred Term	Placebo N = 2200	M ≤ 5 mg N = 2450	M = 10 mg N = 2400	M = 15 mg N = 325	Total M N = 5175	COX N = 2225
Any potential abuse AE	517 (23.5%)	600 (24.5%)	519 (21.6%)	69 (21.1%)	1188 (23.0%)	521 (23.4%)
Somnolence	80 (3.6%)	136 (5.6%)	75 (3.1%)	13 (4.0%)	224 (4.3%)	68 (3.1%)
Sedation	98 (4.5%)	118 (4.8%)	87 (3.6%)	13 (4.0%)	218 (4.2%)	114 (5.1%)
Dizziness	339 (15.4%)	358 (14.6%)	362 (15.1%)	43 (13.2%)	763 (14.7%)	334 (15.0%)
Hallucination	1 (< 0.1%)	0	1 (< 0.1%)	0	1 (< 0.1)%	0
Disturbance in attention	0	0	0	0	0	0
Confusional state	0	0	0	0	0	0
Feeling abnormal	4 (0.2%)	3 (0.1%)	0	0	3 (0.1%)	3 (0.1%)
Disorientation	0	0	0	0	0	0
Memory impairment	1 (< 0.1%)	1 (< 0.1%)	1 (< 0.1%)	0	2 (< 0.1%)	1 (< 0.1%)
Psychomotor hyperactivity	0	0	0	0	0	0
Mood altered	0	0	0	0	0	0
Mania	0	0	1 (< 1%)	0	1	0
Delusion of grandeur	1 (< 0.1%)	0	0	0	0	0
Feeling drunk	0	0	0	0	0	0
Feeling jittery	0	0	1 (< 0.1%)	0	1 (< 0.1%)	0
Daydreaming	0	0	0	0	0	0
Euphoric mood	0	0	0	0	0	0
Elevated mood	0	0	0	0	0	1 (< 0.1%)
Mood swings	1 (< 0.1%)	0	0	0	0	0
Inappropriate affect	0	0	0	0	0	1 (< 0.1%)

M = Mepro.
Source: Appendix Table AE3.1.

Other than dizziness, somnolence, and sedation, few other events were reported. The rate of potential drug abuse AEs was similar across treatment groups. The 1 case of mania (Patient 2003X-0601, study MP2003X) in a patient treated with Mepro 10 mg did not appear to be due to drug abuse. This case is summarized in Section 2.5.

All overdoses were also reviewed to see if any of these were potentially due to drug abuse, and no cases were identified (see Section 5.3.1).

No cases of drug abuse were reported in any Phase 2/3 studies or Phase 1 studies.

> **NOTE:** The selection of AEs shown in Table AII5-3 is arbitrary, based on clinical judgment, and can vary from company to company. This should not be a concern. As long as it is clear what terms were selected, reviewers can determine for themselves what terms to include, exclude, or add for their own analysis. If the drug is marketed, any postmarketing cases of drug abuse should be summarized in this section.

5.5 Withdrawal and Rebound

5.5.1 Clinical Studies

The *residual effect* of Mepro is estimated to be approximately 7 days. The residual effect is defined as the period when Mepro levels are still detectable. This estimate is based on the elimination of the drug. Based on the 7-day residual effect period of Mepro, the posttreatment period was defined as > 7 days after the last Mepro dose.

AEs that occurred > 7 days after the last Mepro dose or worsened in severity > 7 days after the last dose of Mepro were analyzed.

> **NOTE:** In Section 1.2.2, a treatment-emergent AE was defined as (1) an AE that occurred during the treatment period or the period of residual effect of the drug; or (2) an AE present at baseline that worsened in intensity during the treatment period or period of residual effect. For drugs that are cleared quickly, the time of residual effect should be negligible and close to the time

of the last dose. In such cases, the period of residual effect is not important in the determination of treatment-emergent AEs, and the posttreatment period is defined as the period after the last dose of study medication. For drugs that are cleared slowly and have persistent and relevant drug levels, the period of residual effect becomes an important consideration in the determination of treatment-emergent AEs and in defining the posttreatment period. In evaluating the potential for withdrawal/rebound, it is found that a drug with a long residual effect, has a lower potential for withdrawal/rebound effects, whereas a drug with a short residual effect has a greater potential for rebound/withdrawal effects.

All SAEs reported up to 30 days after the last dose were also reviewed.

Appendix tables PTAE1.1, PTAE1.2, and PTAE1.3 summarize the posttreatment AEs that occurred > 7 days after the last dose of study medication for controlled Phase 2/3 studies, all Phase 2/3 studies, and Phase 1 studies, respectively. The intensity of posttreatment AEs can be found in Appendix PTAE2.1, PTAE2.2, and PTAE2.3 for controlled Phase 2/3 studies, all Phase 2/3 studies, and Phase 1 studies, respectively.

Table AII5-4 is a summary of those posttreatment AEs with a rate of ≥ 1% (in the total Mepro group) for controlled Phase 2/3 studies. Posttreatment AE information was available for 80.1%, 85.0%, and 85.9% of placebo, Mepro, and COX patients, respectively.

The Mepro and COX treatment groups showed a higher rate of pain-related (including headache) and arthritis-related (including arthralgias) AEs posttreatment compared to placebo. In the Mepro group, the rates of these events appeared to be dose related. These findings were not unexpected because both Mepro and COX are effective in the treatment of arthritis and also in the control of pain. Therefore, increases in these types of events are expected when effective treatment is stopped. Furthermore, these events were not considered to be withdrawal or rebound events because these events were either mild or moderate in intensity and none were serious. No SAEs or deaths considered to be due to withdrawal/rebound were reported during the posttreatment period.

Table AII5-4 Posttreatment Adverse Events With a Rate of ≥ 1% (in the Total Mepro Group) That Occurred > 7 Days after the Last Mepro Dose—Controlled Phase 2/3 Studies

AE Preferred Term	Placebo N = 1763	M ≤ 5 mg N = 2124	M = 10 mg N = 1998	M = 15 mg N = 276	Total M N = 4398	COX N = 1911
Any posttreatment AE	389 (22.1%)	658 (31.0%)	829 (41.5%)	116 (42.0%)	1603 (36.4%)	764 (40.0%)
Headache	92 (5.2%)	168 (7.9%)	182 (9.1%)	26 (9.4%)	376 (8.5%)	136 (7.1%)
Arthralgias	71 (4.0%)	176 (8.3%)	174 (8.7%)	25 (9.1%)	375 (8.5%)	140 (7.3%)
Pain	37 (2.1%)	100 (4.7%)	116 (5.8%)	19 (6.9%)	235 (5.3%)	96 (5.0%)
Arthritis	21 (1.2%)	70 (3.3%)	102 (5.1%)	16 (5.8%)	188 (4.3%)	71 (3.7%)
Dizziness	35 (2.0%)	45 (2.1%)	38 (1.9%)	5 (1.8%)	88 (2.0%)	38 (2.0%)
Insomnia	23 (1.3%)	26 (1.2%)	18 (0.9%)	3 (1.1%)	47 (1.1%)	19 (1.0%)
Nasopharyngitis	19 (1.1%)	19 (0.9%)	20 (1.0%)	3 (1.1%)	42 (1.0%)	17 (0.9%)

M = Mepro.
Source: Appendix Table PTAE1.1.

The safety database was also searched for any term included in the MedDRA SMQ *Drug withdrawal*, and no AE term included in this SMQ was found.

➡ **NOTE:** If the drug is marketed, any relevant postmarketing withdrawal or rebound information should be summarized in this section.

5.6 Effects on Ability to Drive or Operate Machinery or Impairment of Mental Ability

5.6.1 Nonclinical Studies
No relevant adverse central nervous system, coordination, or eye effects were observed in nonclinical studies (see Appendix NONCLINOV1.0).

5.6.2 Clinical Studies
In determining the potential risk of Mepro on driving, operating machinery, or impairment of mental activity, 4 main areas were evaluated: (1) central nervous system effects and mental impairment, (2) coordination abnormalities, (3) visual disturbances, and (4) accident-related events.

Search criteria included the following terms from controlled Phase 2/3 studies:

- For mental impairment, the MedDRA HLTs *Confusion and disorientation, Disturbances in consciousness NEC, Memory loss (excl dementia),* and *Mental impairment (excl dementia and memory loss).*

- For coordination-related events, the MedDRA HLT *Cerebellar coordination and balance disturbances* and *Vertigos NEC.*

- For visual impairment events, the MedDRA HLGT *Vision disorders.*

- For accident-related events, the MedDRA PTs *Accident, Accident at work, Accident at home, Road-traffic accident,* and *Fall.*

If the same PT term was reported more than once, or more than one PT was reported in an HLT or HLGT, the subject was counted only once for that PT, HLT, or HLGT.

The results of the analysis can be found in Appendix DRIVE1.1 and are summarized in Table AII5-5.

There were no differences seen across treatment groups. Only 1 SAE considered treatment related occurred. This was a case of memory loss reported in a placebo patient (Patient 3002-1901 from study MP3002), which is discussed in Section 2.5.

5.7 Summary of Safety in Special Groups and Situations

Higher Mepro plasma levels were found in females versus males, in subjects with mild-to-moderate hepatic impairment, and in subjects who received Mepro and concomitant administration of fluconazole. Both the rates and attributable risk ratios of common potential adverse reactions were greater in females than males in both the Mepro and COX groups compared to placebo with the exception of PUBs. Females exposed to Mepro were expected to be

Table AII5-5 Summary of Adverse Events Associated with Mental Impairment, Coordination, Visual Disturbance, and Accidental Injuries—Controlled Phase 2/3 Studies

	Placebo N = 220	M ≤ 5mg N = 2450	M = 10mg N = 2400	M = 15mg N = 325	Total M N = 5175	COX N = 2225
Confusion and disorientation (HLT)	2 (0.1%)	1 (< 0.1%)	1 (< 0.1%)	1 (0.3%)	3 (0.1%)	2 (0.1%)
Disturbances in consciousness NEC (HLT)	11 (0.5%)	15 (0.6%)	12 (0.5%)	1 (0.3%)	28 (0.5%)	9 (0.4%)
Memory loss (excl dementia) (HLT)	15 (0.7%)	15 (0.6%)	19 (0.8%)	2 (0.6%)	36 (0.7%)	13 (0.6%)
Mental impairment (excl dementia and memory loss) (HLT)	7 (0.3%)	7 (0.3%)	5 (0.2%)	1 (0.3%)	13 (0.3%)	9 (0.4%)
Cerebellar coordination and balance disturbances (HLT)	2 (0.1%)	5 (0.2%)	2 (0.1%)	0	7 (0.1%)	4 (0.2%)
Vertigos NEC (HLT)	2 (0.1%)	3 (0.1%)	2 (0.1%)	0	5 (0.1%)	3 (0.1%)
Vision disorders (HLGT)	20 (0.9%)	29 (1.2%)	19 (0.8%)	2 (0.6%)	50 (1.0%)	24 (1.1%)
Accident (PT)	4 (0.2%)	5 (0.2%)	7 (0.3%)	0	12 (0.2%)	7 (0.3%)
Accident at home (PT)	0	0	0	0	0	0
Accident at work (PT)	0	0	0	1 (0.3%)	1 (< 0.1%)	1 (< 0.1%)
Road traffic accident (PT)	2 (0.1%)	0	1 (< 0.1%)	1 (0.3%)	2 (< 0.1%)	0
Fall (PT)	9 (0.4%)	5 (0.2%)	5 (0.2%)	2 (0.6%)	12 (0.2%)	9 (0.4%)

M = Mepro.

Source: Appendix Table DRIVE1.1.

at greater risk for PUBs than males due to the higher plasma levels seen in females receiving the same dose as males. Also in a subgroup analysis for age, the rate and attributable risk for PUBs showed no relevant differences between the elderly and nonelderly subjects treated with Mepro. There are insufficient data at this time to determine if the risk for PUBs in females and the elderly is any different with Mepro use compared to other NSAIDs. No differences in the risk profile or attributable risk ratios for the common potential adverse drug reactions were seen between Caucasians and Blacks; there were too few other races to determine if the risk profile of these events differed in other racial groups. Caucasians appear to have an increased risk of developing photosensitivity reactions, but more data are required to better characterize this finding. One case of SJS was reported in an Asian female who tested positive for the B*1502 allele of HLA-B, a gene associated with an increased risk for Stevens-Johnson syndrome in subjects exposed to phenytoin and carbamazepine. The case was further confounded by the concomitant use of penicillin, a drug associated with the development of SJS. However, based on the available case information, attribution to Mepro cannot be entirely ruled out. No regional differences in the rates and attributable risk ratios were seen for the common potential adverse drug reactions in North Americans compared to Europeans.

The lowest recommended dose of 5 mg is recommended for initiating treatment for females, for patients with mild-to-moderate hepatic impairment, and for patients taking fluconazole.

Lithium levels were increased with concomitant administration of Mepro. Patients taking lithium should be closely monitored when Mepro is introduced or withdrawn. There was no observable change in the PK profile of patients receiving methotrexate, digoxin, or warfarin, and the international normalized ratio showed no clinically relevant change with concomitant administration of Mepro and warfarin. Mepro's PK profile was unchanged whether the drug was given with or without food.

Mepro was not mutagenic or clastogenic. Three females exposed to Mepro and 1 female partner of a male exposed to Mepro became pregnant. No adverse pregnancy outcomes considered related to Mepro were identified. However, the small number of pregnancies and the short duration of fetal exposure to drug preclude an assessment of pregnancy risk to humans exposed to Mepro at this time.

In view of the known effects of NSAIDs on the fetal cardiovascular system (risk of closure of the ductus arteriosus), use in the last trimester of pregnancy should be avoided. The onset of labor may be delayed and the duration increased with an increased bleeding tendency in both mother and child. Mepro should not be used during the first 2 trimesters of pregnancy or labor unless the potential benefit to the patient outweighs the potential risk to the fetus.

In rat breast milk, Mepro drug concentration was 1.5 times greater than in plasma. There is no clinical information regarding Mepro's effect on lactation or whether the drug is excreted in human milk. For this reason, potential risk to the lactating mother and nursing infant cannot be determined at this time.

There were only 2 cases of overdose reported. In 1 overdose, 1.5 times the maximum recommended 10 mg Mepro dose was taken; in the second, 12 times the maximum recommend dose was ingested. Both patients fully recovered with no adverse residual effects reported in either case. The information on Mepro overdose and its treatment remains limited at this time.

Based on nonclinical and clinical data, the potential for Mepro abuse is low. No withdrawal or rebound effects were observed when Mepro treatment was stopped.

Mepro showed no adverse effects on mental ability, coordination, or vision; therefore the ability to drive or operate machinery should not be impaired.

■ 6 Postmarketing Data

The drug is not marketed in any country, therefore there are no postmarketing data.

> ➡ **NOTE:** If the drug is marketed, this section should summarize any relevant safety information reported after marketing including serious adverse reaction report, any potentially serious drug interactions, and any findings in subgroups. An estimate of exposure and the methodology used in the calculation of exposure are also required.[1]

> ➡ **NOTE:** This concludes the IAS. Once completed, the information from the IAS is used for the registration dossier's, benefit-risk section,[1,2] the overview of safety,[1] the risk management plan/the risk evaluation and management strategy (REMS),[13,14] the company core data sheet (CCDS)/the company core safety information (CCSI),[15] and prescribing information (e.g., package insert, (PI) and summary of product characteristics (SmPC)).[16,17] The key risks and key aspects of the risk management plan for Mepro are summarized in Appendix I; and the CCSI for Mepro is provided in Appendix III.

References

1. International Conference on Harmonisation of Technical Requirements for Registration of Pharmaceuticals for Human Use. *The Common Technical Document for the Registration of Pharmaceuticals For Human Use—Efficacy—M4E (R1). Clinical Overview and Clinical Summary of Module 2 Module 5: Clinical Study Reports.* Geneva, Switzerland: ICH Secretariat; September 2002. http://www.ich.org/cache/compo/276-254-1.html. Accessed May 4, 2010.

2. Center for Drug Evaluation and Research, Food and Drug Administration, Department of Health and Human Services. *Guideline for the Format and Content of the Clinical and Statistical Sections of an Application.* July 1988. http://www.fda.gov/downloads/Drugs/GuidanceComplianceRegulatory Information/Guidances/UCM071665.pdf. Accessed May 4, 2010.

3. *Guidance for Industry—Drug-Induced Liver Injury: Premarketing Clinical Evaluation.* Washington, DC: US Department of Health and Human Services, Food and Drug Administration, Center for Drug Evaluation and Research (CDER), Center for Biologics Evaluation and Research (CBER). July 2009. http://www.fda.gov/downloads/Drugs/GuidanceCompliance RegulatoryInformation/Guidances/UCM174090.pdf. Accessed May 4, 2010.

4. *Supplementary Suggestions for Preparing an Integrated Summary of Safety Information in an Original NDA Submission and for Organizing Information in Periodic Safety Updates (Leber guidelines)*. Rockville, MD: US Food and Drug Administration; 1987.

5. The Consensus Committee of the American Autonomic Society and the American Academy of Neurology. Consensus statement on the definition of orthostatic hypotension, pure autonomic failure, and multiple system atrophy. *Neurology*. 1996;46:1470.

6. International Conference on Harmonisation of Technical Requirements for Registration of Pharmaceuticals for Human Use. *Clinical Evaluation of QT/QTc Interval Prolongation and Proarrhythmic Potential for Non-Antiarrhythmic Drugs E14*. Geneva, Switzerland:ICH Secretariat; May 2005. http://www.ich.org/cache/compo/276-254-1.html. Accessed May 4, 2010.

7. Center for Drug Evaluation and Research, Food and Drug Administration, Department of Health and Human Services. *Guideline for Conducting a Clinical Safety Review of a New Product Application and Preparing a Report on the Review*. February 2005. http://www.fda.gov/downloads/Drugs/Guidance ComplianceRegulatoryInformation/Guidances/ucm 072974.pdf. Accessed May 4, 2010.

8. International Conference on Harmonisation of Technical Requirements for Registration of Pharmaceuticals for Human Use. *The Extent of Population Exposure to Access Clinical Safety for Drugs Intended for Long-Term Treatment of Non-life-threatening Conditions E1*. Geneva, Switzerland: ICH Secretariat; October 1994. http://www.ich.org/cache/compo/276-254-1.html. Accessed May 4, 2010.

9. Proposed NSAID package insert labeling template1. http://www.fda.gov/downloads/Drugs/DrugSafety/download/ucm106230.pdf. Accessed May 4, 2010.

10. Locharernkul C, Loplumlert J, Limotai C, et al. Carbamazepine and phenytoin induced Stevens-Johnson syndrome is associated with HLA-B*1502 allele in Thai population. *Epilepsia*. 2008; 49:2087–2091.

11. International Conference on Harmonisation of Technical Requirements for Registration of Pharmaceuticals for Human Use. The *Nonclinical Evaluation of the Potential for Delayed Ventricular Repolarization (QT Interval Prolongation) by Human Pharmaceuticals S7B*. Geneva, Switzerland: ICH Secretariat; May 2005. http://www.ich.org/cache/compo/276-254-1.html. Accessed May 4, 2010.

12. Center for Drug Evaluation and Research, Food and Drug Administration, Department of Health and Human Services. *Draft Guidance: Reviewer Guidance Integration of Study Results to Assess Concerns About Human Reproductive and Developmental Toxicities*. October 2001. http://www.fda.gov/downloads/GuidanceComplia nceRegulatoryInformation/Guidances/UCM07924 0.pdf. Accessed May 4, 2010.

13. *Volume 9A of the Rules Governing Medicinal Products in the European Union—Guidelines on Pharmacovigilance for Medicinal Products for Human Use*. Vol. 9A. September 2008. http://ec.europa.eu/enterprise/sectors/pharmaceuticals/documents/eudr alex/index_en.htm. Accessed May 4, 2010.

14. *The Food and Drug Administration Amendments Act*. Public Law 110-85, September 27, 2007. http://frwebgate.access.gpo.gov/cgi-bin/getdoc. cgi?dbname=110_cong_public_laws&docid=f: publ085.110. Accessed May 4, 2010.

15. International Conference on Harmonisation of Technical Requirements for Registration of Pharmaceuticals for Human Use. *Clinical Safety Data Management: Periodic Safety Update Reports for Marketed Drugs E2C(R1)*. Geneva, Switzerland: ICH Secretariat; November 2005. http://www.ich.org/cache/compo/276-254-1.html. Accessed May 4, 2010.

16. Code of Federal Regulations. PART 201—LABELING, Subpart B–Labeling Requirements for Prescription Drugs and/or Insulin, Sec. 201.57 Specific requirements on content and format of labeling for human prescription drug and biological products described in 201.56 (b)(1). April 2009. http://www.accessdata.fda.gov/scripts/cdrh/cfdocs/cfcfr/CFRSearch.cfm?fr=201.57. Accessed May 4, 2010.

17. A Guideline on the Summary of Product Characteristics. September 2009. http://ec.europa.eu/enterprise/sectors/pharmaceuticals/documents/eudralex/vol-2/index_en.htm. Accessed May 4, 2010.

III

Company Core Safety Information for MEPRO (Meproamine Dihydroacetate)

→ **NOTE:** This is the initial company's core safety information (CCSI) for MEPRO and includes nonclinical and clinical study results as well as class effects of nonsteroidal anti-inflammatory drugs. Once marketed, the CCSI is expected to change based on new safety information gained from postmarketing experience. The format of the CCSI was based in part on the European Union's *A Guideline on the Summary of Product Characteristics* (SPC or SmPC), and class labelling from the FDA's template for nonsteroidal anti-inflammatory drugs.[1,2] The CCSI is prepared by the company, and should not be confused with prescription information/product labelling (also referred to as the summary of product characteristics, the data sheet, or package insert). Prescription information/product labelling requires approval by the regulatory authorities in each country. The CCSI is required for the preparation of the Periodic Safety Update Report for Marketed Products (PSUR). The CCSI is used to determine which events are listed or unlisted. Listed events are those whose nature, severity, specificity, and outcome are consistent with the information in the CCSI. Unlisted events are those whose nature, severity, specificity, and outcome are inconsistent with the information in the CCSI.[3,4] The approved prescription information/product labelling for each country may be different in format and content, and is the reference document used to determine whether an adverse event is expected or not expected in a specific country. It is in the language of the country, whereas the CCSI is almost always in English.

1 Name of the Medicinal Product

MEPRO 5 mg

MEPRO 10 mg

2 Qualitative and Quantitative Composition

meproamine dihydroacetate; 5 mg/tablet

meproamine dihydroacetate; 10 mg/tablet

3 Pharmaceutical Form

For oral administration:

5 mg—Mauve film-coated tablets engraved "MEPRO 5" around 1 face and having a score line on the reverse.

10 mg—Robin blue film-coated tablet engraved "MEPRO 10" around 1 face and having a score line on the reverse.

4 Clinical Particulars

4.1 Therapeutic Indications

MEPRO tablets are indicated for the relief of the signs and symptoms of rheumatoid arthritis.

4.2 Posology and Method of Administration

For oral administration:

A MEPRO 5-mg or 10-mg tablet is administered according to a once-daily regimen in the morning.

4.2.1 Dosage

Adults: The recommended dosage of MEPRO is 5 mg or 10 mg daily in a single morning dose. Undesirable effects may be minimized by using the lowest effective dose necessary to control symptoms.

4.2.2 Special Populations
4.2.2.1 Elderly

The elderly are at increased risk of serious consequences or adverse reactions. If use of MEPRO is considered necessary, start treatment with 5 mg once daily. The patient should be monitored regularly for gastrointestinal (GI) perforations, ulcers, and bleeds (PUBs) during nonsteroidal anti-inflammatory drug (NSAID) therapy.

4.2.2.2 Females

Females showed approximately 50% higher C_{max} values compared to males given a single dose of MEPRO 5 mg. MEPRO should be introduced to females using the lowest effective dose.

4.2.2.3 Children and Adolescents

The safety and efficacy of MEPRO have not been adequately evaluated in individuals < 18 years old.

4.2.2.4 Persons With Hepatic Impairment

MEPRO metabolism is reduced in the presence of mild-to-moderate hepatic impairment. Patients with mild-to-moderate hepatic impairment should receive the 5-mg dose and be monitored routinely. Patients with severe hepatic impairment were not studied.

4.2.2.5 Persons With Renal Impairment

No difference in the PK profile of subjects with normal and mild-to-moderate renal impairment was observed, and no dose adjustment is necessary. Patients with severe renal impairment were not studied.

4.3 Contraindications

MEPRO is contraindicated in patients with known hypersensitivity to meproamine dihydroacetate.

MEPRO should not be given to patients who have experienced asthma, urticaria, or allergic-type reactions after taking aspirin or other NSAIDs. Severe, rarely fatal, anaphylactic-like reactions to NSAIDs have been reported in such patients.

MEPRO is contraindicated for the treatment of perioperative pain in the setting of coronary artery bypass graft surgery.

4.4 Special Warnings and Special Precautions for Use

4.4.1 Cardiovascular Effects

Clinical trials of several cyclooxygenase-2 (COX-2) selective and nonselective NSAIDs of up to 3 years' duration have shown an increased risk of serious cardiovascular (CV) thrombotic events, myocardial infarction, and stroke, which can be fatal. All NSAIDs, both COX-2 selective and nonselective, may have a similar risk. Patients with known CV disease or risk factors for CV disease may be at greater risk. To minimize the potential risk for an adverse CV event in patients treated with an NSAID, the lowest effective dose should be used for the shortest duration possible. Physicians and patients should remain alert for the development of such events, even in the absence of previous CV symptoms. Patients should be informed about the signs and/or symptoms of serious CV events and the steps to take if they occur.

There is no consistent evidence that concurrent use of aspirin mitigates the increased risk of serious CV thrombotic events associated with NSAID use. The concurrent use of aspirin and an NSAID does increase the risk of serious GI events.

Two large, controlled, clinical trials of a COX-2 selective NSAID for the treatment of pain in the first 10–14 days following coronary artery bypass graft surgery found an increased incidence of myocardial infarction and stroke.

4.4.2 Hypertension

NSAIDs, including MEPRO, can lead to onset of new hypertension or worsening of preexisting hypertension, either of which may contribute to the increased incidence of CV events. Patients taking thiazides or loop diuretics may have impaired response to these therapies when taking NSAIDs. NSAIDs, including MEPRO, should be used with caution in patients with hypertension. Blood pressure (BP) should be monitored closely during the initiation of NSAID treatment and throughout the course of therapy.

4.4.3 Congestive Heart Failure and Edema

Fluid retention and edema have been observed in some patients taking NSAIDs. MEPRO should be used with caution in patients with fluid retention or heart failure.

4.4.4 Gastrointestinal Effects—Risk of Ulceration, Bleeding, and Perforation

NSAIDs, including MEPRO, can cause serious GI adverse events including inflammation, bleeding, ulceration, and perforation of the stomach, small intestine, or large intestine, which can be fatal. These serious adverse events can occur at any time, with or without warning symptoms, in patients treated with NSAIDs. Only 1 in 5 patients who develop a serious upper GI adverse event on NSAID therapy is symptomatic. Upper GI ulcers, gross bleeding, or perforation caused by NSAIDs occur in approximately 1% of patients treated for 3–6 months, and in about 2–4% of patients treated for 1 year. These trends continue with longer duration of use, increasing the likelihood of developing a serious GI event at some time during the course of therapy. However, even short-term therapy is not without risk.

NSAIDs should be prescribed with extreme caution in those with a prior history of ulcer disease or GI bleeding. Patients with a *prior history of peptic ulcer disease and/or GI bleeding* who use NSAIDs have a greater than tenfold increased risk for developing a GI bleed compared to patients with neither of these risk factors. Other factors that increase the risk for GI bleeding in patients treated with NSAIDs include concomitant use of oral corticosteroids or anticoagulants, longer duration of NSAID therapy, smoking, use of alcohol, older age, and poor general health status. Most spontaneous reports of fatal GI events are in elderly or debilitated patients and, therefore, special care should be taken in treating this population.

To minimize the potential risk for an adverse GI event in patients treated with an NSAID, the lowest effective dose should be used for the shortest possible duration. Patients and physicians should remain alert for signs and symptoms of GI ulceration and bleeding during NSAID therapy and promptly initiate additional evaluation and treatment if a serious GI adverse event is suspected. This should include discontinuation of the NSAID until a serious GI adverse event is ruled out. For high-risk patients, alternate therapies that do not involve NSAIDs should be considered.

4.4.5 Renal Effects

Long-term administration of NSAIDs has resulted in renal papillary necrosis and other renal injury. Renal toxicity has also been seen in patients in whom renal prostaglandins have a compensatory role in the maintenance of renal perfusion. In these patients, administration of an NSAID may cause a dose-dependent reduction in prostaglandin formation and, secondarily, in renal blood flow, which may precipitate overt renal decompensation. Patients at greatest risk of this reaction are those with impaired renal function, heart failure, liver dysfunction, those taking diuretics and ACE inhibitors, and the elderly. Discontinuation of NSAID therapy is usually followed by recovery to the pretreatment state.

4.4.6 Advanced Renal Disease

No information is available from controlled clinical studies regarding the use of MEPRO in patients with advanced renal disease. Therefore, treatment with MEPRO is not recommended in those patients with advanced renal disease. If MEPRO therapy must be initiated, close monitoring of the patient's renal function is advisable.

4.4.7 Anaphylactoid Reactions

As with other NSAIDs, anaphylactoid reactions may occur in patients without known prior exposure to MEPRO. MEPRO should not be given to patients with the aspirin triad. This symptom complex typically occurs in asthmatic patients who experience rhinitis with or without nasal polyps or who exhibit severe, potentially fatal bronchospasm after taking aspirin or other NSAIDs. Emergency help should be sought in cases where an anaphylactoid reaction occurs.

4.4.8 Skin Reactions

NSAIDs, including MEPRO, can cause serious skin adverse events such as exfoliative dermatitis, Stevens-Johnson Syndrome (SJS), and toxic epidermal necrolysis, which can be fatal. These serious events may occur without warning. Patients should be informed about the signs and symptoms of serious skin manifestations, and use of the drug should be discontinued at the first appearance of rash or any other sign of hypersensitivity.

4.4.9 Precautions
4.4.9.1 General

MEPRO cannot be expected to substitute for corticosteroids or to treat corticosteroid insufficiency. Abrupt discontinuation of corticosteroids may lead to disease exacerbation. Patients on prolonged corticosteroid therapy should have their therapy tapered slowly if a decision is made to discontinue corticosteroids.

The pharmacological activity of MEPRO in reducing fever and inflammation may diminish the utility of these diagnostic signs in detecting complications of presumed noninfectious, painful conditions.

4.4.9.2 Hepatic Effects

Borderline elevations of one or more liver tests may occur in up to 15% of patients taking NSAIDs, including MEPRO. These laboratory abnormalities may progress, may remain unchanged, or may be transient with continuing therapy. Notable elevations of ALT or AST (approximately three or more times the upper limit of normal) have been reported in approximately 1% of patients in clinical trials with NSAIDs. In addition, rare cases of severe hepatic reactions, including jaundice and fatal fulminant hepatitis, liver necrosis, and hepatic failure, some of them with fatal outcomes, have been reported.

A patient with symptoms and/or signs suggesting liver dysfunction, or in whom an abnormal liver test has occurred, should be evaluated for evidence of the development of a more severe hepatic reaction while on therapy with MEPRO. If clinical signs and symptoms consistent with liver disease develop, or if systemic manifestations occur (e.g., eosinophilia, rash, etc.), MEPRO should be discontinued.

4.4.9.3 Hematological Effects

Anemia is sometimes seen in patients receiving NSAIDs, including MEPRO. This may be due to fluid retention, occult or gross GI blood loss, or an incompletely described effect upon erythropoiesis. Patients on long-term treatment with NSAIDs, including MEPRO, should have their hemoglobin or hematocrit checked if they exhibit any signs or symptoms of anemia.

NSAIDs inhibit platelet aggregation and have been shown to prolong bleeding time in some patients. Unlike aspirin, their effect on platelet function is quantitatively less, of shorter duration, and reversible. Patients receiving MEPRO who may be adversely affected by alterations in platelet function, such as those with coagulation disorders or patients receiving anticoagulants, should be carefully monitored.

4.4.9.4 Preexisting Asthma

Patients with asthma may have aspirin-sensitive asthma. The use of aspirin in patients with aspirin-sensitive asthma has been associated with severe bronchospasm, which can be fatal. Since cross reactivity, including bronchospasm, between aspirin and other nonsteroidal anti-inflammatory drugs has been reported in such aspirin-sensitive patients, MEPRO should not be administered to patients with this form of aspirin sensitivity and should be used with caution in patients with preexisting asthma.

4.5 Interaction With Other Medications and Other Medicinal Products and Other Forms of Interaction

4.5.1 ACE Inhibitors

Reports suggest that NSAIDs may diminish the antihypertensive effect of ACE inhibitors. This interaction should be given consideration in patients taking NSAIDs concomitantly with ACE inhibitors.

4.5.2 Aspirin

As with other NSAIDs, concomitant administration of meproamine dihydroacetate and aspirin is not generally recommended because of the potential of increased adverse effects.

4.5.3 Furosemide

Clinical studies, as well as postmarketing observations, have shown that NSAIDs can reduce the natriuretic effect of furosemide and thiazides in some patients. This response has been attributed to inhibition of renal prostaglandin synthesis. During concomitant therapy with NSAIDs, the patient should be observed closely for signs of renal failure, as well as to ensure diuretic efficacy.

4.5.4 Lithium

NSAIDs have produced an elevation of plasma lithium levels and a reduction in renal lithium clearance. Mean steady-state plasma concentration of lithium increased 20% with concomitant MEPRO administration. These effects have been attributed to inhibition of renal prostaglandin synthesis by the NSAID. Thus, when NSAIDs and lithium are administered concurrently, subjects should be observed carefully for signs of lithium toxicity.

4.5.5 Methotrexate

The PK effects of methotrexate were evaluated in 12 subjects given a single dose of methotrexate 7.5 mg alone and then given in combination with a single dose of MEPRO 10 mg. The PK profile of methotrexate was essentially unchanged with concomitant administration of MEPRO. NSAIDs have been reported to competitively inhibit methotrexate accumulation in rabbit kidney slices. This may indicate that they could enhance the toxicity of methotrexate. Caution should be used when NSAIDs are administered concomitantly with methotrexate.

4.5.6 Warfarin

The PK effects of warfarin were evaluated in 12 subjects given a 5 mg dose of warfarin for 7 days, and then given warfarin 5 mg in combination with MEPRO 10 mg for 7 days. The PK profile of warfarin was essentially unchanged with concomitant administration of MEPRO. The effects of warfarin and NSAIDs on GI bleeding, however, are synergistic, such that users of both drugs together have a risk of serious GI bleeding higher than users of either drug alone.

4.5.7 Fluconazole

A 3-period crossover drug interaction study was conducted in 12 subjects to evaluate the PK effects of fluconazole and MEPRO after a single dose of fluconazole 150 mg, a single dose of MEPRO 10 mg, and a single dose of fluconazole 150 mg given in combination with a single dose of MEPRO 10 mg. The results of the study showed a 1.5 times increase in MEPRO plasma concentrations and no clinically relevant changes in the PK profile of fluconazole. This was not unexpected and considered to be due to fluconazole's competitive inhibition of MEPRO metabolism via the P-450 2C9 pathway.

4.5.8 Digoxin

The PK profile of digoxin was evaluated in 12 subjects given digoxin 0.25 mg once daily for 7 days alone and then given in combination with MEPRO 10 mg daily for an additional 7 days. There were no relevant changes in the PK profile of digoxin with concomitant MEPRO administration.

4.6 Fertility, Pregnancy, and Lactation

4.6.1 Pregnancy

Congenital abnormalities have been reported in association with NSAID administration in humans; however, these are low in frequency and do not appear to follow any discernible pattern. In view of the known effects of NSAIDs on the fetal cardiovascular system (risk of closure of the ductus arteriosus), use in the last trimester of pregnancy should be avoided. The onset of labor may be delayed and the duration increased with an increased bleeding tendency in both mother and child. NSAIDs should not be used during the first 2 trimesters of pregnancy or labor unless the potential benefit to the patient outweighs the potential risk to the fetus.

4.6.2 Lactation

It is unknown whether MEPRO is excreted in human breast milk. Animal studies have shown excretion of meproamine dihydroacetate in the breast milk of rats. Nursing is not recommended during MEPRO treatment.

4.6.3 Fertility

No safety findings were identified from nonclinical or clinical data suggesting an adverse effect on fertility.

4.7 Effects on Ability to Drive and Use Machines

Undesirable effects such as dizziness, drowsiness, fatigue, and visual disturbances are possible after taking NSAIDs. If affected, patients should not drive or operate machinery.

4.8 Undesirable Effects

4.8.1 Clinical Trials

Table AIII4-1 shows the rates of adverse drug reactions (ADRs) in patients who participated in controlled Phase 2/3 studies for the treatment of rheumatoid arthritis. Duration of exposure ranged from 6 weeks to 1 year. The table includes all ADRs with a rate of ≥ 1% in the total MEPRO group.

Most of the ADRs were related to the GI tract and all were dose related. Onset of GI events excluding PUBs ranged in general between 1 to 3 weeks. The time to onset of PUBs occurred between 4 and 36 weeks. All PUBs and anemias secondary to GI bleeding were serious adverse events and led to discontinuation; otherwise the remaining ADRs in general mild-to-moderate in severity and resolved without sequealae. All subjects who received MEPRO recovered without sequelae.

Nonserious photosensitivity reactions were observed in 5 patients who received MEPRO. All were Caucasian and received MEPRO for 3 or more months. One patient discontinued treatment. All cases resolved including the 4 patients who continued treatment.

➡ **NOTE:** What to include in this section is typically the company's decision, unless regulatory agencies request certain AEs be listed.

Table AIII4-1 **Summary of Adverse Drug Reactions With a Rate of ≥ 1%[a]—Controlled Phase 2/3 Studies**

Adverse Reaction Terms— MedDRA Preferred Term	Placebo N = 2200	M ≤ 5 mg[b] N = 2450	M = 10 mg N = 2400	M = 15 mg N = 325	Total M N = 5175	COX N = 2225
Epigastric discomfort	24 (1.1%)	164 (6.7%)	180 (7.5%)	29 (8.9%)	373 (7.2%)	200 (9.0%)
Nausea	68 (3.1%)	142 (5.8%)	170 (7.1%)	28 (8.6%)	340 (6.6%)	276 (12.4%)
Abdominal pain upper	66 (3.0%)	123 (5.0%)	180 (7.5%)	29 (8.9%)	332 (6.4%)	185 (8.3%)
Dyspepsia	44 (2.0%)	100 (4.1%)	142 (5.9%)	21 (6.5%)	263 (5.1%)	231 (10.4%)
Vomiting	64 (2.9%)	105 (4.3%)	132 (5.5%)	21 (6.5%)	258 (5.0%)	174 (7.8%)
Anaemia	11 (0.5%)	37 (1.5%)	50 (2.1%)	9 (2.8%)	96 (1.9%)	129 (5.8%)
PUBs	1 (< 0.1%)	17 (0.7%)	41 (1.7%)	10 (3.1%)	68 (1.3%)	96 (4.3%)

M = MEPRO; GI = gastrointestinal; PUBs = perforations, ulcers, and bleeds.
[a] Rate ≥ 1% in the total Mepro group.
[b] Only 25 subjects received MEPRO doses < 5 mg.

Some companies will include all adverse events that reached a certain percentage, e.g., ≥ 1% or more regardless of the rate in placebo. Others will include any adverse events where the rate is greater than placebo regardless of what the difference is. For this CCSI only those events considered to be ADRs were included in this section. This determination was based on rates in the MEPRO group that were at least twice the placebo rate and evidence of a dose response. The one case of mania summarized in the IAS (see Appendix II) and considered a potential adverse drug reaction is not included in the CCSI because only one case was reported and it was unclear whether the event was due to the patient's job loss, Mepro, or a combination of both. The one case of Stevens-Johnson syndrome (SJS) reported in the IAS is also not included in this section of the CCSI although it is included in Section 4.4.8 as part of class labelling. This event occurred in an Asian female who tested positive for the B*1502 allele of HLA-B, a gene associated with an increased risk for SJS in subjects exposed to phenytoin and carbamazepine. The subject was also started on penicillin 7 days before developing SJS. Although a potential relationship to MEPRO cannot be ruled out, there are also alternative reasons for this event and for these reasons the case is not included. Note, however, that the health authorities might not agree with these assessments and want these cases included in prescribing information/product labelling; if so, these cases should also be added to the CCSI. Assuming the health authorities agree with the company's assessments, these cases even if not included in this initial CCSI still need to be actively tracked. Consequently, as part of MEPRO's risk management plan (see Appendix I), special questionnaires were developed for potential SJS and mania cases to ensure that complete and relevant information is collected for each new case reported. If well-documented cases of SJS and or mania are subsequently reported and a causal relationship suspected, the CCSI will have to be revised to include these events.

4.8.2 Postmarketing Data
MEPRO is not marketed in any country at this time.

➡ **NOTE:** This is the initial CCSI based on information from nonclinical and clinical studies and class labelling. Once the drug is marketed, new safety information from postmarketing sources will be added as appropriate.

4.9 Overdose

Overdose information is limited. Only 2 cases of overdose were reported. In 1 overdose, 1.5 times the maximum recommended 10-mg MEPRO dose was taken; in the second, 12 times the maximum recommended dose was ingested. Both patients fully recovered with no adverse residual effects reported in either case.

No specific information is available regarding the treatment of MEPRO overdose, and there is no known antidote. In cases of overdose, routine supportive and symptomatic care is recommended. Gastric lavage, administration of activated charcoal, and use of an osmotic cathartic may be indicated depending on the time and extent of the overdose, but this has not been prospectively studied. Forced diuresis, alkalinization of urine, hemodialysis, or hemoperfusion may not be useful due to MEPRO's high protein binding.

■ 5 Pharmacologic Properties

5.1 Pharmacodynamic Properties

In nonclinical studies, inhibition of the COX-2_β receptor showed significant decreases in inflammatory biomarkers and decreases in the signs and symptoms of inflammation in rats, mice, dogs, rabbits, mini pigs, and monkeys. Significantly less ($p \leq 0.05$) inhibition of renal and GI prostaglandins was seen in these same species with MEPRO treatment compared to those treated with active comparators that were nonselective or selective COX-2 NSAIDs. Correspondingly, significantly lower rates ($p \leq 0.05$) of GI events including PUBs, renal toxicity, and fluid retention were also seen with treatment with MEPRO compared to nonselective and selective COX-2 NSAIDs.

5.2 Pharmacokinetic Properties

MEPRO is completely (> 99%) absorbed after oral administration and is approximately 99.4% protein bound.

No differences in apparent volumes of distribution after intravenous and oral administration are observed.

MEPRO crosses the blood–brain barrier.

Peak concentration is generally attained within 1.4–1.5 hours.

Half-life is approximately 24 hours.

Pharmacokinetic properties show linearity across the dose range of 1.25 mg to 15 mg/day.

MEPRO is almost completed metabolized in the liver to 3 inactive metabolites (the major metabolite is 6'-carboxy-meproamine) via the P450 2C9 pathway.

Studies with radio-labeled drug have demonstrated that up to 95% of the orally administered dose is recovered in urine. Very little (< 1%) is excreted unchanged in urine. Urinary excretion is in the form of inactive metabolites.

5.3 Preclinical Safety

Nonclinical data revealed no special hazard for humans based on studies of safety, pharmacology, repeated dose toxicity, genotoxicity, and carcinogenic potential. An increased incidence of ventricular septal heart defects and embryo lethality were noted in rabbits treated through organogenesis. A dose-dependent increase in skeletal abnormalities was seen in rats during organogenesis. An increase in pre-and postimplantation losses was seen in rats treated through the late gestation and lactation period. These findings occurred at doses that far exceeded recommended human doses.

■ 6 Pharmaceutical Particulars

6.1 List of Excipients

5 mg—Maize starch, magnesium stearate, pregelatinized maize starch. Film coating: hypromellose, and macrogol 400.

10 mg—Maize starch, acacia, magnesium stearate, sodium lauryl sulphate. Film coating: hypromellose, macrogol 400, Opaspray M-1-7111B.

6.2 Incompatibilities

Not applicable.

6.3 Shelf Life

5 mg: 5 years
10 mg: 5 years

6.4 Special Precautions for Storage

Store below 25°C.

6.5 Nature and Contents of Container

5 mg—Polypropylene container with polyethylene cap. Pack sizes: 100, 1000 tablets.

10 mg—Polypropylene container with polyethylene cap. Pack sizes: 100, 500 tablets.

Glass bottle with screw cap—Pack sizes: 50, 100 tablets.

6.6 Special Precautions for Disposal

No special requirements.

References

1. *A Guideline on the Summary of Product Characteristics*. September 2009. http://ec.europa.eu/enterprise/sectors/pharmaceuticals/documents/eudralex/vol-2/index_en.htm. Accessed April 21, 2010.

2. Proposed NSAID package insert labeling template1. http://www.fda.gov/downloads/Drugs/DrugSafety/download/ucm106230.pdf. Accessed April 21, 2010.

3. International Conference on Harmonisation of Technical Requirements for Registration of Pharmaceuticals for Human Use. *Clinical Safety Data Management: Periodic Safety Update Reports for Marketed Drugs E2C(R1)*. Geneva, Switzerland:ICH Secretariat; November 2005. http://www.ich.org/cache/compo/276-254-1.html. Accessed April 21, 2010.

4. *Volume 9A of The Rules Governing Medicinal Products in the European Union—Guidelines on Pharmacovigilance for Medicinal Products for Human Use*. September 2008. http://ec.europa.eu/enterprise/sectors/pharmaceuticals/documents/eudralex/vol-9/index_en.htm. Accessed April 21, 2010.

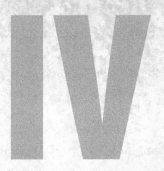

6-Month Periodic Safety Update Report—Mepro

Periodic Safety Update Report for:
Meproamine Dihydroacetate (MEPRO)
6-Month Report
Period Covered by Report:
November 1, 2008–January 31, 2009
International Birth Date: July 31, 2008
Date of Report: February 16, 2009

➡ **NOTE:** The following is an example of a PSUR based on postmarketing data for the fictitious drug Mepro. Although this is the second PSUR, it is the first to have postmarketing safety information. This example is based on the International Conference on Harmonisation (ICH) Guideline, *Clinical Safety Data Management: Periodic Safety Update Reports for Marketed Drugs E2C(R1)*.[1] This is a simple report with only a few cases included. As marketing authorization is granted in more countries and the drug is on the market longer, the number of cases and the complexity of the PSURs are expected to increase. But this example should be at least a starting point in understanding how to prepare a PSUR. A generic format was used for this report. Check your country's regulations and guidance documents regarding specific content and format requirements. As mentioned in previous sections of the book, the following caveats should be understood:

- *Caveat No. 1*—Be sure to follow the regulations and guidance documents relevant to your own country because these can differ across countries.
- *Caveat No. 2*—Regulations keep changing and new guidances are issued over time. What is relevant today can be outdated tomorrow.
- *Caveat No. 3*—There are many approaches in the way data can be analyzed, summarized, displayed, and interpreted. Some of the approaches included in this example may not be the best fit for your drug. Or different ways of data summarization not mentioned here will be required. Some may also disagree with the approaches that are recommended.

Contents

Executive Summary

This is the second periodic safety update report (PSUR) for meproamine dihydroacetate (MEPRO), referred to in this report as Mepro. This report summarizes safety information received by the Global Pharmacovigilance Department of Brie Pharmaceuticals from November 1, 2008 to January 31, 2009.

Mepro is approved and marketed in one country— the United States. The international birth date, i.e., date of first market authorization, is July 31, 2008. Mepro is currently under authorization review in the European Union using the centralized authorization procedure.

During the reporting period of this PSUR, there were no rejections of marketing authorization applications, no license suspensions, and no restrictions in the distribution of Mepro for safety or efficacy reasons.

The company's core safety information (CCSI) used as the reference safety information for the reporting period for this PSUR was based on the core data sheet in effect at the start of this period. There were no changes made to the core data sheet during this period.

Exposure to Mepro during this period is estimated to be 1479.5 person-years exposure based on 540,000 tablets sold and the assumption that a person took at least 1 Mepro tablet once a day.

During this reporting period, Brie Pharmaceuticals received 34 cases, including 41 adverse event terms. The majority of events were spontaneously reported, nonserious, and listed. Approximately half of the adverse event terms were gastrointestinal related.

There were no initial reports with a fatal outcome received during this reporting period.

There was one unlisted serious case received during the period covered in this report. This was a case of mania reported in a 36-year-old Caucasian female with a history of manic-depressive illness. Two weeks after starting Mepro 5 mg, she stopped taking her lithium because she felt she didn't need it anymore. Nineteen days later she was hospitalized with an acute manic attack. It is unclear whether the event was due to Mepro alone, stopping lithium, or a combination of the 2 events. This is the second case of mania reported (the first case was reported during clinical development). Close monitoring for mood disorders is part of the Mepro risk management plan.

Study MP4001, "A Prospective, Randomized, Double-Blind Active-Control Study Evaluating the Safety of Mepro Compared to COX," in 15,000 patients (10,000 to be randomized to Mepro and 5,000 to COX), and also part of the risk management plan, was initiated during the reporting period of this PSUR.

There was 1 intentional overdose. The patient ingested a total of 100 mg of Mepro. The patient initially had upper abdominal pain, nausea, and vomiting but made a full recovery after treatment with gastric lavage and activated charcoal.

No late-breaking news affecting the risk profile of Mepro was received.

Overall, the adverse events received during the reporting period of this PSUR showed no change in the characteristics or severity of listed events. Since this is the first PSUR containing adverse event data, a change in frequency of listed events could not be evaluated.

Based on the information received to date, no new drug-related risks were identified. The benefit–risk profile remains essentially unchanged. No changes were made to the CCSI or are planned at this time.

1 Introduction

This is the second periodic safety update report (PSUR) for meproamine dihydroacetate (MEPRO), referred to in this report as Mepro. This report summarizes safety information received by the Global Pharmacovigilance Department of Brie Pharmaceuticals from November 1, 2008 to January 31, 2009.

➥ **NOTE:** The currently mandated postmarketing periodic report in the United States is the Periodic Adverse Experience Report (PADER), which is different in content and format from the PSUR that is used in the European Union and elsewhere.[2,3] The PSUR is likely to replace the PADER in the future, and the FDA currently accepts the PSUR format in lieu of the PADER with several modifications. The United States requires that PSURs be submitted quarterly for the first 3 years and then annually thereafter.[2,4] The European Union requires submission of the PSUR every 6 months until 2 full years of marketing experience has been gained, then annually for the following 2 years, and at 3-year intervals thereafter. Another difference is the United States requires inclusion of cases from patients/consumers and other nonhealthcare professionals (i.e., not medically confirmed) whether the reports are listed or unlisted events. In Volume 9A of *The Rules Governing Medicinal Products in the European*

Union—Guidelines on Pharmacovigilance for Medicinal Products for Human Use, it is stated that medically unconfirmed serious and nonserious (listed and unlisted) reactions should be included in an annex (i.e., appendix to the PSUR). Furthermore, according to *Volume 9A*, non-medically confirmed cases should not be discussed in the text of the PSUR unless the case is judged to be important to include.[3] There are other differences as well and the regulations governing the European Union and the United States should be reviewed and followed for the respective regions.[2–4]

1.1 Therapeutic Class

Mepro belongs to the therapeutic class of anti-inflammatory and antirheumatic agents, nonsteroids (M01A).

1.2 Pharmacology

Mepro is a new-generation, nonsteroidal anti-inflammatory drug (NSAID) that preferentially inhibits the cyclooxygenase 2-beta ($COX-2_\beta$) receptor. In nonclinical studies, inhibition of the $COX-2_\beta$ receptor showed significant decreases in inflammatory biomarkers and decreases in the signs and symptoms of inflammation in rats, mice, dogs, rabbits, mini pigs, and monkeys. Significantly less ($p \leq 0.05$) inhibition of renal and gastrointestinal prostaglandins was seen in these same species with Mepro treatment compared to those treated with active comparators that were nonselective or selective COX-2 NSAIDs. Correspondingly, significantly ($p \leq 0.05$) lower rates of gastrointestinal perforations, ulcers, and bleeds (PUBs), renal toxicity, and fluid retention were also seen with treatment with Mepro compared to nonselective and selective COX-2 NSAIDs.

1.3 Indication

Mepro is indicated for the relief of the signs and symptoms of rheumatoid arthritis.

1.4 Dosage Recommendation

The recommended dose is 5 mg or 10 mg given once daily.

■ 2 Worldwide Market Authorization Status

Mepro is approved and marketed in one country—the United States. The international birth date, i.e., the date of first market authorization, is July 31, 2008.

■ 3 Update of Regulatory Authority or Marketing Authorization Holder Actions Taken for Safety Reasons

During the reporting period of this PSUR, there were no rejections of marketing authorization applications, no license suspensions, and no restrictions in the distribution of Mepro for safety or efficacy reasons.

Mepro is currently under authorization review in the European Union using the centralized authorization procedure.

■ 4 Changes to Reference Safety Information

The company's core safety information (CCSI) used as the reference safety information for the reporting period for this PSUR was based on the core data sheet in effect at the start of this period. There were no changes made to the core data sheet during this period, and a copy is included in Appendix 1.

■ 5 Patient Exposure

5.1 Clinical Studies

Study MP4001, "A Prospective, Randomized Double-Blind Active-Control Study Evaluating the Safety of Mepro Compared to COX," was the only clinical study ongoing during the reporting period of this PSUR. A total of 30 patients were enrolled. The study is blinded so only an estimate of exposure can be made. Based on the 2:1 randomization ratio of this study, it is estimated that 20 patients were exposed to Mepro and 10 to COX. This study is discussed further in Sections 7.2.1 and 8.3.

5.2 Market Experience

The total number of Mepro tablets sold from November 1, 2008, to January 31, 2009 was 540,000. Mepro exposure in person-years exposure (PYE) was estimated based on the assumption that a patient took at least 1 tablet once a day. PYE was calculated as follows:

Number of tablets sold = 540,000 = Number of persons who took at least 1 Mepro tablet per day = Number of persons-days.

PYE = Number of person-days/(365 days per year) = (540,000 person-days)/(365 days per year) = 1,479.5 PYE

■ 6 Presentation of Individual Case Histories

6.1 General Considerations

Adverse reaction terms were coded using MedDRA version 12.0.

If a case included more than 1 MedDRA Preferred Term (PT), the most medically important term (primary PT) was listed first and included under the primary System Organ Class (SOC) for that term.

If a case was received from any of the following sources, it was included in the report:

- Spontaneous reports from health professionals, patients/consumers, and other nonhealthcare professionals
- Reports from regulatory agencies
- Brie-sponsored studies
- The literature
- Other sources, including:
  - Exchange of reports on adverse reactions in the framework of contractual agreements
  - Data from special registries
  - Reports from poison control centers
- Epidemiological databases

Literature searches were done at least weekly. The databases searched were EMBASE and MEDLINE. Search terms included:

- Mepro
- Meproamine dihydroacetate

- Adverse event, adverse reaction, adverse drug reaction
- Lack of effect, lack of efficacy
- Interaction
- Overdose, abuse, misuse, medication error, prescription error
- Pregnancy, lactation
- Withdrawal, rebound

All cases regardless of source were medically reviewed.

6.2 Cases Presented as Line Listings

Line listings were prepared in accordance with the International Conference on Harmonisation (ICH) Guideline, *Clinical Safety Data Management: Periodic Safety Update Reports for Marketed Drugs E2C(R1).*[1]
Listings can be found in the following appendices:

- Appendix 2—All serious adverse reaction reports from spontaneous reporting (confirmed by a healthcare professional), received from a regulatory agency, or reported from the literature.
- Appendix 3—Nonserious unlisted adverse reaction reports from spontaneous reporting (confirmed by a healthcare professional), or reported from the literature.
- Appendix 4—Nonserious listed adverse reaction reports from spontaneous reporting (confirmed by a healthcare professional).
- Appendix 5—All serious adverse reactions from Brie-sponsored studies considered drug related by either the investigator or Brie Pharmaceuticals.
- Appendix 6—Serious and nonserious (listed and unlisted) adverse reactions from spontaneous reporting by patients/consumers and other nonhealthcare professionals that were not confirmed by a healthcare professional (i.e., medically unconfirmed cases).

➡ **NOTE:** Remember, as discussed previously, there is a difference in reporting requirements between the United States and the European Union regarding inclusion/exclusion of cases from patients/consumers and other nonhealthcare professional reports (i.e., not medically confirmed). These differences can cause confusion and considerably more work for the MAH when preparing reports for the same drug in different regions.

6.2.1 Overview of Cases
During this reporting period, Brie Pharmaceuticals received 34 cases, including 41 adverse event terms. The majority of events were spontaneously reported, nonserious, and listed. Table AIV6-1 summarizes the source and seriousness of reports.

6.3 Cases Presented as Summary Tabulations

Table AIV6-2 summarizes by source the 41 adverse reaction terms reported from the 34 cases received.

➡ **NOTE:** There are many ways to present these data. It is the authors' preference to use the format shown in Table AIV6-2 and group serious and nonserious AEs in the same table because the reporting rate of the same event regardless of seriousness may help in signal detection. Also note, this summary tabulation includes both medically confirmed and unconfirmed adverse reactions, because the United States is the only country marketing the drug. If the PSUR was also for the European regulatory authorities, this table would be split into 2 separate tables—1 that contained only medically confirmed cases (for the European Union) and one that contained both (i.e., Table AIV6-2) for the United States. In preparing summary tabulations, it should also be noted that nonserious listed events should be included.[1] The determination of listed events was based on the CCSI presented in Appendix III.

6.4 Marketing Authorization Holder's Analysis of Individual Case Histories

6.4.1 Initial Reports With Fatal Outcome by Primary SOC
There were no initial reports with a fatal outcome received during this reporting period.

6.4.2 Other Serious Events From Spontaneous Reporting Sources by Primary SOC
There was 1 unlisted serious case received during the period covered in this report. This was a case of mania (BRI08006) reported in a 36-year-old Caucasian female with a history of manic-depressive illness. She started Mepro 5 mg on November 3, 2008. On November 17, 2008, the patient stopped taking her lithium because she felt she didn't need it anymore. Nineteen days later, on December 6, 2008, she was hospitalized with an acute manic attack.

Brie Pharmaceuticals comment: It is unclear whether the manic attack was due to the patient stopping her lithium, due to Mepro alone, or a combination of these 2 actions. This is the second report of mania. The first was reported in a clinical study (Patient 2003X-0601 from Study MP2003X) and occurred in a 48-year-old Caucasian male with no other explanations for the event. This case was summarized in the integrated analysis of safety (IAS). Because of this 1 case, as part of the risk management program, a questionnaire was developed and call center and drug safety personnel were trained to capture complete information on any reports of changes in mood. Mood-related events will continue to be closely monitored.

➡ **NOTE:** Even though this case was summarized in the IAS, it was not included in the CCSI (see Appendix III). This event is therefore an unlisted event.

6.5 Follow-up on Serious Reports From Previous PSURs

No follow-up reports were received from the previous PSUR, because this is the first PSUR that includes adverse event information.

Table AIV6-1 **Number of Cases Received During Reporting Period—All Sources**

Spontaneous Reports			Regulatory Authorities			Studies		Literature			Other[a]			Total		
S	NS	Tot	S	NS	Tot	S	Tot	S	NS	Tot	S	NS	Tot	S	NS	Tot
3	30	33	1	0	1	0	0	0	0	0	0	0	0	4	30	34

[a] Includes information from other sources such as special registries, contractual partners, etc.; S = serious; NS = nonserious; Tot = total.

Table AIV6-2 **Summary Tabulation of Adverse Events—All Sources**

Adverse Reaction Terms by MedDRA SOC and PT	Spontaneous Reports	Regulatory Authorities	Literature	Studies	Other[a]	Total
Blood and Lymphatic Disorders						
Anaemia	1					1
Eye Disorders						
Cataract	1					1
Vision blurred	1					1
Gastrointestinal Disorders						
Abdominal pain upper	3					3
Dyspepsia	4					4
Epigastric distress	4					4
Nausea	6					6
PUBs[b]	2 (2)					2 (2)
Vomiting	2					2
General Disorders and Administrative Site Conditions						
Drug interaction	1					1
Injury, Poisoning, and Procedural Complications						
Intentional overdose		1 (1)				1 (1)
Investigations						
Antipsychotic drug level increased	1					1
Nervous System Disorders						
Dizziness	4					4
Headache	3					3
Pregnancy, Puerperium, and Perinatal Conditions						
Feeding disorder neonatal	1					1
Psychiatric Disorders						
Mania	1 (1)					1(1)
Skin and Subcutaneous Tissue Disorders						
Increased tendency to bruise	1					1
Photosensitivity reaction	2					2
Rash	1					1
Vascular Disorders						
Hypertension	1					1

[a] Includes information from other sources such as special registries, contractual partners, etc.

[b] PUBs = perforations, ulcers, and bleeds.

The number in parentheses = serious events. *Italicized terms* = unlisted events.

■ 7 Studies

7.1 Newly Analyzed Studies

7.1.1 Clinical Studies
No new clinical studies were analyzed during this reporting period.

7.1.2 Nonclinical Studies
No new nonclinical studies were analyzed during this reporting period.

7.2 Targeted New Safety Studies

7.2.1 Clinical Studies
Study MP 4001, "A Prospective, Randomized Double-Blind Active-Control Study Evaluating the Safety of Mepro Compared to COX," is part of Brie Pharmaceuticals Company's risk management program and postapproval commitment to the FDA. The following are the key aspects of the study:

- Total number of patients to be randomized: 15,000 patients.
  - 10,000 patients to receive Mepro (5,000 at 5 mg and 5,000 at 10 mg)
  - 5,000 subjects to receive COX 25 mg
- Study duration: 3 years.
- Number and location of study sites: 400 sites in the United States, Canada, and the European Union.
- End points:
  - Primary end points:
    - ≥ 30% reduction in the risk of ischemic strokes and cardiovascular ischemic events compared to COX.
    - ≥ 30% reduction in the risk of PUBs compared to COX.
  - Secondary end points: ≥ 30% reduction in hypertension, renal disease, and congestive heart failure compared to COX.
- Enrollment period: Estimated to be 18 months.
- First patient randomized: January 7, 2009.
- Other study features: The number of Caucasians will be limited to ≤ 50% of patients randomized in order to determine the safety profile in other races.

7.2.2 Nonclinical Studies
No new nonclinical targeted safety studies were started or were ongoing during the reporting period of this PSUR.

7.3 Published Studies

No published studies were found during the reporting period of this report.

7.4 Other Studies

No other studies were ongoing or started during this PSUR's reporting period.

■ 8 Other Information

8.1 Efficacy-Related Information

No reports were received regarding lack of efficacy.

8.2 Late-Breaking Information

No late-breaking information was received after the data lock date of January 31, 2009.

8.3 Risk Management Plan

The risk management program established for Mepro includes the following:

- Routine postmarketing pharmacovigilance.
- Development of questionnaires and training of call center personnel and drug safety associates to ensure complete collection of information reported during calls to the manufacturer for the following events:
  - Any cases of mania or changes in mood
  - Photosensitivity reactions
  - Any serious skin condition suggestive of erythema multiforme, Stevens-Johnson syndrome, or toxic epidermal necrolysis
  - Any cases of aplastic anemia, agranulocytosis, hepatotoxicity, renal toxicity, torsades de pointes/QT prolongation (although no safety signals were identified during clinical development)
- Because the results of the IAS suggested a better safety profile for Mepro compared to COX, it was decided to conduct a prospective, randomized, double-blind, active-controlled study to evaluate ischemic stroke/ischemic cardiovascular risk and PUBs as the primary end points. Secondary end points include evaluation of risk of hypertension,

renal disease, and congestive heart failure. Study MP 4001, "A Prospective, Randomized Double-Blind Active-Control Study Evaluating the Safety of Mepro Compared to COX," was initiated during this reporting period. Enrollment and details of this study are provided in Sections 5.1 and 7.2.1, respectively.

8.4 Risk–Benefit Analysis Report

No separate risk-benefit analysis report was done during the reporting period of this report.

■ 9 Overall Safety Evaluation

9.1 Review by System Organ Class

In this section, reactions that were serious and unlisted, listed events that were inconsistent with the CCSI, and those considered medically important (based on clinical judgment) are summarized by SOC. If a case had more than one adverse event term, the most clinically important event was listed first and included under the primary SOC for that term.

9.1.1 Eye Disorders
9.1.1.1 PTs Vision Blurred, Cataract
Blurry vision, without pain, was reported in a 15-year-old Caucasian female (BRI09001) who was taking Mepro 5 mg for 21 days for treatment of juvenile rheumatoid arthritis. A subsequent eye exam revealed a small cataract in her left eye. She was taking no other medication at the time. There was no history of eye pain or inflammation, no trauma, and no other causes that could explain the cataract.

Brie Pharmaceuticals comment: This is the first report of cataract. Follow-up information regarding medical history, especially any history of inflammation, concomitant drugs including the use of herbal/nutraceuticals products, and history of trauma was requested. Note that iritis/uveitis and cataracts are well described in juvenile rheumatoid arthritis and are felt to be a consequence of chronic eye inflammation and part of the inflammatory process of juvenile rheumatoid arthritis.

9.1.2 Gastrointestinal Disorders
9.1.2.1 PTs Gastric Ulcer, Duodenal Ulcer
Two cases of gastrointestinal ulcers were reported. A duodenal ulcer was reported in a 57-year-old Caucasian male

(BRI09008) 4 weeks after starting Mepro 10 mg. The patient admitted having 4 beers before his GI complaints began. A 45-year-old Black male (BRI08003) was diagnosed with a gastric ulcer after complaining of upper abdominal pain 3 weeks after starting Mepro 5 mg. The patient was taking ibuprofen (dose unknown) for a toothache for 5 days prior to the onset of his abdominal pain. He was unaware that Mepro was also an NSAID and that he should not have taken both. Both ibuprofen and Mepro were stopped. Both patients' ulcers resolved without sequelae.

The other GI-related events reported during this period were nonserious and listed events.

Brie Pharmaceuticals comments: No change in the GI risk profile was identified during the reporting period of this PSUR. The two cases of ulcers occurred in patients exposed to other substances (i.e., alcohol, NSAID) associated with an increased risk of PUBs. There were no reports of PUBs in females or the elderly during this reporting period.

9.1.3 Injury, Poisoning, and Procedural Complications
9.1.3.1 PT Intentional Overdose
There was one intentional overdose reported (BRI09023). This case is discussed in Section 9.3.

9.1.4 Psychiatric Disorders
9.1.4.1 PT Mania
One case of mania (serious and unlisted) was reported. This case is summarized and discussed in Section 6.4.2.

9.1.5 Skin and Subcutaneous Tissue Disorders
9.1.5.1 PT Increased Tendency to Bruise
A nonserious case of easy bruising was reported by an 83-year-old Caucasian female (BRI09019) who was taking Mepro 5 mg for 2 weeks and noticed bruising of her arms and legs after very little trauma to her extremities. She admitted to having very fragile skin. Because of the pain relief she was receiving with Mepro, she decided to continue treatment.

9.1.5.2 PT Photosensitivity Reaction
Two cases of photosensitivity reaction were reported. Both occurred in Caucasians after 78 and 84 days of treatment, respectively. One occurred in a 33-year-old female (BRI09010) and the other (BRI09018) in a 57-year-old male. Both were nonserious and resolved within 2 weeks of occurrence. Mepro treatment was continued without interruption in both cases.

9.1.5.3 PT Rash
A nonserious case of rash was reported (BRI09024) in a 27-year-old Caucasian female. The rash was described as

red flat patches on arms and legs that were not pruritic. No other information is available at this time.

Brie Pharmaceuticals comment: The 2 cases of photosensitivity reaction described in this section are similar to the 5 cases reported during clinical development. All cases occurred in Caucasians. In the subjects from clinical trials, onset occurred after 3 or more months of exposure. These 2 cases occurred slightly earlier, i.e., 78 and 84 days after starting Mepro.

9.2 Drug Interactions

There was one case (BRI09004) of a drug interaction reported during this period. The case was reported by a healthcare professional and involved a 37-year-old Caucasian female with manic-depressive disorder who developed elevated levels of lithium after taking 5 mg of Mepro for 21 days. She had to stop her lithium for 2 weeks.

Brie Pharmaceuticals comment: The finding of elevated lithium levels with concomitant Mepro use is already listed in the CCSI.

9.3 Experience With Overdose

One report (BRI09023) was received from the FDA of an intentional overdose. This occurred in a 28-year-old Caucasian male who was despondent over his girlfriend leaving him. He took 10, 10-mg Mepro tablets, for a total dose of 100 mg. The subject had nausea, vomiting, and upper abdominal pain. He underwent gastric lavage and received activated charcoal. He was admitted to the hospital for observation and suicide precautions. The patient recovered without any sequelae.

9.4 Drug Abuse or Misuse

There were no reports received regarding drug abuse or misuse.

9.5 Positive or Negative Experiences During Pregnancy and Lactation

One consumer nursed her baby (BRI08001) and complained the infant would not breastfeed. The mother was informed that breastfeeding while taking Mepro was not recommended.

Brie Pharmaceuticals comment: The current CCSI states that breastfeeding is not recommended.

9.6 Special Patient Groups

9.6.1 Pediatric Patients

A case of blurry vision and cataract was reported in a 15-year-old female with juvenile rheumatoid arthritis (BRI09001). This case is discussed in Section 9.1.

9.6.2 Elderly

There were no serious adverse reactions reported in individuals ≥ 65 years old. One case of easy bruising in an 83-year-old female (BRI09019) is discussed in Section 9.1.

9.6.3 Patients With Hepatic or Renal Impairment

No reports were received from patients with known hepatic or renal impairment.

9.6.4 Those Using Mepro Off Label (Unapproved Indications)

Case BRI09001, regarding blurry vision and cataract in a 15-year-old female with juvenile rheumatoid arthritis, was discussed in Section 9.1. Treatment of Mepro for juvenile rheumatoid arthritis is currently under review by the FDA but is not an approved indication at this time.

9.7 Effects of Long-Term Treatment

Mepro has been marketed for only the past 3 months. All long-term data come from clinical trials that showed no unexpected safety findings after long-term (i.e., ≥ 6 months) treatment.

9.8 Patient/Consumer and Other Nonhealthcare Professional Reports

A line listing of patient/consumer and other nonhealthcare professional reports can be found in Appendix 6.

9.9 Prescription Errors/Medication Errors

No cases of medication or prescription errors were received during the reporting period of this report.

■ 10 Conclusion

Overall, the adverse events received during the reporting period of this PSUR showed no change in the characteristics or severity of listed events. Because this is the first PSUR containing adverse event data, a change in frequency of listed events could not be evaluated.

Based on the information received to date, no new drug-related risks were identified. The benefit–risk profile remains essentially unchanged. No changes were made to the CCSI or are planned at this time.

■ 11 Appendices

* = Confirmed by a Healthcare Professional;

** = Unconfirmed by a Healthcare Professional;

*** = MedWatch 3500A Forms for Nonserious Expected Adverse Reaction Reports were not included based on a waiver received from the FDA;

= For US only[2,4]

References

1. International Conference on Harmonisation of Technical Requirements for Registration of Pharmaceuticals for Human Use. ICH Harmonised Tripartite Guideline. *Clinical Safety Data Management: Periodic Safety Update Reports for Marketed Drugs E2C(R1)*. Geneva, Switzerland: ICH Secretariat; November 2005. http://www.ich .org/cache/compo/276-254-1.html. Accessed April 21, 2010.

2. Code of Federal Regulations. Part 314—Application for FDA Approval to Market a New Drug, Subpart B–Applications, Sec. 314.80 Postmarketing reporting of adverse drug experiences. April 2009. http://www.accessdata.fda.gov/scripts/cdrh/ cfdocs/cfcfr/CFRSearch.cfm?fr=314.80. Accessed April 21, 2010.

3. *The Rules Governing Medicinal Products in the European Union—Guidelines on Pharmacovigilance for Medicinal Products for Human Use*. Vol. 9A. September 2008. http://ec.europa.eu/enterprise/ sectors/pharmaceuticals/documents/eudralex/ index_en.htm. Accessed April 21, 2010.

4. *Draft Guidance: Guidance for Industry Postmarketing Safety Reporting for Human Drugs and Biological Products including Vaccines*. Washington, DC: US Department of Health and Human Services, Food and Drug Administration, Center for Drug Evaluation and Research (CDER) Center for Biologics Evaluation and Research (CBER); March 2001. http://www.fda .gov/BiologicsBloodVaccines/GuidanceCompliance RegulatoryInformation/Guidances/Vaccines/ucm0748 50.htm. Accessed April 21, 2010.

APPENDIX

V

Clinically Significant Criteria for Laboratory, Vital Signs, Body Weight, Body Mass Index, and Electrocardiogram Parameters

NOTE: In this appendix, suggested clinically significant criteria are provided for laboratory, vital signs, body weight, body mass index, and electrocardiogram (ECG) parameters. These criteria are used in the identification of subjects with potentially important findings. For some of these parameters, there is little published information regarding the criteria to use for determining clinically significant or markedly abnormal changes. Many of the criteria suggested in this appendix are based on clinical judgment, which is subjective. Because there is no one standard, there may be disagreement among various reviewers as to what constitutes a clinically significant change. Until standard criteria are established, the best that can be done is to clearly show what criteria were used. If a reviewer disagrees with the criteria used, the data can be reanalyzed based on the reviewer's preferred criteria. The criteria for most of the clinically significant changes, unless otherwise specified, include subjects with normal baseline values who had clinically significant treatment values. Although the suggested criteria are for subjects with normal baseline values, it is important to review *all* subjects with abnormal baseline values that had a clinically significant treatment value to ensure that no important finding was inadvertently overlooked.

■ Suggested Criteria for Clinically Significant Changes—Hematology Parameters

Table AV-1 is a summary of suggested clinically significant criteria for hematology parameters.

Table AV-1 **Suggested Clinically Significant Hematology Criteria*[1]**

Parameter	Clinically Significant Values (US Conventional Units)[a]	Clinically Significant Values (International System of Units—SI)[a]
Hemoglobin (Hb)	≤9.5g/dL (F)	≤95 g/L (F)
	≤11.5 g/dL (M)	≤115 g/L (M)
Hematocrit (Hct)	≤32% (F)	≤0.32 (F)
	≤37% (M)	≤0.37 (M)
White blood cells (WBC)	≤2.8×10³/cells/mm³	≤2.8×10⁹/L
Platelet count	≤75×10³/mm³	≤75×10⁹/L
	≥700×10³/mm³	≥700×10⁹/L

F = females; M = males.

[a] Clinically significant criteria—a normal baseline value and a clinically significant treatment value.

* Some criteria based on clinical judgment.

Table AV-2 **Suggested Clinically Significant Clinical Chemistry Criteria (Excluding Liver Function Tests)* [1-3]**

Parameter	Clinically Significant Value US Conventional Units[a]	Clinically Significant Value International System of Units (SI)[a]
Albumin	<2.5 g/dL	<25 g/L
Calcium	<7 mg/dL	<1.75 mmol/L
	>12 mg/dL	>3.0 mmol/L
Chloride	<90 mEq/L	<90 mmol/L
	>115 mEq/L	>115 mmol/L
Cholesterol	>300 mg/dL	>7.8 mmol/L
Creatinine	>2.0 mg/dL	177 µmol/L
Creatine kinase	>3×ULN	>3×ULN
Glucose	<50 mg/dL	<2.8 mmol/L
	>250 mg/dL	>13.9 mmol/L
High-density lipoprotein cholesterol	<45 mg/dL	<1.2 mmol/L
Low-density lipoprotein cholesterol	>160 mg/dL	>4.1 mmol/L
Phosphorus	<2.0 mg/dL	<0.6 mmol/L
	>5.0 mg/dL	>1.6 mmol/L
Potassium	<3.0 mEq/L	<3.0 mmol/L
	>5.5 mEq/L	>5.5 mmol/L
Protein, total	<4.5 g/dL	<45 g/L
Sodium	<130 mEq/L	<130 mmol/L
	>150 mEq/L	>150 mmol/L
Triglycerides	>300 mg/dL	>3.4 mmol/L
Blood urea nitrogen	>30 mg/dl	>10.7 mmol/L
Uric acid	>8.0 mg/dL (F)	>476 µmol/L (F)
	>10.0 mg/dL (M)	>595 µmol/L (M)

F = females; M = males.

* Some criteria based on clinical judgment.

[a] Clinically significant criteria—normal baseline value and a clinically significant treatment value.

Suggested Criteria for Clinically Significant Clinical Laboratory Changes (Excluding Liver Function Tests)

Table AV-2 is a summary of suggested criteria for clinically significant laboratory changes (excluding liver function tests).

Suggested Criteria for Evaluation of Drug-Induced Liver Injury

Based on the FDA guidance document for evaluation of drug-induced liver injury (DILI), the following analyses and conventions are recommended[4]:

- The rate of subjects with a normal baseline ALT value and a treatment value $\geq 3 \times$ upper limit of normal (ULN), $\geq 5 \times$ ULN, $\geq 10 \times$ ULN, and $\geq 20 \times$ ULN*

- The rate of subjects with a normal baseline AST value and a treatment value $\geq 3 \times$ ULN, $\geq 5 \times$ ULN, $\geq 10 \times$ ULN, and $\geq 20 \times$ ULN*

- The rate of subjects with normal baseline ALT and AST values with treatment values that were $\geq 3 \times$ ULN, $\geq 5 \times$ ULN, $\geq 10 \times$ ULN, and $\geq 20 \times$ ULN* for both ALT and AST

- The rate of subjects with a normal baseline total bilirubin level (TBL) and a treatment value above normal (H).

- The rate of subjects with a normal baseline TBL and a treatment value $> 2 \times$ ULN

- The rate of subjects with normal baseline alkaline phosphatase (ALP) values and a treatment value $> 1.5 \times$ ULN

- The rate of subjects with a normal baseline ALT value and TBL, and treatment values of:
  - $ALT > 3 \times ULN + TBL > 1.5 \times ULN$
  - $ALT > 3 \times ULN + TBL > 2 \times ULN$

- The rate of subjects with a normal baseline AST and TBL, and treatment values of:
  - $AST > 3 \times ULN + TBL > 1.5 \times ULN$
  - $AST > 3 \times ULN + TBL > 2 \times ULN$

- The rate of subjects with normal ALT, ALP values and TBLs at baseline who met the following criteria for Hy's Law during treatment:
  - $ALT > 3 \times ULN + ALP < 2 \times ULN + TBL \geq 2 \times ULN$

- The rate of subjects with normal AST, ALP values, and TBLs at baseline who met the following criteria for Hy's Law during treatment:
  - $AST > 3 \times ULN + ALP < 2 \times ULN + TBL \geq 2 \times ULN$

- The rate of any subject with normal ALT or AST values at baseline and $> 3 \times$ ULN of ALT or AST and the MedDRA PTs *Nausea, Vomiting, Anorexia, Abdominal pain,* or *Fatigue* within +/− 14 days of the abnormal ALT or AST values. If the patient reported the same PT more than once or reported more than 1 PT, e.g., *Nausea* and *Vomiting*, the subject is counted only once.

➡️ **NOTE:** +/− 14 days was added by the authors to identify cases with a temporal association to the abnormal aminotransferase values, and also to ensure cases are included even if laboratory changes and adverse events are not evaluated/reported at the same time. The selection of +/−14 days is arbitrary. One factor to consider is the time between study visit evaluations.

Suggested Criteria for Clinically Significant Changes in Urinalysis Parameters

Table AV-3 summarizes the suggested criteria for clinically significant changes in urinalysis parameters.

Table AV-3	Clinically Significant Urinalysis Criteria*[1]
Laboratory Parameter	**Criteria[a]**
Protein	Increase of ≥ 2 units from baseline
Glucose	Increase of ≥ 2 units from baseline
Ketones	Increase of ≥ 2 units from baseline
Occult blood	Increase of ≥ 2 units from baseline
RBCs	Increase of ≥ 10 cells/hpf from baseline
WBCs	Increase of ≥ 20 cells/hpf from baseline
Casts	Increase of ≥ 2 units from baseline

hpf = high powered field.
* Some criteria based on clinical judgment.
[a] Clinically significant criteria = a normal baseline value and a clinically significant treatment value.

* If a subject had more than 1 treatment value within the same category, e.g., $\geq 10 \times$ ULN, the subject was only counted once for that category. If a subject had treatment values in more than one category, the subject was counted in the worst (i.e., the most extreme) category.

■ Suggested Criteria for Changes in Vital Signs, Body Weight, and Body Mass Index

Table AV-4 summarizes the suggested criteria for clinically significant changes in vitals signs, body weight, and body mass index.

■ Suggested Criteria for Clinically Significant Changes—ECG Parameters (Excluding QTc)

Table AV-5 is a summary of suggested clinically significant criteria for ECG parameters (excluding QTc).

Table AV-4 Suggested Clinically Significant Criteria for Vital Signs, Body Weight, and Body Mass Index*[1]

Parameter	Clinically Significant Value[a]	Change From Baseline[a]
Heart rate	≥ 120 bpm	Increase of ≥ 15 bpm
	≤ 50 bpm	Decrease of ≥ 15 bpm
Systolic blood pressure	≥ 180 mmHg	Increase of ≥ 20 mmHg
	≤ 90 mmHg	Decrease of ≥ 20 mmHg
Diastolic blood pressure	≥ 105 mmHg	Increase of ≥ 15 mmHg
	≤ 50 mmHg	Decrease of ≥ 15 mmHg
Respiratory rate	≥ 30 bpm	Increase of ≥ 10 bpm
	≤ 8 bpm	Decrease of ≥ 4 bpm
Body temperature	≥ 38.3°C (101°F)	Increase of ≥ 1°C (2°F)
	≤ 96.8°F (36°C)	Decrease of ≥ 1°C (2°F)
Body weight	None specified	Increase ≥ 7%
	None specified	Decrease ≥ 7%
Body mass index	None specified	Increase to a higher BMI category[b]

bpm = beats per minute or breaths per minute; mmHg = millimeters of mercury.

* Some criteria based on clinical judgment.

[a] To be counted in the rate, the subject had to have a clinically significant treatment value (if specified) and the magnitude of change from baseline shown for each parameter.

[b] BMI categories include < 18.5, 18.5 to 25, > 25.

Table AV-5 Suggested Clinically Significant Criteria for ECG Parameters (Excluding QTc)*[1]

ECG Parameter	Clinically Significant Change
Heart rate	≥ 120 bpm during treatment and an increase of ≥ 15 bpm from baseline
	≤ 50 bpm during treatment and a decrease of ≥ 15 bpm from baseline
PR interval	< 120 ms (< 0.12 s) during treatment and a normal baseline value
	> 210 ms (> 0.21 s) during treatment and a normal baseline value
QRS complex	> 110 ms (> 0.11 s) during treatment and a normal baseline value

bpm = beats per minute; ms = milliseconds; s = seconds.

*Some criteria based on clinical judgment.

■ Suggested Criteria for QT (Corrected) Interval Changes

Categorical/Clinically Significant Shifts

QT interval—corrected (QTc) categorical/clinically significant shifts are based on the International Conference on Harmonisation guidance document, *The Clinical Evaluation of QT/QTc Interval Prolongation and Proarrhythmic Potential for Non-Antiarrhythmic Drugs E14,* and include the following[5]:

■ Subjects with normal baseline values and a treatment value > 450 milliseconds, > 480 milliseconds and > 500 milliseconds. If a subject had more than 1 treatment value within the same category, e.g., > 450 milliseconds, the subject is counted only once for that category. If a subject had treatment values in more than one category, the subject is counted in the worst (i.e., the most extreme) category.

■ Subjects with above normal baseline values and a treatment value > 450 milliseconds, > 480 milliseconds, and > 500 milliseconds. If a subject had more than 1 treatment value within the same category, e.g., > 450 milliseconds, the subject is counted only once for that category. If a subject had treatment values in more than one category, the subject is counted in the worst (i.e., the most extreme) category.

■ Subjects with normal baseline values and an increase during treatment of > 30 milliseconds and > 60 milliseconds from baseline. If a subject had more than 1 treatment value within the same category, e.g., > 30 milliseconds, the subject is counted only once for that category. If a subject had treatment values in both categories, the subject is counted in the worst (i.e., the most extreme) category.

■ Subjects with above normal baseline values and an increase during treatment of > 30 milliseconds and > 60 milliseconds from baseline. If a subject had more than 1 treatment value within the same category, e.g., > 30 milliseconds, the subject is counted only once. If a subject had treatment values in both categories, the subject is counted in the worst (i.e., the most extreme) category value.

References

1. *Supplementary Suggestions for Preparing an Integrated Summary of Safety Information in an Original NDA Submission and for Organizing Information in Periodic Safety Updates (Leber guidelines).* Rockville, MD: US Food and Drug Administration; 1987.

2. Center for Drug Evaluation and Research, Food and Drug Administration, Department of Health and Human Services. *Reviewer Guidance Conducting a Clinical Safety Review of a New Product Application and Preparing a Report on the Review.* February 2005. http://www.fda.gov/downloads/Drugs/Guidance ComplianceRegulatoryInformation/Guidances/ucm 072974.pdf. Accessed May 4, 2010.

3. Fischbach FT, Dunning MB. *A Manual of Laboratory and Diagnostic Tests.* 8th ed. Philadelphia, PA: Lippincott Williams & Wilkins; 2009.

4. Guidance for Industry—Drug-Induced Liver Injury: Premarketing Clinical Evaluation. US Department of Health and Human Services, Food and Drug Administration, Center for Drug Evaluation and Research (CDER), Center for Biologics Evaluation and Research (CBER). July 2009. http://www.fda.gov/downloads/Drugs/Guidance ComplianceRegulatory Information/ Guidances/ UCM174090.pdf. Accessed May 4, 2010.

5. International Conference on Harmonisation of Technical Requirements for Registration of Pharmaceuticals for Human Use. *The Clinical Evaluation of QT/QTc Interval Prolongation and Proarrhythmic Potential for Non-Antiarrhythmic Drugs E14.* Geneva, Switzerland: ICH Secretariat; May 2005. http://www.ich.org/cache/compo/276-254-1.html. Accessed May 4, 2010.

Index